Hand
Card

Basic Science and
Clinical Aspects
of Cardiovascular
Pharmacology

Handbook of Cardiac Drugs

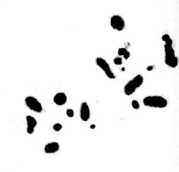

Basic Science and Clinical Aspects of Cardiovascular Pharmacology

Ralph E. Purdy, Ph.D.
Associate Professor, Department of Pharmacology,
University of California, Irvine,
California College of Medicine, Irvine, California

Robert J. Boucek, M.D.
Professor of Medicine, Section of Cardiology,
Loma Linda University School of Medicine;
Director, Cardiovascular Research, Loma Linda
University Medical Center and Pettis Memorial
Veterans Administration Hospital, Loma Linda,
California

Foreword by **Paul M. Vanhoutte, M.D., Ph.D.**
Professor of Physiology and Pharmacology
and Consultant, Departments of
Physiology and Biophysics,
Mayo Medical School and Mayo Graduate
School of Medicine, Rochester, Minnesota

Little, Brown and Company
Boston/Toronto

Copyright © 1988 by Ralph E. Purdy and Robert J. Boucek

First Edition
Second Printing
All rights reserved. No part of this book may be
reproduced in any form or by any electronic or
mechanical means, including information storage
and retrieval systems, without permission in
writing from the publisher, except by a reviewer
who may quote brief passages in a review.

Library of Congress Catalog Card No. 88-80818

ISBN 0-316-72245-6

Printed in the United States of America

FG

To those who have given so generously:

Dr. Carl Riedesel, whose example convinced me to enter the field of science.

Dr. John Bevan, who kindly provided me with rich experiences and opportunities to learn cardiovascular pharmacology.

In memory of Dr. Che Su, whose friendship I treasured and whose scientific rigor was exemplary to all.

Leslie, Chris, and Colin, with whom I find great joy in sharing everything.

R.E.P.

To Irish, whose emotional commitment and intellectual companionship made possible our academic adventure.

R.J.B.

Contents

Foreword	xv
Preface	xvii
Acknowledgments	xix

1. Congestive Heart Failure — 1
In collaboration with Robert J. Boucek, Jr., M.D., Associate Professor of Pediatric Cardiology, Vanderbilt University School of Medicine

Definition	1
Compensatory Responses	1
Treatment of Acute Heart Failure	4
Diuretics	7
Vasodilator Therapy	8
Morphine Sulfate	8
Organic Nitrates	9
Sodium Nitroprusside (Nipride)	10
Digitalis Glycosides	12
Dobutamine Hydrochloride	23
Dopamine Hydrochloride	25
Norepinephrine Bitartrate	26
Treatment of Chronic Congestive Heart Failure (Left Ventricular Systolic Dysfunction)	26
Therapeutic End Points—Digitalis	27
Diuretics	28
Hydralazine	31
Minoxidil	31
Phentolamine	31
Prazosin Hydrochloride	32
Captopril and Enalapril Maleate	32
Digoxin	34
Digitoxin	35
Deslanoside	35
Digitalis Toxicity	36
Digitalis-Drug Interactions	42
Nonglycoside Inotropic Agents	47
Treatment of Chronic Congestive Heart Failure (Left Ventricular Diastolic Dysfunction)	50

2. Cardiac Arrhythmias — 54
In collaboration with Vilma I. Torres, M.D., Assistant Professor of Medicine and Director, Clinical Electrophysiology Laboratories, Loma Linda University School of Medicine

Clinical Guides to Therapy for the Arrhythmias	54

viii   Contents

Overview of Electrical and Mechanical Properties of the Heart ... 59

Cardiac Electrical Activation and the Myocardial Contractile Response ... 62

Cardiac Action Potential ... 63

Mechanisms of Arrhythmia: Automaticity and Abnormalities of Conduction and Refractoriness ... 69

Arrhythmogenic Properties of Digitalis ... 73

Classification of Antiarrhythmic Agents ... 75

Drug Actions Responsible for Opposing Arrhythmias ... 76

Effects of Class I Antiarrhythmic Agents on Cardiac Action Potential ... 78

Basis for the Antiarrhythmic Action of Class II Drugs — Beta Blockers ... 82

Basis for the Antiarrhythmic Action of Class III and IV Drugs ... 83

Antiarrhythmic Properties of Adenosine Triphosphate and Adenosine ... 84

Properties of Individual Class Ia Antiarrhythmic Drugs ... 86
   Quinidine ... 86
   Procainamide Hydrochloride ... 90
   p-Amino-*N*-(2-diethylamino ethyl) Benzamide ... 93
   Disopyramide Phosphate ... 95

Properties of Individual Class Ib Antiarrhythmic Drugs ... 98
   Lidocaine Hydrochloride ... 98
   Phenytoin Sodium (Dilantin, Diphenylan) ... 100
   Mexiletine Hydrochloride ... 102
   Tocainide Hydrochloride ... 104

Properties of Individual Class Ic Antiarrhythmic Drugs ... 106
   Encainide ... 106
   Flecainide Acetate ... 108
   Lorcainide Hydrochloride (Investigational) ... 110

Properties of Individual Class II Antiarrhythmic Drugs ... 112
   Atenolol ... 114
   Pindolol ... 115
   Propranolol Hydrochloride ... 116
   Timolol Maleate ... 117
   Esmolol ... 118

Properties of Individual Class III Antiarrhythmic Drugs	119
Amiodarone Hydrochloride	119
Bretylium Tosylate	122
Properties of Individual Class IV Antiarrhythmic Drugs	124
Diltiazem Hydrochloride	126
Verapamil Hydrochloride	126
Appendix: Antiarrhythmic Drug Interactions	128

3. Arterial Hypertension   141

Pathophysiology of Primary (Essential) Hypertension	141
Arterial Hypertension Types	145
Treatment of Primary (Essential) Hypertension	148
Emergencies of Hypertension (Blood Pressure Reduction in Hours)	152
Urgencies of Hypertension	153
Resistant Hypertension	154
Antihypertensive Drugs as Monotherapy or Combined Therapy	154
Individual Thiazide Diuretic Drugs	159
Chlorothiazide: Diuril, SK-Chlorothiazide	159
Hydrochlorothiazide: Esidrix, Hydrodiuril, Oretic, Generic	160
Bendroflumethiazide: Naturetin	160
Benzthiazide: Aquatag, Exna, Proaqua, Generic	160
Cyclothiazide: Anhydron	160
Hydroflumethiazide: Diurcardin, Saluron, Generic	161
Methyclothiazide: Aquatensen, Enduron, Generic	161
Polythiazide: Renese	161
Trichlormethiazide: Metahydrin, Naqua, Generic	162
Individual Thiazidelike Diuretic Drugs	162
Chlorthalidone: Hygroton, Generic	162
Indapamide: Lozol	162
Metolazone: Diulo, Zaroxyolyn	163
Quinethazone: Hydromox	163
Loop Diuretics	163
Furosemide: Lasix, SK-Furosemide	164
Ethacrynic Acid: Edecrin	165
Bumetanide: Bumex	165
Potassium-Sparing Diuretics	166
Spironolactone: Aldactone, Generic	167

Amiloride: Mirador	**168**
Triamterene: Dyrenium	**168**
Fixed Combinations of Potassium-Sparing and Thiazide Diuretics	**168**
Spironolactone and Hydrochlorothiazide Tablets	**169**
Amiloride and Hydrochlorothiazide Tablets	**169**
Triamterene and Hydrochlorothiazide Capsules	**169**
Diuretic Drug Interactions	**169**
Sympathetic Depressant Drugs — Beta Adrenoceptor Blockers, Beta Blockers	**171**
Individual Beta Blockers	**178**
Acebutolol: Sectral	**178**
Atenolol: Tenormin	**179**
Labetalol: Normodyne, Trandate	**179**
Metoprolol: Lopressor	**179**
Nadolol: Corgard	**180**
Oxprenolol: Trasicor, Slow-Trasicor	**180**
Pindolol: Visken	**181**
Propranolol: Inderal, Inderal LA, Detensol, Generic	**181**
Timolol: Blocadren	**182**
Fixed Dose Combinations of Beta Blockers and Diuretics	**182**
Atenolol and Chlorthalidone Tablets: Tenoretic	**182**
Metoprolol Tartrate and Hydrochlorothiazide Tablets: Lopressor HCT	**183**
Nadolol and Bendroflumethiazide Tablets: Corzide	**183**
Pindolol Hydrochloride and Hydrochlorothiazide Tablets: Viskenzide	**183**
Propranolol Hydrochloride and Hydrochlorothiazide Tablets: Inderide	**183**
Timolol Maleate and Hydrochlorothiazide Tablets: Timolide	**183**
Beta Blockers — Drug Interactions	**183**
Sympathetic Nervous System Depressant Drugs	**186**
Properties of Individual Sympathetic Nervous System Depressant Drugs	**187**
Reserpine: Sandril, Serpasil, SK-Reserpine, Generic	**187**
Diupres-250–500	**189**
Diutensin-R	**189**
Hydromox-R	**189**
Hydropres-25–50	**190**
Metatensin	**190**
Naquival	**190**
Regroton	**190**
Demi-Regroton	**190**
Renese-R	**190**

Salutensin	190
Salutensin-Demi	190
Serpasil-Esidrix No. 1, No. 2	190
Guanethidine: Ismelin	191
Guanadrel: Hylorel	192
Alpha-Methyldopa: Aldomet	194
Clonidine: Catapres	195
Guanabenz: Wytensin	197
Guanfacine (Investigational Drug)	198
Prazosin: Minipress	199
Fixed Dose Combinations of Sympathetic Depressant Drugs and Diuretics	201
Clonidine Hydrochloride and Chlorthalidone Tablets: Combipres	201
Methyldopa and Chlorothiazide Tablets: Aldoclor	201
Methyldopa and Hydrochlorothiazide Tablets: Aldoril	202
Sympathetic Nervous Tissue Depressant-Drug Interactions	202
Vasodilators	204
Individual Vasodilator Agents	206
Hydralazine: Apresoline, Generic	206
Minoxidil: Loniten	207
Angiotensin-Converting Enzyme Inhibitors	208
Individual Angiotensin-Converting Enzyme Inhibitors	210
Captopril: Capoten	210
Enalapril	211
Angiotensin-Converting Enzyme Inhibitors—Drug Interactions	212
Calcium (Ca^{2+}) Channel Antagonists	213
Individual Calcium (Ca^{2+}) Channel Antagonists	215
Diltiazem: Cardizem	215
Nifedipine: Adalat, Procardia	215
Verapamil Hydrochloride: Calan, Isoptin	216

4. Angina, Ischemia, and Myocardial Injury and Infarction   218

Anatomic Considerations of Coronary Artery Blood Flow	218
Physiologic Considerations of Coronary Artery Blood Flow	219
Role of the Autonomic Nervous System	220
Adaptation to Coronary Artery Stenosis-Subendocardial Region Vulnerability	222
Myocardial Ischemia and Reperfusion	223

Drug Treatment of Myocardial Ischemia and Infarction	230
Sublingual Nitroglycerin	234
Isosorbide Dinitrate	234
Erythrityl Tetranitrate	235
Lingual Nitroglycerin Aerosol	235
Buccal Nitroglycerin	235
Oral Nitroglycerin	235
Isosorbide Dinitrate	236
Pentaerythritol Tetranitrate	236
Topical Nitroglycerin	237
Nitroglycerin-Containing Discs or Patches	237
Intravenous Nitroglycerin	237
Beta-Adrenergic Receptor Antagonists: Beta Blockers	239
Individual Beta Blockers	243
Propranolol Hydrochloride	243
Acebutolol Hydrochloride	244
Atenolol	244
Metoprolol Tartrate	244
Nadolol	245
Pindolol	245
Timolol Maleate	245
Ca^{2+} Channel Blockers in the Treatment of Ischemic Heart Disease	246
Individual Ca^{2+} Channel Blockers	250
Nifedipine	250
Verapamil Hydrochloride	251
Diltiazem	252
Prostaglandin-Related Agents	253
Dipyridamole	253
Epoprostenol Sodium	255
5. Hyperlipidemia and Hypercholesterolemia	**258**
Theories of Atherosclerosis Pathogenesis	258
Plasma Lipoproteins	261
Lipoproteins and Atherosclerosis	265
Genetic Basis for Atherosclerosis	268
Identifying High Risk Factors for Coronary Artery Disease	268
Elevated Levels of Plasma Cholesterol and/or Triglyceride	271
Dietary Modulation of Hyperlipoproteinemia	272
Drug Management of Hyperlipoproteinemia	277

Niacin: Mediated Reduction of Very Low Density Lipoproteins and Low Density Lipoproteins	279
Clofibrate (Atromid-S): Mediated Reduction in Low Density Lipoproteins and Type III Hyperlipoproteinemia	283
Gemfibrozil (Lopid): Mediated Reduction of Hypertriglyceridemia-Hyperlipidemia	286
Cholestyramine Resin (Questran): Modulation of Cholesterol Absorption and Low Density Lipoproteins	288
Colestipol Hydrochloride (Colestipol): Modulation of Low Density Lipoprotein-Receptor Activity	290
Probucol (Lorelco): Mediated Reduction in Low Density Lipoproteins and High Density Lipoproteins	292
Mevinolin: A Drug That Inhibits Cholesterol Synthesis	294
Hormonal Therapy in the Management of Hyperlipoproteinemia	296
Norethindrone Acetate (Aygestin, Norlutate)	296
Oxandrolone (Anavar)	297
Ethinyl Estradiol	297
Dextrothyroxine Sodium (Choloxin)	298

6. Intravascular Thrombogenesis and Thrombolysis — 304

Intravascular Blood Coagulation: Thrombogenesis	304
Intravascular Thrombolysis	306
Convergence of Tissue Kinins, Complement Activation, Thrombogenesis, and Thrombolysis	307
Blood Platelets	308
Aspirin	309
Dipyridamole	309
Sulfinpyrazone	312
Thrombus	313
Anticoagulants	315
Heparin	316
Individual Antithrombotic Drugs	319
Heparin Calcium	319
Heparin Sodium	319
Treatment of Heparin-Mediated Response or Toxicity	319
Protamine Sulfate	319
Vitamin K Antagonists	320
Dicumarol (Abbott)	324
Warfarin Sodium	324
Therapy of Overdose of Vitamin K Antagonists (Phytonadione, K_1)	325

Menadiol Sodium Diphosphate, Vitamin K_4	326
Clinical Use of Antithrombotic Drugs	327
Diagnosis of Deep Vein Thrombosis	327
Diagnosis of Pulmonary Embolism	328
Coronary Artery Disease — Myocardial Infarction	329
Coronary Artery Disease — Unstable Angina Pectoris	331
Valvular Heart Disease and Atrial Fibrillation	333
Cerebrovascular Disease	333
Thrombolytics	334

Drug Evaluations
   Streptokinase
   Urokinase
   t-PA
	345
	345
	346
	346

Therapy Directed Towards Limiting Myocardial Reperfusion Injury and Thrombogeneity	347
Index	355

Foreword

In our Western society, the major cause of mortality and morbidity remains the failure of the cardiovascular system to provide an adequate supply of blood to all tissues. Thus, hypertension, hyperlipidemia, atherosclerosis, angina pectoris, myocardial infarction, arrhythmias, and heart failure remain major problems for a large portion of the population.

Physicians, whether in general or specialized practice, are confronted daily with the need to prescribe drugs to relieve cardiovascular symptoms or to prevent their complications. This task is not simple because each of the many drugs available is chemically and pharmacologically distinct. Furthermore, the growing use of multiple drugs increases considerably the chance of interaction between the different therapeutic agents given to the patient. Thus, the amount of data and facts, both basic and clinical, the physician should know to fully understand the complexity of cardiovascular pharmacology has increased exponentially in the last decade, to a point that is almost impossible to overlook.

The pressure for information regarding cardiac drugs is most intense in emergency situations where global information on cardiovascular pharmacodynamics and pharmacokinetics must be available to the primary care physician in a comprehensive but readily available format. Meeting this challenge is difficult and has been the primary concern of the authors of *Handbook of Cardiac Drugs: Basic Science and Clinical Aspects of Cardiovascular Pharmacology*. Indeed, Drs. Purdy and Boucek have made every possible effort to provide physicians both with solid, indepth coverage of the theories and immediate access to therapeutic facts. They said to me: "We held in our minds the image of a physician in the emergency room at 2:00 A.M., confronted with a situation requiring a rapid response. We believe that the physician will be able to pick up our book and go straight to the section that provides the information needed in capsule form. However, if additional information is required, the physician can return to our book the next day and read on the particular subject in depth." It is remarkable how well the authors have achieved their goal of continued accessibility and comprehensiveness.

The key to the success of the book is the organization and harmony of the individual chapters, an extensive table of contents, and a first-class index. The book is a scholarly written, complete overview of cardiovascular pharmacology that provides easy retrieval of the clinically important facts. This book will be a great help not only to practicing physicians applying cardiovascular pharmacology but also to medical students learning to understand it.

Paul M. Vanhoutte, M.D., Ph.D.

Preface

Because of the mercurial expressions and the potential lethality of certain cardiovascular diseases, physicians and other health care professionals are often required to diagnose and identify an effective therapeutic strategy under stressful and time-limited conditions. In this setting the pragmatics of cardiovascular pharmacology require rapid access to information for appropriate drug selection in managing acute expressions of congestive heart failure, cardiac dysrhythmia, arterial hypertension, myocardial ischemia, and intravascular thrombogenesis. In writing this book we kept in mind the emergency room or intensive care unit at 2:00 A.M. with a particular cardiovascular crisis where superb cross-indexing to drugs and their dosages, modes of administration, adverse reactions, and drug interactions could spell the difference between success and failure — between life and death for the patient. Thereafter, we have provided an extensive review of the pathophysiology and diagnosis, as well as nuances of the selected drugs, for retrospective and scholarly survey under more quiet and thoughtful conditions.

Direction for drug management of chronic cardiac diseases with its own set of nuances was another objective of the book. Here, knowledge of the pathophysiology of the chronic disease extends the understanding of drugs in palliating, modulating, preventing, or even reversing a chronic disease. In achieving this objective we have provided insights into an ever-expanding data base from which effective therapeutic strategies for managing chronic expressions of heart failure, arrhythmias, hypertension, and ischemic heart disease can be arranged by cardiologists, internists, and family practitioners.

In considering therapeutic choices for managing acute and chronic expressions of cardiac disease, special attention was given to age-related differences in drug response. Because of these differences in target organ response and in the transport, distribution, and elimination of drugs, guidance in selecting drugs and proper doses is essential information for a successful practice of both pediatric and geriatric cardiology. In addition, the multi-system diseases of many geriatric patients lead to "polypharmaceutics" and the ever-present but often overlooked possibility of noxious drug interactions.

A contemporary thrust in adult cardiology is the prevention of target organ deterioration from hypertension, hyperlipidemia, ischemia, and intravascular thrombus formation. While preventive cardiology is and has been a focus of pediatricians, adult- and geriatric-oriented clinicians are latter-day enthusiasts. Therefore, preventive cardiology is included as part of the chapters on hypertension, hyperlipidemia, atherogenesis, myocardial ischemia, myocardial reperfusion injury, intravascular thrombogenesis, and vascular restenosis following angioplasty or bypass grafting.

A listing of selected literature citations is included at the end of each chapter to provide ready entry into the key considerations of the pathophysiology and pharmacology of the major cardiac diseases. The list is not encyclopedic for the subject material. References recognized as standards by the medical community were used as sources for specific drug information. For example, dosages and administration modes were taken from the *United States Pharmacopeia Drug Information* and the *AMA Drug Evaluations*. These references, along with *EDI Drug Interactions*, were used to identify relevant drug interactions. Finally, Goodman and Gilman's *The Rational Basis for Therapeutic Practice* was used as a general source of drug information.

If improved clarity in understanding and managing exceedingly complex cardiac diseases comes from our efforts, then the book will have achieved its main purpose. A functionally effective book on the basic and applied science of cardiovascular pharmacology will provide a unique resource for house staff, cardiac fellows, family physicians, internists, and medical and surgical cardiologists.

R. E. P.
R. J. B.

Acknowledgments

We thank Drs. Frank C. Boucek and Mark M. Boucek for their review and helpful criticisms of Chapter 1. We also thank Elizabeth Anne Shirley, M.S., M.P.H., R.D., for her critical review of Chapter 5. We gratefully acknowledge the excellent work of Ms. Kathy Huettl and Ms. Cherie Jameison in preparing the first typed copies of Chapters 1 through 3. In addition, we single out Ms. Linda Relph for special recognition. She not only prepared the first typed copies of Chapters 4 through 6 but also drew all illustrations and prepared the many subsequent drafts of all the chapters. Ms. Relph's tireless efforts were essential to the completion of the book, and we are grateful to her.

Handbook of Cardiac Drugs

Basic Science and Clinical Aspects of Cardiovascular Pharmacology

Notice
The indications and dosages of all drugs in this book have been recommended in the medical literature and conform to the practices of the general medical community. The medications described do not necessarily have specific approval by the Food and Drug Administration for use in the diseases and dosages for which they are recommended. The package insert for each drug should be consulted for use and dosage as approved by the FDA. Because standards for usage change, it is advisable to keep abreast of revised recommendations, particularly those concerning new drugs.

1

Congestive Heart Failure

Definition

Congestive heart failure (CHF) is a complex clinical response to a cardiac output that is inadequate for the metabolic needs of tissues. The initial clinical manifestations may be fatigability, a diminished exercise tolerance or dyspnea with mild effort, peripheral edema, or a combination of these. Occasionally CHF presents as an acute respiratory distress.

Acute respiratory distress secondary to pulmonary congestion is a common presentation of acute left heart failure and represents a major therapeutic challenge in cardiology. In pulmonary congestion (or peripheral edema), the basic phenomenon of fluid moving from blood to extracellular spaces on the arterial side and returning on the venous side of the capillary bed is altered. Under normal conditions, hydrostatic pressure exceeds colloid osmotic pressure on the arterial side, and a pressure gradient is created that drives fluid from the blood compartment. The reverse is true on the venous side, where a lower hydrostatic pressure allows the colloid osmotic pressure to move fluid back to the blood compartment. In CHF, elevation of venous hydrostatic pressure caused by increases in plasma volume raises the hydrostatic-colloid pressure ratio, and fluid remains in the extracellular compartment.

The determinants of cardiac output under normal, healthful conditions, along with pharmacologic modifiers, are summarized in Fig. 1-1. These determinants are the preload and the afterload to the heart coupled with the myocardial contractility and the heart rate.

Compensatory Responses

Once initiated, CHF sets in motion autoregulatory processes mediated in large measure by autonomic nervous and neurohumoral activities. These autoregulatory processes provide avenues for therapeutic palliation when a cure is not possible.

The transmitter substances and hormones associated with primary compensatory neurohumoral activities profoundly affect:

circulatory fluid volume and venous constriction (preload)
cardiac rate (chronotropy) and rhythmicity
contractile properties of the heart (inotropy)
arterial and arteriolar contraction (afterload) of the heart

SYMPATHETIC NERVOUS SYSTEM

An increased filling pressure (preload) enhances adrenergic (sympathetic) release and reduces clearance of catecholamines,

Written in collaboration with Robert J. Boucek, Jr., M.D., Associate Professor of Pediatric Cardiology, Vanderbilt University School of Medicine, Nashville, TN

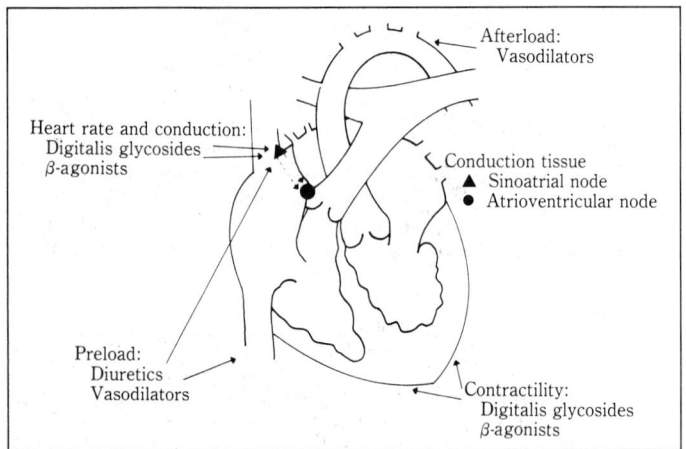

Fig. 1-1. Sites where therapeutic intervention improves cardiac function.

thereby raising arterial levels of norepinephrine and dopamine. In the early stages of CHF, increased catecholamine levels stimulate myocardial adrenergic β-receptor (adrenoceptor) activities to maintain cardiac output (inotropy) as well as arterial and β-adrenoceptor activities to raise vascular tone (afterload).

Data from endomyocardial biopsies indicate that the down-regulation of β-adrenoceptors begins with mild to moderate ventricular dysfunction; thereafter a reduced myocardial β-adrenoceptor density is related to the degree of heart failure. Most important, β-adrenoceptor "down-regulation is associated with pharmacologically specific impairment of the β-agonist-mediated contractile response" [10]. In later stages of CHF, high levels of norepinephrine are released from the heart, but the density and contractile response of cardiac adrenoceptors are reduced. As a consequence, a patient in end-stage CHF with a dilated heart and low stroke volume experiences limited inotropic benefits from released norepinephrine. At this stage, elevated plasma norepinephrine levels improve cardiac output **only** by increasing the heart rate (chronotropy). Plasma norepinephrine levels are high in patients with progressive CHF; therefore the absolute plasma norepinephrine level may be a better guide to prognosis than depressed hemodynamic indices of cardiac performance [5].

NEUROHUMORAL SYSTEMS

Coincident with or following the sympathetic nervous system response to CHF is a set of secondary compensatory responses involving the atrial natriuretic peptide (ANP), renal processes, and arginine vasopressin as they affect preload, afterload, heart rate, and myocardial contractility.

Plasma ANP arising from secretory cells located in both atria is released by changes in right atrial, pulmonary artery wedge, and mean arterial pressures and by increases in heart rate and plasma volume. ANP links the heart, kidneys, adrenals, blood vessels, and brain in a complex hormonal system involved in volume and pressure homeostasis. It blocks the adrenal glands' production of aldosterone, has the potential for interfering with the renin-angiotensin system and the arginine vasopressin system, and may be involved in clinical conditions associated with fluid retention. The diuretic and natriuretic actions of ANP are mainly due to its vasorelaxing effect on renal arteries and arterioles and to increases in glomerular filtration rate and filtration fraction.

In CHF, plasma ANP concentrations are directly related to cardiac filling pressure and inversely related to the left ventricular ejection fraction. Even though ANP can increase the glomerular filtration rate at doses that decrease blood pressure and total renal blood flow, the hormone is ineffective in producing natriuresis in patients with CHF [3]. Interestingly, injection of a synthetic analogue of ANP in patients with chronic CHF causes considerable reductions in (1) mean systemic arterial pressure, (2) pulmonary mean and diastolic pressures, and (3) right atrial pressure. In turn, these reductions increase cardiac output [8].

In the more advanced stages of CHF with high levels of sympathetic tone, the activation of the renin-angiotensin system appears to dominate effects of ANP and, in fact, contributes substantially to the progression of CHF. The direct effects of increased sympathetic tone and activation of the renin-angiotensin system are to (1) increase total peripheral resistance; (2) cause venoconstriction, thereby reducing venous capacitance; and (3) increase plasma volume. Increased peripheral resistance alone reduces cardiac output, and all three extracardiac effects contribute to cardiac dilatation: increased peripheral resistance by reducing cardiac emptying during systole so that the ventricular volume at diastole is greater; both the reduced venous capacitance and increased plasma volume by increasing venous return to the heart and thus the preload of ventricular filling during diastole.

Arginine vasopressin (AVP) levels are also increased with CHF. The role of AVP in osmoregulation remains intact in CHF, but the absolute AVP level for a given serum osmolality is high. The hyponatremia in some patients with severe CHF may be due in part to an increased neurohypophyseal secretion of AVP. AVP may also contribute to vasoconstriction in CHF. A variable relationship exists between AVP level and urinary osmolality in CHF.

ROLE OF THE KIDNEY

Abnormal sodium (Na^+) levels and water retention are phenomena of early as well as advanced stages of CHF. Initially, the afferent signal(s) for Na^+ retention may arise from low-pressure, volume-sensitive receptors in the thorax or volume receptors in the atria and ventricles. In advanced CHF, signals for Na^+ and water retention arise from (1) the reduced renal blood, secondary to decreased cardiac output; (2) the increased renal vascular resistance from sustained sympathetic stimulation, particularly at the level of the afferent and efferent arterioles; and (3) elevated circulating angiotensin II, secondary to sympathetic stimulation of the juxtaglomerular cells with the attending release of renin. Angiotensin may participate with sympathetic stimulation in increasing renal vascular resistance. Other factors, such as increased circulating vasopressin levels, contribute to the alteration of kidney function. Each of these signals operates to reduce glomerular filtration. However, through adjustments at the level of afferent and efferent arterioles, the kidney maintains glomerular filtration at or near normal levels by increasing the filtration fraction.

ROLE OF PROSTAGLANDINS

While CHF activates the sympathetic and neurohumoral systems, in advanced CHF counterregulatory hormonal factors that modulate vasoconstrictive and Na^+-retaining properties of the sympathetic and renin-angiotensin systems are also activated. Production of vasodilator prostaglandins, such as prostaglandin E_2 (PGE_2) and prostacyclin (PGI_2), is activated in severe CHF. Increases in PGE_2 reduce impedance to the left ventricular (LV) outflow as well as enhance Na^+ excretion. As a result of counterregulatory prostaglandin factors, patients with CHF are particularly susceptible to clinical deterioration when given nonsteroidal anti-inflammatory drugs (e.g., indomethacin). Drugs such as captopril, on the other hand, enhance PGE_2 production, since both captopril and PGE_2 reduce left ventricular impedance in CHF.

CARDIAC DILATATION

Cardiac chamber size affects sarcomere length and, ultimately, wall stress. Initially, enlargement of the heart serves a beneficial purpose by increasing the cardiac output according to the Frank-Starling law, which equates increased heart size and sarcomere length with greater systolic contraction. However, according to the law of Laplace, the mechanical efficiency of the heart is also a function of heart size; that is, at a given ejection pressure, the wall tension developed during systole increases with ventricular radius. Thus, in a markedly dilated heart, loss of mechanical efficiency not only offsets the benefits gained from the Frank-Starling effect, but also contributes to the impairment of pump function. As a consequence, the Frank-Starling curve for the failing heart is flatter than the normal curve (Fig. 1-2), and, in acute congestive heart disease, the heart operates in the plateau region, even at rest. Additional cardiac chamber dilation causes the heart to operate on the descending limb of the Frank-Starling curve, that is, to decompensate.

Treatment of Acute Heart Failure

CAUSES

CHF may appear acutely, or it may develop over weeks or months. In either scenario, therapeutic management is directed

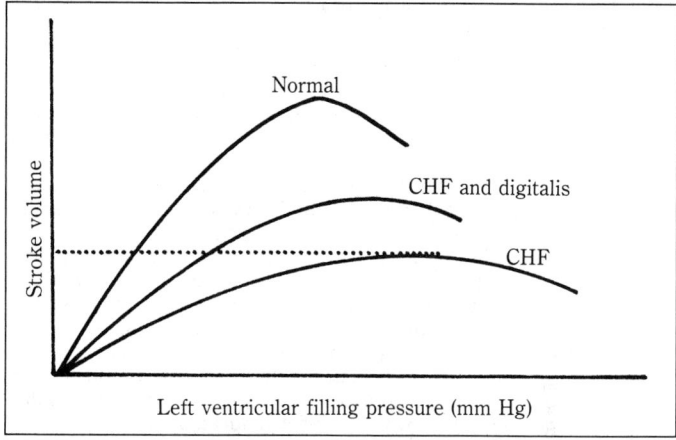

Fig. 1-2. The Frank-Starling relationship between stroke volume and left ventricular filling pressure in normal and failing heart and in the failing heart during therapy with digitalis. Peak of the curve for congestive heart failure (*CHF*) is indicated by dotted line.

toward modifying preload, afterload, heart rate, or myocardial contractility. The focus of therapy, however, is influenced by the acuteness or the chronicity of CHF. In infancy and childhood, a rapid onset of CHF may be the presenting sign of congenital anomalies associated with abnormal preload or afterload (Table 1-1). In pediatric patients the overall incidence of CHF is highest in infancy; however, there are numerous causes in childhood and adolescence (Table 1-1). Congenital heart disease, acquired myocardial dysfunction (infectious or toxic in origin), and valvular incompetence are the major causes in children and adolescents.

Acute CHF in adults (Table 1-2) is most commonly due to myocardial dysfunction secondary to myocardial infarction (MI). In such cases, the severity of the failure (Killip classification [13]) bears a direct relationship to the mortality rate, as shown in Table 1-3.

Patients with MI and pulmonary edema require hemodynamic monitoring by Swan-Ganz catheter in the pulmonary artery as well as a catheter in a peripheral artery in order to assess therapy and reduce the mortality rate.

THERAPEUTIC END POINTS

The following end points are sought in the management of acute heart failure:

Relief of dyspnea by reducing pulmonary edema
Improvement of cardiac output by decreasing preload, afterload, or both; by increasing myocardial contractility; and by reducing heart rate
Improvement of oxygen delivery to the tissue

Table 1-1. Causes of acute heart failure in the pediatric population

I. Congenital anomalies
   A. Associated with abnormal preload
      1. Extracardiac: patent ductus arteriosus; aortic septal defect; truncus arteriosus; arteriovenous (AV) fistula (cerebral, hepatic)
      2. Intracardiac: ventricular septal defect; single ventricle; AV canal; atrial septal defect; common atrium; anomalous pulmonary venous return
      3. Inflow lesions: mitral stenosis; cor triatriatum; pulmonary vein stenosis; total anomalous pulmonary venous connection with obstructed common pulmonary vein; tricuspid atresia with small foramen ovale
   B. Associated with abnormal afterload — obstruction to blood (outflow lesions): pulmonic or aortic stenosis or atresia; coarctation of aorta; hypoplastic aorta; hypoplastic left heart with constricted ductus arteriosus

II. Primary myocardial dysfunction
   A. Congenital
      1. Endocardial fibroelastosis
      2. Cardiac artery anomalies
   B. Metabolic
      1. Glycogen storage disease
      2. Hypocalcemia; hypoglycemia
   C. Acquired
      1. Myocarditis
      2. Nutritional

III. Secondary myocardial dysfunction
   A. Arrhythmia
   B. Hypertension
   C. Renal disease
   D. Hyperthyroidism
   E. Respiratory distress

IV. Disturbed myocardial oxygen supply or cardiac filling
   A. Severe anemia
   B. Severe hypoxemia and acidemia
   C. Pericardial effusion
   D. Tension pneumothorax

MODULATION OF PRELOAD AND AFTERLOAD

Depressed cardiac output can be improved by drugs that modify the preload, the afterload, or both. Drugs acting primarily on the venous side or on blood volume decrease central venous and pulmonary wedge pressure, leading to the mobilization of edematous fluid, which in turn reduces pulmonary congestion and associated dyspnea. Drugs acting on the arterial side decrease total peripheral resistance and allow more rapid and complete cardiac emptying during systole and therefore an increase in cardiac output.

Decreasing venous return by rotating tourniquets, phlebotomy, or IV diuretics is a means of acutely lowering preload in acute pulmonary edema. Phlebotomy should be used only in patients

Table 1-2. Causes of acute heart failure in adults

Condition	Disease
Excessive afterload	Hypertension
	Mitral or aortic valve stenosis
Excessive preload	Valvular regurgitation
	Arteriovenous shunt
Myocardial dysfunction	Ischemia secondary to coronary artery disease
	Infarction with reduced pump function
	Cardiomyopathy: idiopathic; alcoholic nutritional deficiency (e.g., severe thiamine deficiency)
	Toxic assault (e.g., doxorubicin)
	Thyrotoxicosis, hypothyroidism
Inflow obstruction	Inflammatory chronic pericarditis
Cor pulmonale	Dilatation and failure of the right heart caused by chronic pulmonary obstruction disease

with a hemoglobin level higher than 11 mg/dl who are free of hypotension. (Approximately 250 ml of blood may be removed in a standard blood donor bag setup under constant arterial pressure monitoring.)

DIURETICS

Diuretic IV therapy for children and adolescents [1] is as follows:

Furosemide: 1 mg/kg; repeat 1–2 times/day for 2–3 days
Side effects and treatment: dilutional hyponatremia; fluid restriction, furosemide

In adults, diuretics reduce preload. Patients who have not taken diuretics may obtain relief from acute dyspnea by the diuresis obtained from 20–40 mg of furosemide (IV) or 25–50 mg of ethacrynic acid. Diuretics must, however, be used with caution in patients with acute CHF.

Table 1-3. Mortality and Killip classification of congestive heart failure (CHF)

Classification	Clinical findings	Short-term mortality (%)
I (uncomplicated)	No CHF	6
II (mild to moderate)	Bibasilar rales and/or S3	17
III (severe)	Rales above tip of scapula, S3 gallop, frank pulmonary edema	38
IV (cardiogenic shock)	Reduced peripheral perfusion, mental confusion, diaphoresis, hypotension (<90 mm Hg systolic)	81

The diuretic effect on preload (blood volume) and on serum potassium (K^+) must be closely monitored in pediatric and adult patients with acute pulmonary edema. Preload is assessed from the pulmonary artery diastolic pressure (obtained from a Swan-Ganz catheter).

Reduction of preload in acute CHF (in pediatric and adult populations) has three benefits: First, central venous pressure is lowered, creating pressure gradients at the venous side of the capillary bed that favor mobilization of edematous fluid from the extracellular to the intravascular compartment and subsequent urinary elimination. Second, venous return to the heart is reduced, lowering ventricular end-diastolic volume, which in turn decreases the work of the heart and myocardial oxygen consumption. Third, a reduced central venous pressure favors clearance of pulmonary lymph.

The capacity of diuretics to reduce intravascular volume also limits the usefulness of these agents. If diuresis is too vigorous, venous return to the heart, and therefore cardiac output, is substantially reduced, and CHF may be exacerbated. Thus, the dose of diuretic must be titrated to obtain the lowest possible intravascular volume with little or no reduction in cardiac output.

In general, diuretic therapy is not accompanied by increases in cardiac output, unless an elevated systemic arterial pressure is lowered and systemic peripheral resistance is reduced.

VASODILATOR THERAPY

Vasodilator therapy may be used if the patient is normotensive or hypertensive. In children and adolescents [1], vasodilators are usually reserved for cases with unsatisfactory response to inotropic and diuretic therapy.

Children, adolescents:
  Isoproterenol hydrochloride, 0.01–0.50 µg/kg/min IV.
  Sodium nitroprusside, 0.5–3.0 µg/kg/min IV.
  Hydralazine, 0.5–1.0 mg/kg IV q6–8h.
Adults:
  Morphine sulfate, 5–10 mg IV.
  Nitroglycerine, 15 µg/min IV.
  Sodium nitroprusside, 0.5 µg/kg/min IV (beginning infusion rate).

Morphine Sulfate

Morphine sulfate relieves respiratory distress secondary to bronchospasm in the acute pulmonary edema of CHF. Morphine sulfate also relieves pain and anxiety and induces sedation. In addition, the drug dilates peripheral arteriolar and venous channels and reduces pre- and afterloading of the heart to increase cardiac output. Although useful in the acute stages of pulmonary edema, morphine sulfate is soon exchanged for other vasodilators.

An IV injection of morphine sulfate greatly reduces heart rate, cardiac index, stroke index, and arterial pressure. Cardiac filling pressure (pulmonary wedge pressure) is also reduced. Oxygen consumption is considerably reduced, reflecting sedation and analgesia [18].

The drug is available as morphine sulfate injection, 2, 4, 8, 10, and 15 mg/ml, and may be administered by intramuscular (IM) injection of 5–20 mg every 4 hours as needed. An initial IM dose of 5–10 mg, based on a body weight of 70 kg, is recommended. Subcutaneous injection may also be used. However, the IM route is preferred when multiple doses are anticipated. If the IV route is necessary, morphine sulfate should be administered in 4- to 10-mg doses diluted in 4–5 ml of water and injected over a period of 4–5 minutes. Lower doses (2 mg IV) injected slowly are recommended in low output states especially in geriatric (>65 years) patients. The IM route may not be desired in patients with myocardial infarction because of the release of creatine kinase from skeletal muscle. Greater risk of adverse reactions —respiratory depression, hypotension, peripheral circulatory collapse — accompanies the use of the IV route.

Because of its potential depressive effect on respiration, extreme caution must be used when giving morphine sulfate to patients with any form of respiratory impairment: for example, asthma, chronic obstructive pulmonary disease, cor pulmonale, hypoxia, or hypercapnia.

Organic Nitrates

Coincident with the use of morphine sulfate, patients with moderate acute CHF are usually given organic nitrates, either IV, sublingually, or transdermally. Nitrates dilate the venous capacitance vessels and large arteries such as the epicardial coronary and pulmonary arteries, with lesser effect on systemic arterial resistance vessels (arterioles). Thus, these agents decrease central venous, pulmonary capillary wedge, and right atrial pressures and are particularly effective in reducing pulmonary congestion. Under some circumstances, they may improve myocardial perfusion by a combination of coronary artery vasodilation and decreased left ventricular end-diastolic pressure.

The organic nitrates share with other venodilators the capacity to induce orthostatic hypotension. Used alone, the organic nitrates may have their greatest benefit in patients with mild to moderate left ventricular failure, elevated pulmonary capillary wedge pressure, and near-normal cardiac output. Not generally recognized is a heparin resistance induced by parenterally administered organic nitrates and a marked increase in sensitivity (to heparin) upon discontinuing IV nitrates. Patients requiring IV nitroglycerin and heparin infusions should be monitored by measurements of the activated partial thromboplastin time, particularly when the dose of nitrates is altered.

DIRECTIONS FOR IV NITROGLYCERIN INFUSION

1. Dissolve 50 mg nitroglycerin in 250 ml 5% D/W (done in pharmacy).

2. Monitor arterial pressure of frequent intervals with Dinamap measurements.
3. With low cardiac output, insert Swan-Ganz catheter to follow pulmonary capillary wedge pressure (PCWP). A thermodilution catheter should be used to obtain repeated cardiac output (CO) measurements.
4. Calculate body surface area (BSA) from the height and weight.
5. Obtain baseline heart rate and hemodynamics:

Cardiac output (CO) — 3.5–5.0 liter/min

Cardiac index (CI) (2.4–4 liter/min/m^2) = CO/BSA (m^2) (BSA = body surface area; calculated from height and weight charts)

Stroke volume (SV) (70–130 ml/contraction = CO/heart rate

Stroke volume index (SI) (35–70 ml/contraction/m^2) = SV/BSA

Rate-pressure product (R-PP) (72–96 mm Hg × beat/min) = Systolic pressure × heart rate ÷ 100

Systemic vascular resistance (SVR) (1130 ± 78 dyne/second/cm^{-5}) = (mean arterial pressure [MAP] − central venous pressure [CVP]) × 80 ÷ CO (80 is a constant converting R units to dyne/second/cm^{-5}) or (20 resistance units) = MAP/CO

Pulmonary vascular resistance (PVR) (<160 dyne/second/cm^{-5}) = (mean pulmonary artery pressure [MPAP] − pulmonary capillary wedge pressure [PCWP]) × 80 ÷ CO or (2 resistance units) = MPAP − PCWP/CO

Left ventricular end diastolic pressure (LVEDP) (<10 mm Hg) = mean PCWP

6. Begin infusion at 10 μg/min with infusion pump. In a solution of 50 mg in 250 ml 5% D/W, 3 ml/hr will deliver about 10 μg/min. Increase infusion in 3 ml/hr increments until MAP reaches 75–80 mm Hg. Overshooting is fine tuned with smaller increments
7. Another goal is an optimal PCWP of about 18 mm Hg.
8. Repeat calculations every 15 minutes during infusion.

Sodium Nitroprusside (Nipride)

IV sodium nitroprusside is a potent, immediate-acting organic nitrate that acts equally on venous and arterial circuits to reduce both pre- and afterloading of the heart. Sodium nitroprusside is more potent in reducing afterload than is nitroglycerin. Central venous, pulmonary capillary wedge, left ventricular end-diastolic, and systemic arterial pressures are decreased. Pulmonary congestion and dyspnea are reduced, and cardiac output may increase, provided that left ventricular end-diastolic pressure and volume are markedly reduced. Sodium nitroprusside increases forward stroke volume in mitral and aortic regurgitation.

Sodium nitroprusside has a brief action, and the pharmacologic response essentially ends as the IV infusion is stopped because the drug is rapidly converted to thiocyanate.

According to Cohn and colleagues [4], a short-term (48-hour) infusion of sodium nitroprusside started after 9 hours from the onset of pain significantly improved the survivor rate of patients with MI at 13 weeks. They caution that the drug had a deleterious effect (on survival) when the infusion was started within 9 hours of onset of the acute pain and that sodium nitroprusside should not be used in patients with low left ventricular filling pressure.

The drug (50-mg vial) is dissolved in 2–3 ml of D/W. The solution is then diluted to 250 ml with 5% D/W and promptly wrapped in aluminum foil. Sodium nitroprusside deteriorates with exposure to light and should be used within 4 hours after preparation. In an aqueous solution, sodium nitroprusside yields a nitroprusside ion that reacts within minutes with a variety of inorganic and organic substances to form a colored solution (blue, green, or dark red). If colored solutions develop, the infusion should be replaced.

DOSAGE AND ADMINISTRATION

After preparing the solution, the time of preparation should be noted to prevent administration for longer than 4 hours. The sodium nitroprusside infusion fluid should not be employed as a vehicle for other drugs. The **average dose** is 3µg/kg/min (usual range of 0.5–10.0 µg/kg/min). Usually, 3 µg/kg/min lowers arterial pressure 30–40% below pretreatment diastolic levels. Infusion rate is then adjusted to lower the diastolic pressure below 90 mm Hg. At no time should the infusion rate reduce systolic blood pressure below 90 mm Hg.

ADVERSE EFFECTS

Sodium nitroprusside should be used with great **caution** in patients with a history of inadequate cerebral circulation.

The drug can cause the following **adverse effects:** nausea, retching, diaphoresis, apprehension, headaches, restlessness, muscle twitching, retrosternal discomfort, palpitations, and abdominal pain.

OVERDOSAGE

The first sign of **overdosage** is profound hypotension and metabolic acidosis. This may be followed by dyspnea, headache, vomiting, dizziness, ataxia, and loss of consciousness. If these symptoms and/or signs appear, sodium nitroprusside infusion should be immediately discontinued.

Massive overdosage may produce signs similar to those of cyanide poisoning: coma, imperceptible pulse, absent reflexes, widely dilated pupils, pink color, hypotension, and shallow breathing. If massive overdosage has occurred, do the following:

Discontinue sodium nitroprusside.
Administer amyl nitrite inhalations for 15–30 seconds each minute until 3% sodium nitrite solution is prepared for IV administration.
Give sodium nitrite (3%) solution at a rate not exceeding 2.5–5.0 ml/min up to a total dose of 10–15 ml with careful blood pressure monitoring.

Then inject sodium thiosulfate (IV) 12.5 gm in 50 ml of 5% D/W over a 10-minute period.

Monitor patient for reappearance of overdose signs.

If overdose signs reappear, then repeat the sodium nitrite and sodium thiosulfate injections in one-half the above dose.

Arterial pressure drops with sodium nitrite and sodium thiosulfate may be corrected with vasopressor agents.

CALCULATION OF SODIUM NITROPRUSSIDE INFUSION RATES

The following formula is useful for calculating dosage of any drug given by an intravenous infusion pump set at milliliters per hour (ml/hr) [12]:

$\mu g/min/kg = (16.7) (ml/hr) (mg/ml) \div kg$

where $\mu g/min/kg$ is dose given by the infusion pump in ml/hr, 16.7 is the constant used to convert hours to minutes and milligrams to micrograms, mg/ml is the drug concentration in the infusion bottle, and kg is the patient's weight.

The following equation is useful in ordering solution and calculating the rate of the infusion to give a certain dosage of drug:

$ml/hr = (\mu g/min/kg) (kg) \div 16.7 (mg/ml)$

BETA BLOCKER AFTER ACUTE MYOCARDIAL INFARCTION AND CONGESTIVE HEART FAILURE

Patients (30–69 years old) in the Beta Blocker Heart Attack Trial (BHAT) (see Chap. 4) were randomly assigned to placebo (1921 patients) or propranolol hydrochloride, 180–240 mg daily (1916 patients), 5–21 days after MI. The beta blocker did not worsen the CHF and did not decrease the total mortality but significantly reduced the occurrence of sudden death [2].

MODULATION OF MYOCARDIAL CONTRACTILITY

Digitalis Glycosides

Positively inotropic agents should be used with caution in acute CHF secondary to myocardial infarction in order to avoid additional ischemic myocardial injury. These agents enhance contractility, increase cardiac output, and lead to reflex systemic vasodilation. When they are used, the lowest dose that produces the desired effect should be employed with guidance from hemodynamic monitoring.

The most widely used positively inotropic drug is digitalis, but its usefulness in acute CHF is limited because of its restricted potency when compared with nonglycosidic positively inotropic agents. However, the effect of digitalis on the autonomic nervous system and on sinoatrial (SA) and atrioventricular (AV) activities may be important in a clinical setting of atrial fibrillation with rapid ventricular response as a complication of MI.

After IV administration of digitalis (digoxin), the concentration declines rapidly so that within 15 minutes only 6% may be found

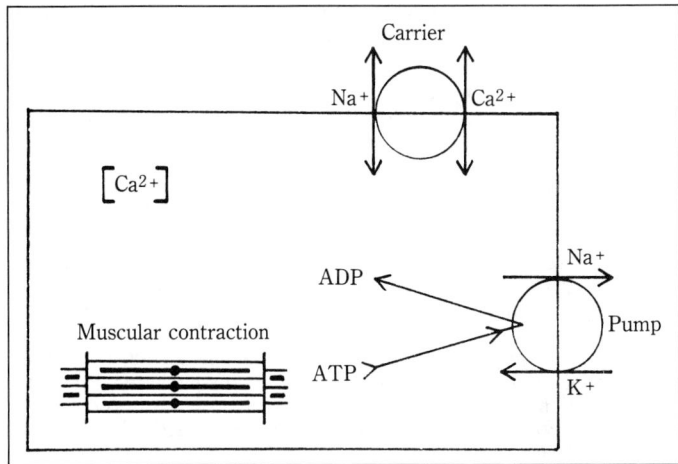

Fig. 1-3. Cardiac membrane mechanisms regulating free cytosolic calcium: Na^+-K^+ ATPase pump; Na^+-Ca^{2+} exchange carrier. (ADP = adenosine diphosphate; ATP = adenosine triphosphate.)

in plasma. The distribution is such that the highest concentration occurs in the kidney, followed by that in cardiac muscle. Because of differences in tissue mass, skeletal muscle binds more digoxin than does cardiac muscle, but the concentration is lower in skeletal than in cardiac muscle. Reduced skeletal muscle mass (because of aging or inanition) or lowered renal function will produce higher plasma digoxin levels for a given IV dose. A large plasma volume and interstitial fluid space will lower serum digoxin levels when compared to values calculated on the basis of dose estimates based on milligrams per kilogram body weight.

Mechanism of Action

Even with knowledge gained after years of research, the mechanism of digitalis-mediated myocardial inotropy remains unknown. Nevertheless, certain aspects of the mechanism are known. Digitalis has no direct effect on the intracellular mechanisms of oxygen utilization, substrate metabolism, or other factors involved in the generation of high-energy phosphate. Instead, digitalis appears to act by altering ionic fluxes across the cardiac cell membrane.

Two membrane components of prime importance in this process are the Na^+ pump, which extrudes Na^+ and transports K^+ into the cell, and the Na^+-Ca^{2+} exchange carrier, which mediates the coupled exchange transport of Na^+ and Ca^{2+} across the membrane (Fig. 1-3). The direction of exchange via this carrier is determined by the relative concentrations of the two ions on either side of the cell membrane. In the most likely sequence of events, digitalis binds to and inhibits Na^+-K^+ adenosinetriphosphatase (ATPase) located in the cell membrane. The activity of this enzyme generates the energy for the Na^+ pump. Thus, inhibition of the enzyme decreases pump activity and therefore the rate of extrusion of Na^+ from the cell. All of the Na^+ that enters during the first phase of the action potential is pumped out, but at a slower rate.

As a consequence, the Na^+ concentration on the inner side of the cell membrane $[NA_i]$ is transiently higher during each heartbeat and is available for exchange with extracellular CA^{2+} via a Na^+-Ca^{2+} exchange carrier, by an electrogenic Ca^{2+} influx, or both. Ca^{2+} binds to troponin and initiates the interaction of actin and myosin. Intracellular Ca^{2+} ($[Ca_i]$) becomes transiently elevated during each heartbeat. Peak $[Ca_i]$ initiates and determines the force of cardiac contraction. Presumably, the transiently higher $[Ca_i]$ caused by digitalis facilitates this process. A possible additional mechanism for controlling $[Ca_i]$ concentration has also been identified. Increased $[Ca_i]$ stimulates release of stored Ca^{2+} from the sarcoplasmic reticulum, further increasing the concentration of $[Ca_i]$. In summary, a digitalis-mediated transient elevation of $[Na_i]$ during systole ultimately leads to transiently elevated $[Ca_i]$ levels and thus to increased strength of myocardial contraction (positive inotropy).

Inotropic Action of Digitalis and the Frank-Starling Relationship

The inotropic action of digitalis is independent of the relationship between cardiac output (stroke volume) and left ventricular end-diastolic volume (the Frank-Starling relationship). Provided the diseased heart has residual contractile reserve, digitalis increases contractility at any level of cardiac dilatation (see Fig. 1-2). The Frank-Starling curve for severe congestive disease has a shallow slope, and the heart operates at the peak of the curve in order to maintain resting cardiac output. Digitalis generates a new, steeper Frank-Starling curve. Moreover, the greater strength and rate of systolic ejection increases the efficiency of left ventricle emptying and reduces heart size at the beginning of diastole; that is, left ventricular end-diastolic volume decreases, allowing the heart to utilize the residual reserve and operate on the more favorable ascending part of the Frank-Starling curve. With marked cardiac dilatation, reduction in heart size and improved mechanical efficiency become an important component of the successful treatment of CHF with digitalis.

Digitalis and the Sympathetic Nervous System

A positively inotropic effect of digitalis is not always paralleled by or proportionate to a reduced heart rate caused by atrioventricular blocking (dromotropic effect). Indeed, the digitalis-mediated inotropic and dromotropic effects may be modified by the autonomic nervous system environment. An elevated sympathetic activity in CHF is reduced as the cardiac output improves with digitalis. In addition, digitalis directly stimulates afferent receptors in the heart wall, carotid sinus, nodosa ganglion, and central vagal nuclei to increase afferent input to the medullary vasomotor control center and decreases sympathetic nerve traffic from the central nervous system.

Reduction of sympathetic tone reverses many of the adverse hemodynamic aspects of CHF. Peripheral resistance, and thus afterload on the heart, is reduced, increasing cardiac output;

venodilation reduces central venous pressure. Moreover, reduced sympathetic stimulation in the kidney, combined with improved renal perfusion, increases urine formation, which leads to a decline in plasma volume and contributes to a reduction in central venous pressure. As a consequence, cardiac preload is reduced, and venous hydrostatic pressure falls below colloid osmotic pressure sufficiently to allow the mobilization of edematous fluid. The degree to which all of these hemodynamic changes occur depends on the pathophysiology of the particular patient. The ideal therapeutic response is rarely achieved with digitalis alone; agents with other modes of action — diuretics and vasodilators — are usually required for optimum control of CHF.

Vagal Effects of Digitalis

Digitalis decreases heart rate by (1) acting directly on the sinoatrial node (chronotropic effect) (2) slowing the conduction of impulses through the AV node (dromotropic effect), and (3) altering several membrane properties of the atrial myocardium. In the therapeutic concentration range, these effects are mediated by the vagus nerve (although, in toxic concentrations, digitalis may elicit the same effects by acting directly on atrial tissue). As previously noted, digitalis stimulates the afferent receptors of the baroreceptor reflex in the aortic arch and carotid sinus, the nodosa ganglion, and the central vagal nuclei. Such stimulations have opposite effects on the outflow nerve traffic of the parasympathetic and sympathetic nervous systems: The former is increased; the latter, decreased. However, the increased parasympathetic or vagal stimulation to the heart appears to be more important, since blockade of the parasympathetic system with atropine nearly eliminates digitalis-induced cardiac slowing. The vagus nerve has little or no effect on the function of the ventricles.

Vagal stimulation releases acetylcholine, which in turn stimulates muscarinic receptors throughout the atria. The resulting atrial cell membrane response accounts, in part, for behavioral changes in the different types of atrial tissue. Vagal stimulation increases the background outward potassium (K^+) current (i_{ki}) and decreases inward Ca^{2+} current (i_{si}) via Ca^{2+} channels. In the SA node the increase in i_{ki} underlies a reduction in the rate of diastolic depolarization. Thus, the time required for the membrane potential to reach threshold for an action potential is increased, and heart rate is slowed. The action potential of both the SA and the AV node is carried exclusively by Ca^{2+} current. As described below, the decrease of inward Ca^{2+} current prolongs the action potential, contributing to the heart rate slowing.

The vagally mediated reduction in inward Ca^{2+} current has two effects on AV nodal action potential. First, the rate of rise of the 0 phase is slowed. (The 0 phase determines the rate of cell-to-cell conduction.) Thus, the reduced i_{si} decreases the velocity of the impulse conduction through the AV node. Second, the duration of the action potential and the effective refractory period (ERP) are increased. These increases are likely to be linked to the operation of a Ca^{2+}-dependent K^+ channel, although the precise mechanism of action has not been fully elucidated. The action potential, however, is terminated, in part, by an outward K^+ current during phase 3. The K^+ conductance occurs via a Ca^{2+}-dependent K^+

channel. The vagally mediated reduction in inward Ca^{2+} current may prolong the time required for the Ca^{2+} concentration on the interior side of the membrane to reach the level necessary to activate the K^+ channel and prolong phase 2 and thereby the action potential.

Clinically, the action of digitalis is readily appreciated by the slowing of the ventricular rate of patients with atrial fibrillation and in preventing many instances of supraventricular tachycardia.

Benefits of Digitalis-Induced Vagal Stimulation

The actions of digitalis on the SA and AV nodes have important clinical consequences. Slowing of cardiac rate is a useful indicator of digitalis effect. In addition, the slower heart rate, combined with the more rapid rate of systolic contraction, results in a longer period of diastole, a particularly important response in CHF secondary to atherosclerotic coronary artery disease (CAD), in which the risk of ischemic damage to subendocardial muscle mass is proportional to the length of the diastolic interval.

The direct and vagal actions of digitalis have opposite effects on atrial muscle. In the therapeutic plasma concentration range, the vagal action predominates and increases the passive outward K^+ current (i_{ki}), thereby enhancing repolarization during phase 3 of the action potential. By this mechanism, digitalis reduces atrial action potential duration (APD) as well as the ERP. The direct effects of digitalis on atrial muscle resemble those on ventricular muscle (described in the next section) and are a component of digitalis toxicity, namely atrial standstill. The clinical importance of the digitalis effect on vagal actions on atrial muscle is slight. A reduced ERP may be responsible for the increase in rate of atrial impulse generation when digitalis is used to treat atrial flutter or fibrillation. (For a complete description of the electrophysiologic properties of digitalis, see Chap. 2.)

Pharmacologic Properties of the Digitalis Glycosides

All of the digitalis glycosides exhibit similar, if not identical, pharmacologic profiles characterized by the same narrow margin of safety; that is, the therapeutic dose of any glycoside is approximately 30–50% of the toxic dose. Selection of a particular glycoside is based on matching the pharmacokinetic properties of the drug to the needs dictated by the pathophysiology of the patient. For example, a patient with kidney disease may require a glycoside that is eliminated by liver metabolism; another patient with acute heart failure may require a glycoside with a rapid onset of the intravenous route of drug administration. While numerous digitalis glycosides are available, digoxin, digitoxin, and deslanoside are the most commonly used agents and provide a full range of pharmacokinetic choices.

Source and Chemical Characteristics of the Cardiotonic Glycosides

The major cardiotonic glycosides are extracted and purified from plant sources. Digoxin and deslanoside are derived from *Digitalis lanata;* digitoxin, from both *D. lanata* and *D. purpurea.* The

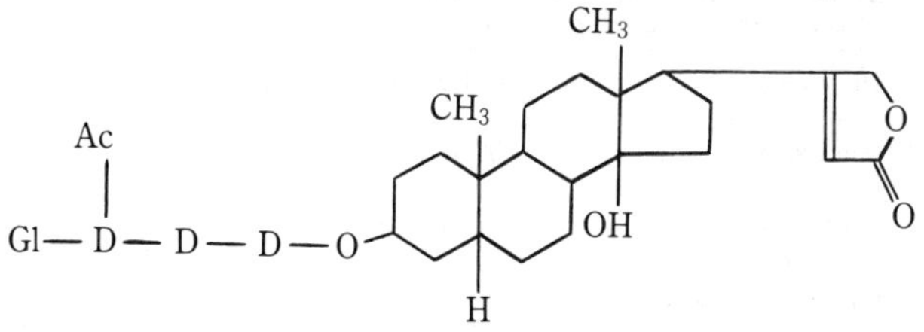

Fig. 1-4. Chemical structure of lanatoside A. (D = digitoxose [a six-carbon-ring glucoselike molecule]; Ac = acetyl; Gl = glucose.) Alkaline hydrolysis removes the acetyl and glucose moieties, yielding digitoxin.

glycosides are composed of a steroid structure with a lactone ring in position 17, called the genin or aglycone, and a sugar moiety of one to three 6-carbon rings called the glycone (Fig. 1-4). The genin confers pharmacologic activity, while the glycone is a major determinant of the pharmacokinetic characteristics of the glycoside. Structurally, digoxin differs from digitoxin by possessing a hydroxyl group in position 12, while deslanoside possesses a terminal glucose molecule on the aglycone.

The major clinical importance of structural differences in the cardiotonic glycosides is their lipid solubility: Digitoxin is the most lipid soluble, digoxin is intermediate, and deslanoside is the least soluble. These differences determine relative rates of gastrointestinal absorption, the degree of plasma protein binding, and the route of elimination of drug from the body.

Pharmacokinetic Properties of the Cardiotonic Glycosides

The more highly lipid soluble the digitalis preparation, the more completely the drug is absorbed after oral administration and the more readily it is reabsorbed from the lumen of renal tubules after entering the glomerular filtrate. Thus unlike the other glycosides, digitoxin is 100% absorbed through the gastrointestinal tract and is not eliminated by the kidney. The other glycosides are less lipid soluble and therefore cannot cross the lipid barrier presented by the tubular epithelial cells. Digitoxin elimination, primarily by liver metabolism, involves conjugation to glucuronic and sulfuric acids as well as the successive hydrolytic removal of sugar molecules. Suprisingly, digitoxin elimination is not impaired by liver disease, and under these clinical conditions the plasma half-life remains unchanged. Digitoxin also undergoes substantial enterohepatic circulation. Though digitoxin is available for IV use, the onset of action after administration by this route is extraordinarily long. Thus this route is not recommended. The binding of the cardiac glycosides to plasma proteins is also directly related to lipophilia: Lipid-soluble digitoxin is more than 90% bound to plasma proteins (primarily albumin), while the binding of the other glycosides is minor or nonexistent.

Digoxin and deslanoside are similar in many of their pharmacokinetic properties, and the following discussion of digoxin elimination applies to deslanoside as well. Digoxin elimination, primarily by the kidney, is closely related to the glomerular

Table 1-4. Pharmacokinetic properties of the cardiotonic glycosides

Property	Digitoxin	Digoxin	Deslanoside
Gastrointestinal absorption	100%	75%	0%
Administration routes	Oral or IV	Oral or IV	IV
Onset of action			
IV	½–2 hr	5–30 min	10–30 min
Oral	1–4 hr	½–2 hr	
Plasma half-life	5–9 days	31–48 hr	33–36 hr
Plasma protein binding	>90%	25%	0%
Excretory pathway	Hepatic	Renal	Renal

filtration rate. Thus, a decrease in the glomerular filtration rate brought about by either disease or aging reduces digoxin elimination and necessitates a reduction of the dose to prevent toxicity.

Table 1-4 lists the important pharmacokinetic properties of the cardiotonic glycosides.

The different bioavailabilities of digoxin from different oral preparations is due, in part, to the less-than-complete absorption of the drug after oral administration and, to a greater extent, to differences between pharmaceutical preparations. Before the problem of variation in bioavailability was recognized in the 1970s, the in vitro, 1-hour dissolution rates of various tablet preparations made in the United States ranged between 4 and 94%. The United States Pharmacopeia has subsequently set the minimum dissolution rate at 65%, dramatically reducing differences in bioavailability among the currently available tablets and capsules. Nevertheless, it is advisable to avoid changing digoxin oral preparations once the patient's condition has been properly stabilized on a given product.

Dosage Options

As noted previously, the therapeutic doses of the digitalis glycosides are between 30 and 50% of the toxic doses. This extremely narrow margin of safety must be an overriding consideration in the therapeutic use of these agents. Given the marked variability in drug response among patients, the heart rate and electrocardiogram (ECG) changes of each patient should be monitored during the initial adjustment of blood levels to the therapeutic range (digitalization). Thereafter, the patients must be monitored intermittently for possible changes in inotropic effects, cardiac rate, or rhythm changes, and drug blood levels should be assayed from time to time to identify a loss of drug effect or the appearance of toxicity.

The **plateau principle** describes the rate of accumulation of drug in the blood stream for the cardiac glycosides eliminated by first-order kinetics. According to this principle, drugs that are infused intravenously at a constant rate achieve a steady-state blood level after five elimination half-lives. Drugs that are

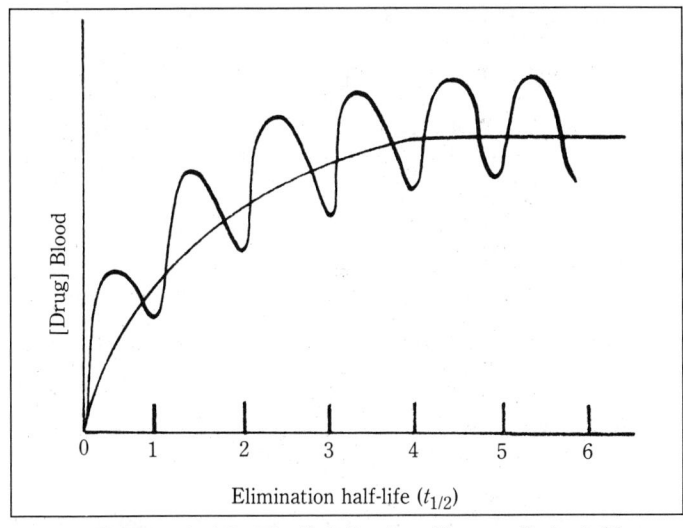

Fig. 1-5. Plateau principle. The digitalis glycosides are eliminated by first-order kinetics; therefore, steady blood levels are achieved after five elimination half-lives.

administered orally, for example, on a once a day schedule, will also achieve a constant mean blood level after five half-lives. However, the daily blood levels may oscillate, first above and then below the mean, with each administration (Fig. 1-5). Maintenance doses are given to maintain the plateau blood levels and are sufficient to replace the amount of drug lost since the last dose. In the case of digitoxin, with a half-life of 7 days, only 10% of the drug eliminated daily must be replaced as a maintenance dose. In the case of digoxin, with a half-life of 1½ days, 35% of the drug must be replaced daily.

If digoxin therapy is initiated using maintenance doses only, the plateau principle dictates that steady-state blood levels will be achieved in five half-lives, or approximately 7 days. This dosage strategy is advantageous in patients who do not require rapid digitalization. It allows daily monitoring of drug effect throughout the digitalization period and, therefore, the most precise determination of correct maintenance dose.

Initiation of digitoxin therapy with maintenance doses only is impractical given the long (7-day) half-life of this agent. Plateau blood levels would be achieved only after 35 days. Thus, a large loading or digitalizing dose must be given. To monitor drug effect and avoid toxicity, the digitalizing dose is always divided and given in several doses during the first day of therapy. Maintenance doses are given daily thereafter.

Acute CHF may necessitate rapid digitalization and digitalizing doses. Because of their rapid onset of action either digoxin or deslanoside may be used, and the dose is divided and given over a period of several hours to monitor drug effect.

Factors Guiding the Selection of Individual Cardiac Glycosides

The pathophysiology of the patient dictates the selection of the cardiac glycoside. In acute CHF, the need may be for a fast-acting and IV-administered drug. It is generally held that the longer half-life of digitoxin increases the risk to the patient when toxicity develops; that is, a longer period will be required for elimination processes to lower the blood concentration of digitoxin out of the toxic range. However, such risks should not be the basis for avoiding its use. Blood levels of digitoxin remain reliably stable in spite of changes in either renal or hepatic status. Moreover, since digitoxin displays marked enterohepatic circulation, steroid-binding ion exchange resins administered in the case of toxicity may be effective in lowering digitoxin blood levels.

Digoxin has the advantage that it can be administered both orally and intravenously, and that it has a rapid onset of action by the latter route. Thus digoxin may be the drug of choice in patients requiring rapid digitalization followed by long-term oral therapy. No difficulty is encountered switching from IV to oral digoxin. Two additional advantages of using digoxin are the availability of radioimmunoassays for the direct measurement of blood levels of the drug and the availability of digoxin antibody preparations for rapid removal of digoxin from the blood in the case of severe toxicity.

Deslanoside, administered only by the IV route, has a rapid onset of action and is used in emergencies in the treatment of acute CHF or supraventricular tachyarrhythmia. However, it is difficult to maintain a stable cardiotonic effect while switching from this agent to an oral glycoside. For that reason, IV digoxin may be preferred.

Digitalization of Children and Adolescents

In practice, less digitalis is required on a kilogram basis for a given serum level and toxicity in premature infants than in children or adults.

Acute digitalization with digoxin: 0.04 mg/kg IV (0.05 mg/kg PO).
½ dose (0.02 mg/kg) immediately.
¼ dose (0.01 mg/kg) 3–12 hours after initial dose.
¼ dose (0.01 mg/kg) 3–12 hours after second dose.
Maximum total dose: 1 mg.
Maintenance: 0.01–0.02 mg/kg/day in two doses 12 hours apart; begin maintenance 12 hours after last digitalizing dose [1].

Digitalization of Geriatric Patients (>65 Years of Age)

Cardiac glycosides are one of the most toxic medications used by elderly patients and are the leading cause of drug reactions and drug-induced hospitalizations in geriatric patients. The increased incidence of toxicity is probably due to altered pharmacokinetics of the drugs (reduced renal function; reduced body water and, concomitantly, unexpectedly high levels of plasma digoxin; increased and more varied half-life).

Formulas are available for calculating the maintenance dose for digitalis in geriatric patients [11] with atrial fibrillation and a fast ventricular response or those with CHF. If the clinical condition requires rapid digitalization, a loading dose (LD) can be estimated from the following formula:

$LD = (V_d \times C_{ss})/F$

where V_d is the distribution volume for digoxin, C_{ss} is the desired serum value (low side of effective dose), and F is the fraction absorbed (0.7 for tablets and 1.0 for IV digoxin).

The volume of digoxin distribution (V_d) can be estimated from the following formula:

V_d (L/70 kg) = 269 + 3.12 (creatinine clearance (Cl_{cr}).

Once calculated, the loading dose is given in three divided doses.

For slow digitalization with digoxin, the plateau principle (see Fig. 1-5) dictates a steady blood level after five elimination half-lives. With a half-life of 1½ days for digoxin, digitalization can be expected within 7 days. Because the sensitivity of the heart to digitalis probably increases in geriatric patients, evidence of toxicity (symptoms and cardiac rate + rhythm) should be assessed at 3 days.

Once it is calculated, the loading dose should be given in three divided doses.

In the elderly patient, other problems exist: (1) Through forgetfulness, the patient may skip an occasional dose. This problem suggests the use of digitoxin, because the concomitant fall in blood concentration is minimal. (2) Cardiac and neural tissue sensitivities to digitalis increase with age. Unfortunately, variations in tissue sensitivity to digitalis must be recognized clinically, since the tissue response is only loosely related to the plasma levels of the glycoside.

Method for Switching from IV to Oral Digitalis

The method for switching from IV to oral digitalis or from one glycoside to another requires knowledge of the pharmacokinetics of the two drugs. For example, a change from digitalis of prompt action, deslanoside, to oral digoxin (capsule form) should begin 6 hours after the last dose of deslanoside to avoid the loss of digitalis effect. And, assuming a daily maintenance dose of 0.25 mg for both glycosides, the patient would receive 0.125 mg of digoxin at 6 and 12 hours after the last dose of deslanoside. Thereafter, 0.375 mg total digoxin is given in divided doses over the period of the next 2 days and 0.25 mg daily thereafter.

Nonglycosidic Drugs to Improve Myocardial Contractility

Mechanism of Action

Most inotropic agents, including digitalis glycosides, increase intracellular levels of free Ca^{2+} to react with contractile proteins in order to generate a greater force of myocardial contraction. Some drugs may also increase contractile protein sensitivity to intracellular Ca^{2+}.

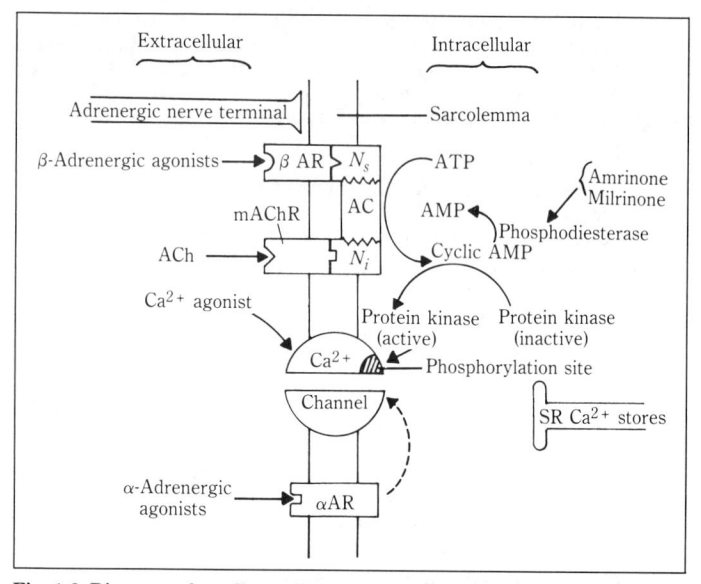

Fig. 1-6. Diagram of cardiac cell membrane showing neurotransmitter receptors and the calcium channel as well as membrane and intracellular components of the second messenger, cyclic adenosine monophosphate (cAMP). Beta receptor agonists increase cAMP concentration by activation of adenylate cyclase (AC) while muscarinic receptor agonists decrease cAMP concentration by inhibiting this enzyme. The concentration of cAMP may also be increased by agents such as amrinone and milrinone that inhibit the cAMP-degrading enzyme phosphodiesterase. When cAMP concentration increases, a protein kinase is activated, which phosphorylates several proteins including the calcium channel. This, in turn, facilitates calcium entry via the calcium channel, causing a positive inotropic response. α-Adrenergic agonists may also cause a positive inotropic response by an effect on the calcium channel. (β AR = beta adrenergic receptor; N_s = regulatory protein linking β AR to AC and mediating stimulation; AC = adenylate cyclase; mAChR = muscarinic acetyl choline receptor; N_i = regulatory protein linking mAChR to AC and mediating inhibition; aAR = alpha adrenergic receptor; ATP = adenosine triphosphate; AMP = adenosine monophosphate; SR = sarcoplasmic reticulum.) (Contributed by Dr. T. W. Smith to W. S. Colucci, R. F. Wright, and E. Braunwald. New positive inotropic agents in the treatment of congestive heart failure. Reprinted, by permission of *The New England Journal of Medicine* [314:290, 1986]).

The catecholamines produce a positively inotropic action by stimulating $β_1$-receptors, which in turn raises the activity of membrane-bound adenylate cyclase and increases intracellular levels of cyclic adenosine monophosphate (cyclic AMP) (Fig. 1-6). Increased cyclic AMP stimulates protein kinases that phosphorylate substances on the cell membrane and the sarcoplasmic reticulum and, in turn, enhances Ca^{2+} flux and raises $[Ca^{2+}]$. Cyclic AMP is degraded by intracellular cyclic nucleotide phosphodiesterases. Inhibition of intracellular cyclic AMP degradation results in changes resembling those produced by stimulating adenylate cyclase. In addition, phoshorylated proteins are returned to a dephosphorylated state by phosphoprotein phosphatases. Inhibition of these phosphatases may mimic an increased intracellular cyclic AMP level.

As summarized in Fig. 1-6, positively inotropic agents may act at various sites to increase levels of cyclic AMP and raise amounts of intracellular Ca^{2+} for binding with troponin C and thus increase contractility of the myocardium.

The myocardium possesses predominantly β_1-adrenoceptors and approximately 15% β_2-adrenoceptors; it also may contain α_1-adrenoceptors. In some animal species, α_1-adrenoceptors are abundant in the myocardium and, when stimulated, increase the rate of contraction. The mechanism of action is unclear (not through the adenylate cyclase as the β_1-adrenoceptor response and does not increase SA node automaticity [chronotropy] or the rate of myocardial relaxation). Myocardial α_1-adrenoceptors may be important to the inotropic mechanism of dobutamine.

Many of the nonglycoside inotropic agents are adrenergic agonists and offer a useful spectrum of pharmacologic activities in addition to their inotropic effect. On the other hand, their long-term use is limited by a β-adrenoceptor down-regulation and consequent loss of hemodynamic effect as tolerance develops. For example, substantial reduction in inotropic effect is observed after 72 hours of IV infusion of β-adrenoceptor agonist, and complete attenuation is observed after 1 month of continuous oral therapy. β-Adrenoceptor agonists may be effective for either short-term or intermittent therapy.

Nonglycosidic Drugs in Children, Adolescents, and Adults

Improved myocardial contractility for severe CHF in children and adolescents [1] may result from IV nonglycosidic inotropic therapy:

Isoproterenol — disadvantages: tachycardia and dysrhythmia
Dopamine — disadvantages: no afterload reduction and possible pulmonary artery constriction
Dobutamine — disadvantages: limited afterload reduction and no renal arterial dilation

Choice of agent is influenced by the following considerations:

1. Afterload reduction desired or pulmonary hypertension present (tachycardia and arrhythmia not a problem) — **isoproterenol**
2. Tachycardia or arrythmia a problem; renal artery vasodilation desired — **dopamine hydrochloride**
3. Increased myocardial contractility as sole objective — **dobutamine hydrochloride**

Dobutamine Hydrochloride

Dobutamine (DBT) is an inotropic agent useful in the short-term treatment of low-output cardiac failure. A synthetic sympathomimetic amine, the drug is a β_1-adrenoceptor agonist with little β_2- or α_1-adrenoceptor agonist action. It elicits predominantly an inotropic response in the heart, having very little chronotropic activity. In acute left ventricular failure, DBT directly increases stroke volume and contractility; indirectly decreases left ventricular end-diastolic pressure, heart size, and cardiac wall tension; and indirectly relieves pulmonary congestion. DBT increases coronary artery perfusion (because of increased cardiac output), decreases left ventricular filling pressure (preload), and reduces systemic vascular resistance (afterload) (by reducing sympathetic drive). DBT has minimal effect on myocardial automaticity.

A number of clinical studies of patients with coronary artery disease without CHF (normal left ventricular ejection fraction) show a 20–40% increase in myocardial oxygen consumption ($M\dot{V}O_2$) as approximated by the heart rate–systolic blood pressure double product [19]. The heart rate–systolic blood pressure double product is a minimal approximation of $M\dot{V}O_2$, since it neglects the contribution of the inotropic state and minimizes contributions other than arterial pressure in determining systolic left ventricular wall stress during systole. Setting aside the limitations of the double product approximations, DBT infusion at rates of 2.5–10.0 μg/kg/min increases the $M\dot{V}O_2$, and in some patients with CAD may induce coronary insufficiency (angina or ECG changes).

DOSAGE FORM AND ADMINISTRATION

DBT is available as lyophilized dobutamine hydrochloride, 250 mg in a 20-ml vial for reconstitution. DBT is incompatible with alkaline solutions and should be reconstituted before administration by addition of either 10 or 20 ml of either sterile water, 5% dextrose injection, 0.9% sodium chloride injection, or sodium lactate injection. Once prepared, the IV solution should never be used for periods longer than 24 hours. The final concentration, 250–5000 μg/ml, is selected on the basis of the fluid needs of the patient. The plasma half-life is 2 minutes.

The rate of infusion that increases cardiac output ranges from 2.5–10.0 μg/kg/min. The infusion should be initiated at 2.5 μg/kg/min and adjusted as needed in a stepwise fashion. Repeated cardiac output measurements are required to control the infusion rate.

INDICATIONS

The prime indication for DBT is inotropic support in the short-term treatment of acute CHF in adults with pulmonary congestion. In patients with rapid ventricular response to atrial fibrillation, digitalis therapy should be used before DBT administration.

CONTRAINDICATION

DBT should not be used if the PCWP and heart size are normal, nor in patients with hypertrophic subaortic stenosis.

ADVERSE EFFECTS

DBT causes a marked increase in either heart rate or blood pressure in a small percentage of patients, but these side effects can be controlled by lowering the dose. DBT may also elicit ventricular ectopic activity. DBT at doses shown to be beneficial hemodynamically maintains oxygen extraction across the coronary circulation so that increased cardiac work is balanced by increased coronary blood flow.

During administration of DBT, the cardiac rhythm and arterial blood pressure should be continuously monitored. In addition, pulmonary wedge pressure and cardiac output should be measured before and while administering DBT.

Dopamine Hydrochloride

Dopamine (DA) is the endogenous precursor of norepinephrine. In low doses (<2 μg/kg/min IV infusion), it stimulates dopamine receptors in the renal and mesenteric vascular beds, causing vasodilation. In doses greater than 2 μg/kg/min, DA stimulates both α_1- and β-adrenoceptors, causing peripheral vasoconstriction and a positively inotropic cardiac response, and induces the local release of norepinephrine. In doses above 4 μg/kg/min, the α_1-adrenoceptor-mediated vasoconstriction, including venoconstriction, predominates over the dopaminergic vasodilator response and may increase cardiac preload. DA may then increase pulmonary congestion. The undesirable side effects of DA may be countered by simultaneous use of a vasodilator such as sodium nitroprusside or nitroglycerine. Dopamine generally does not increase heart rate until doses above 7 μg/kg/min are achieved. At these high levels, DA may induce arrhythmia.

The primary use of DA in CHF is to produce a positively inotropic response, particularly when hypotension requiring vasoconstriction predominates. When blood pressure is near normal, DA may be administered in low doses (3 μg/kg/min) to enhance renal perfusion and dobutamine added to improve inotropy. DA plus sodium nitroprusside (5–20 μg/kg/min) will prevent acute hypertension and an elevation of PCWP. When blood pressure is in the hypotensive or shock range, high-dose DA may be used to increase both cardiac contractility and total peripheral resistance. Sodium nitroprusside may be added as needed; the doses of both agents should be titrated to achieve optimum cardiac output and a mean blood pressure in the range of 70–80 mm Hg.

DOSAGE FORM AND ADMINISTRATION

The drug is available as dopamine hydrochloride injection 40, 80, and 160 mg/ml and must be diluted for infusion using any of the following IV solutions: sodium chloride injection, 5% dextrose injection, 5% dextrose and 0.9% sodium chloride injection, dextrose in 0.45% sodium chloride solution, 5% dextrose in lactated Ringer's solution, sodium lactate (⅙) injection, or lactated Ringer's solution. The amount of dilution depends on the fluid restriction needs of the patient. However, commonly used concentrations are 800 and 1600 μg/ml.

DA infusion is initiated at doses of 2–5 μg/kg/ml and is increased to 20 μg/kg/ml as needed. The usual DA infusion dose range is up to 20 µg/kg/min. Doses greater than 50 µg/kg/ml have been used safely in severe acute CHF.

Norepinephrine Bitartrate

Norepinephrine (NE) is an α- and β-adrenoceptor agonist that causes a powerful vasoconstrictor response and increases myocardial contractility. Use of NE is limited to the acute management of CHF or myocardial depression accompanied by profound hypotension. The objective is to increase cardiac output quickly and to elevate blood pressure into the range that will ensure adequate coronary perfusion (mean blood pressure above 70 mm Hg).

DOSAGE FORM AND ADMINISTRATION

Norepinephrine bitartrate 1 mg/ml is available in 4-ml ampules. One must add 4 ml of solution to 1000 ml of a dextrose-containing solution (dextrose prevents NE oxidation): 5% dextrose solution in distilled water or 5% dextrose in saline solution. One then infuses 2–3 ml of diluted NE (4 µg base/ml) and observes the response. The infusion is adjusted to achieve a low normal blood pressure (80–100 mm Hg, systolic pressure). The average maintenance dose is 2–4 µg/min.

ADVERSE EFFECTS AND CONTRAINDICATIONS

NE can cause bradycardia, extreme hypertension, and increased myocardial work. Blood pressure and ECG must be monitored throughout therapy, and blood pressure must be maintained in the low normal range. Particularly in patients with hypovolemia, NE can cause vasoconstriction, organ ischemia, and oliguria (because of renal vasoconstriction). Consequently, blood volume and electrolyte abnormalities should be corrected promptly before norepinephrine administration. NE administration during cyclopropane or halothane anesthesia is contraindicated because of the possible development of ventricular tachyarrhythmias.

NE is a powerful vasoconstrictor, and its local accumulation at the infusion site can cause tissue necrosis and sloughing. NE should be infused into a large vein to ensure rapid dilution in the blood and to avoid extravasation. Catheter tie-in techniques should also be avoided.

Treatment of Chronic Congestive Heart Failure (Left Ventricular Systolic Dysfunction)

Chronic congestive heart failure (CCHF) is, for the most part, a manifestation of left ventricular systolic dysfunction. However, some 15–30% of patients with CCHF have normal or near-normal systolic function. The following discussion is concerned with CCHF secondary to left ventricular systolic dysfunction. CCHF secondary to left ventricular diastolic dysfunction is discussed at the end of this chapter.

For many years, digitalis plus diuretics was the standard regimen for CCHF. However, current evidence indicates that a beneficial response to digitalis is not a constant in CCHF. Digitalis exerts its greatest benefit in supraventricular tachycardia with a rapid ventricular response, when the ventricles are dilated because of poor LV function (valvular or congenital heart disease), or with a depressed ejection fraction secondary to a severely increased afterload (hypertension). Digitalis has minimal or possibly deleterious effects in CCHF caused by high output, that is, volume overload, myocardial infarction, endocrinopathies (hypo- or hyperthyroidism), infiltrative or inflammatory cardiomyopathies, right inflow tract obstruction (pericarditis), and right heart failure in general.

In the healthy subject, digitalis, while increasing cardiac contractility, may have little effect on cardiac output and may actually increase peripheral resistance. In contrast, in patients with CCHF digitalis increases cardiac output, decreases peripheral resistance, increases venous capacitance, and reduces plasma volume. Thus, inotropic and peripheral arterial effects of digitalis depend on a pathologic myocardial substrate.

Most evidence of improved inotropic function in response to digitalis therapy relates to acute failure, while systolic dimensional changes and time intervals determined from M-mode echocardiography as well as hemodynamic indices suggest a sustained improvement (for 4–6 weeks) of left ventricular function in patients with CCHF. Whether an improved left ventricular function persists with use of digitalis beyond these weeks is uncertain.

THERAPEUTIC END POINTS

The overall goal of digitalis therapy is to improve the quality of life for patients with CCHF. Relief of dyspnea, increase in exercise tolerance, and mobilization of edematous fluid are among the desired responses to therapy. Therapy can be assessed quantitatively by changes in hemodynamic variables, in the ECG, and in the plasma concentrations of glycoside. The following outline summarizes the important therapeutic end points (most are characteristic of low-output CCHF, but not necessarily of other forms of cardiac failure):

I. Improvement of symptoms
   A. Relief of dyspnea at rest, during exercise, or both
   B. Relief of fatigue
   C. Increased exercise tolerance
II. Improvement of cardiac function
   A. Increased cardiac output and stroke volume
   B. Reduced heart rate
   C. Decreased heart size
III. Improved hemodynamics
   A. Decreased peripheral resistance
   B. Decreased venous pressure and increased capacitance
   C. Decreased circulation time

IV. Mobilization of edematous fluid
   A. Increased urine output with concomitant weight loss
   B. Reduction of
      1. Venous engorgement
      2. Edema
      3. Lung congestion
      4. Ascites
      5. Pleural effusions
      6. Liver congestion
V. Electrocardiographic changes
   A. Increased PR interval
   B. ST segment depression
   C. Flattening or inversion of the T wave
   D. Shortening of the QT interval
VI. Measurement of digitalis blood levels by radioimmunoassay (RIA)
   A. Digoxin therapeutic range: 1–2 ng/ml
   B. Digitoxin therapeutic range: 10–30 ng/ml (This includes both free and plasma-protein-bound drug.)

MODULATION OF PRELOAD AND AFTERLOAD

Diuretics

A spectacular advance in the treatment of CCHF was the development of diuretics. In about 40% of patients with CCHF edematous fluid will not be mobilized by bed rest, a low-Na^+ diet, and digitalis. A prerequisite for a rational use of diuretic therapy is knowledge of the nephron and sites where Na^+ is filtered, reabsorbed, and exchanged for K^+. The nephron and sites of Na^+ movements and diuretics are represented in Fig. 3-1.

Children and Adolescents

The following diuretics may be used in the pediatric population [1]:
1. **Furosemide:** drug of choice for parenteral therapy.
   a. **IV:** 1 mg/kg; repeat 1 or 2 times/day for 2–3 days if needed for chronic treatment.
   b. **Oral:** 2–5 mg/kg/day by mouth in 1 or 2 doses.
2. **Hydrochlorothiazide:** 2–5 mg/kg/day by mouth in 1 or 2 doses.
3. **Spironolactone:** 1–2 mg/kg/day by mouth in 1 or 2 doses.

Adults

MILD EDEMA. Bed rest, Na^+ restriction (<1 gm/day), and digitalization may effect the required diuresis.

MODERATE EDEMA. If moderate edema persists in spite of Na^+ restriction and digitalization, diuretic acting on the distal tubular segment (i.e., thiazides at doses of 25–50 mg of hydroclorothiazide daily) should be used intermittently (every other day or 2–3 times per week) to reduce K^+ loss. Long-acting thiazides (i.e., chlorthalidone 25 or 50 mg every other day may be given.

SEVERE EDEMA WITH PULMONARY CONGESTION. If cardiac failure is severe or renal failure is present, furosemide 20–500 mg daily may be administered. Ethacrynic acid, 50 mg daily to 300 mg 2 times/day, may also be used.

INTRACTABLE EDEMA AND SEVERE ANASARCA. Fluid mobilization may require a menu of diuretics. One recommendation is to effect a short-term widespread blocking of Na^+ resorption along the entire tubule by giving acetazolamide (Diamox) (500 mg every 8 hours for 6–8 doses), furosemide (40 mg every 12 hours for 2 days) for the loop, and amiloride (5 mg every 12 hours) for 2 days for the distal tubule (selected because of its striking Mg^{2+}-sparing effect).

Geriatric Patients (>65 Years)

The elderly have a marginally adequate dietary K^+ intake and are more prone to orthostatic hypotension with hypovolemia. Selection of diuretic requires information regarding the patient's creatinine clearance. In general, the thiazides are less effective if the creatinine clearance is less than 30 ml/min. If the clearance is less than 30 ml/min, then furosemide in adequate amounts to induce diuresis will be required.

It should be remembered that diuretic therapy in CCHF at any age stimulates the renin-angiotensin system. Activation of this system raises the level of angiotensin II and increases the afterload and the associated work load of the heart. It should also be remembered that diuretic therapy is not accompanied by increase in cardiac output (although there are exceptions, in which diuretic therapy is associated with a fall in blood pressure and total peripheral resistance).

Side Effects and Treatment

HYPOKALEMIA. Replace with oral potassium chloride (KCl).

HYPOCHLOREMIC ALKALOSIS. Give ammonium chloride orally, if KCl is ineffective.

DILUTIONAL HYPONATREMIA. Fluid restriction, furosemide.

ACUTE Na^+ DEPLETION. Stop diuretic and liberalize Na^+ intake.

VASODILATORS

Vasodilators are a major adjunctive therapy for CCHF. The action site of the various vasodilators varies. Their pharmacologic doses are summarized in Table 1-5.

Standard Dosages

Hydralazine

Give 0.5–5.0 mg/kg/day in three divided doses (maximum of 200 mg/day). Nitrates to reduce preload are required.

Captopril

Give 0.5–6.0 mg/kg/day in two to four divided doses. Make note of **potential neutropenia or proteinuria.**

Therapeutic Effects

The mechanisms of action, pharmacologic properties, and therapeutic uses of the vasodilator agents are discussed further in

Table 1-5. Action and dosage of vasodilators

Agent	Vascular dilatation		Dosage
	Venous	Arteriolar	
Hydralazine	−	+ + +	10–100 mg q6h PO
Minoxidil	−	+ + +	10–40 mg/day PO
Prazosin	+ + +	+ +	1–10 mg q8h PO
Captopril	+ + +	+ +	6.25–50.00 mg q6–8h PO
Enalapril	+ + +	+ +	5–10 mg bid PO

Key: + = mild; + + = moderate; + + + = marked; − = none.

Chap. 3. In the following discussion, the effects of vasodilators on venous and arterial dilation are considered separately. Nevertheless, it will be seen that the most common therapeutic approach utilizes venous and arterial dilation in combination.

The vasodilators have no direct effect on the myocardium; nevertheless, they indirectly improve the functional capacity of the patient and relieve the major symptoms of CCHF. Agents acting primarily on the venous side decrease central venous and pulmonary capillary wedge pressure, leading to the mobilization of edematous fluid, which in turn reduces pulmonary congestion and associated dyspnea. Agents acting primarily on the arterial side decrease total peripheral resistance and afterload on the heart, allow more rapid and complete cardiac emptying during systole, and, therefore, increase cardiac output. The resulting improved tissue perfusion relieves the weakness and fatigue that often accompany CCHF. Special benefit is gained from afterload reduction in patients with mitral or aortic regurgitation. Regurgitation volume is reduced, while forward stroke volume is increased.

Under certain conditions, the benefits of vasodilator therapy are self-limiting. Aggressive venodilation decreases venous return and, ultimately, cardiac output. Since reduced cardiac output may be a component of CCHF, a further reduction must be considered as an adverse drug effect. When using venodilator agents, the therapeutic goal must be to reduce central venous pressure to the lowest level possible consistent with a minimal reduction in cardiac output. The use of dilators acting on the arterial side may be contraindicated in CCHF accompanied by severe hypotension, since blood pressure reduction will lead to tissue underperfusion, particularly in the coronary, cerebral, and renal vascular beds. Similarly, arterial (arteriolar) dilating agents are contraindicated in severe aortic stenosis in which cardiac output is not increased by afterload reduction and blood pressure falls into the hypotensive range. In general, the use of vasodilators acting on the arterial side is associated with reflex tachycardia and plasma volume expansion. However, the incidence and severity of reflex tachycardia is much less in the CCHF patient (exceptions are noted below). On the other hand, plasma volume expansion remains a problem in long-term vasodilator therapy and may necessitate the concomitant use of a diuretic. The selective nature of vasodilators for systemic or pulmonary bed influences their usefulness in treating congenital or acquired structural defects such as ventricular septal defect and CCHF.

Many vasodilators, including nitrates, sodium nitroprusside, hydralazine, and captopril, mediate their effects, in part, by increasing the endogenous production of prostaglandins PGI_2 and PGE_2. The effects of these vasodilators can be attenuated by the concomitant use of indomethacin, a cyclo-oxygenase inhibitor.

Individual Vasodilator Agents

Hydralazine

Hydralazine dilates primarily resistant arterioles, having little effect on capacitance vessels. Thus, orthostatic hypotension is rarely induced by this agent. Hydralazine offers the distinct therapeutic advantage of having its greatest dilator effect on the splanchnic, coronary, cerebral, and renal vascular beds. Cardiac output is increased by this agent, and forward stroke volume is increased in patients with mitral or aortic regurgitation. When used to treat hypertension, hydralazine commonly induces reflex tachycardia, particularly in patients with a small left ventricle. However, this adverse response is generally absent during vasodilator therapy in patients with CCHF and an enlarged heart. The resultant increase in cardiac output in the latter patients reduces the reflex sympathetic tone. Hydralazine is almost always used in combination with an organic nitrate, a diuretic, digitalis, or a combination of these for long-term treatment of CCHF.

In a major Veterans Administration cooperative study [6], the addition of hydralazine and isosorbide dinitrate to the therapeutic regimen of digoxin and diuretics in patients with chronic CHF favorably affected left ventricular function and mortality. However, side effects were common, and one or both drugs were discontinued in 1 of 5 patients.

Minoxidil

Minoxidil, like hydralazine, dilates primarily arterioles and decreases afterloading on the heart. It possesses greater intrinsic vasodilator capacity than hydralazine, and as an antihypertensive agent it is reserved for the treatment of severe hypertension refractory to other therapy. Similarly, minoxidil should be reserved for the treatment of CCHF associated with severe or intractable hypertension. Minoxidil may induce reflex tachycardia (even in the CHF patient) and plasma volume expansion. Dosage must be adjusted to avoid substantial increases in cardiac work, and minoxidil should always be used in combination with a diuretic.

Phentolamine

Phentolamine is an α-adrenergic receptor antagonist and reduces both venous and arterial tone. In addition, it exerts a direct positively inotropic effect on the heart. Thus, it can increase cardiac output by both reducing afterload and increasing cardiac contractility. While phentolamine is available for oral administration, it is administered almost exclusively by IV injection or infusion for the treatment of acute left ventricular failure. Phentolamine has a greater potential than other vasodilators to induce reflex tachycardia and shares with sodium nitroprusside the side effect of orthostatic hypotension. The therapeutic use of phentolamine closely resembles that of sodium nitroprusside in the treatment of acute CHF.

Prazosin Hydrochloride

Prazosin is a selective α^1-adrenergic receptor antagonist that reduces both central venous and systemic arterial pressure, relieves pulmonary congestion, and increases cardiac output. There is some evidence of attenuation of these beneficial hemodynamic effects during long-term prazosin hydrochloride therapy. Prazosin hydrochloride is considered adjunctive therapy in the treatment of CCHF and is almost always used in combination with a diuretic, digitalis, or both. Prazosin hydrochloride may raise serum digoxin levels by reducing the plasma binding as well as the nonspecific tissue binding of the glycoside. The increase in the free digoxin may increase the inotropic or toxic effects of the glycoside.

Captopril and Enalapril Maleate

Captopril and enalapril are inhibitors of angiotensin-converting enzyme (ACEI), an enzyme that converts angiotensin I to angiotensin II. Sustained, increased sympathetic stimulation of the renin-angiotensin-aldosterone system in patients with severe CCHF is a major cause for a high left ventricular afterloading. Such an excessive neurohumoral compensatory mechanism actually enhances and perpetuates left ventricular depression, and pharmacologic blockade of this system produces sustained improvement of left ventricular function.

The magnitude of the hemodynamic effects of the ACEI depend, in part, on the renin-angiotensin-aldosterone system. When this system is activated, the circulating level of angiotensin II increases, which in turn increases vascular tone on both the venous and arterial sides. ACEIs block angiotensin II formation, which accounts, in part, for the vasodilator response of these agents. However, the mechanism of the ACEIs is more complex than this. Catecholamine blood levels are also elevated in CCHF, and these levels are reduced by the ACEIs. Aldosterone levels often are increased in CCHF and are reduced with ACEI therapy.

Chronic blockade of the ACE with captopril may produce sustained improvements in CCHF and renal function. Care must be exercised, however, in initiating therapy with captopril, particularly in patients with severe CCHF (class IV, New York Heart Association functional category). Doses of 6.25 mg every 6–8 hours with close blood pressure monitoring in the sitting and standing positions are in order. Even with sustained improvement in left ventricular function, an increased survival of patients with CHF treated with captopril remains to be reported.

In addition to its striking hemodynamic effects, captopril raises serum digoxin as well as the serum and total K^+ levels. Creatinine, urea, and digoxin clearances are reduced. Captopril may cause fever, myalgia, and arthralgias in patients receiving allopurinol, and caution must be exercised in using captopril and allopurinol in patients with chronic renal failure. Captopril may produce a chronic cough and severe onycholysis.

Comparisons of captopril (150 mg daily) and enalapril (40 mg daily) in patients with severe CCHF revealed similar decreases in systemic blood pressure, but the hypotensive effects were more prolonged with enalapril than with captopril [17]. The sustained hypotension probably accounted for a decline in creatinine clearance and K^+ retention that was greater with enalapril than with captopril.

A multicenter study, the Consensus Trial, a cooperative North Scandinavian enalapril survival study [7] involving 253 patients with CCHF (double-blind, placebo-controlled, and randomized), revealed an overall reduction in 6-month mortality from 44% to 26% (control versus enalapril maleate). The 12-month mortality was also reduced from 52% to 36%. Overall, 33% experienced sudden death; the incidence was similar in the control and treated groups. The severity of heart failure (New York Heart Association functional class) was improved in 42% of the treated group and 22% of the placebo group. Heart size was reduced by 3.2% (control) and 9.6% (enalapril), and heart rate was reduced only in the treated patients.

The following **precautions** are necessary when prescribing ACEI:

Use of K^+-sparing diuretics should be avoided.
Risk of renal dysfunction with marked hypotension, particularly in patients with hyponatremia, must be noted.
Diabetic patients with reduced efferent arteriolar responsiveness may experience hyperkalemia, proteinuria, and plasma accumulation of ACEI.

MODULATION OF MYOCARDIAL CONTRACTILITY

Digitalis Glycoside Dosages

Dosages of all digitalis glycosides must be individually adjusted. Lean body weight provides an initial basis for dose selection. However, the therapeutic response in each patient is the only reliable determinant of final maintenance dose. Generally, smaller doses are required for inducing a positively inotropic response in CCHF than for controlling the ventricular rate in atrial tachyarrhythmia. Before initiating digitalis therapy, it is extremely important to determine whether the patient has taken any cardiotonic glycoside within the previous 2–3 weeks. If so, drug dosage must be appropriately lowered. When digoxin is selected and altered renal function is suspected, a measured increase in creatinine clearance should prompt a downward adjustment of the drug dose. In order to account for differences in bioavailability and plasma half-life, dosage adjustment is also needed when changing from an IV preparation for digitalization to an oral preparation for maintenance. The one exception is changing from IV digoxin to liquid-filled capsules of digoxin, both of which have the same bioavailability.

Digoxin

DOSAGE FORMS AND STRENGTHS AVAILABLE

Capsules: 50, 100, and 200 µg (0.05, 0.1, and 0.2 mg, respectively).
Elixir: 50 µg (0.05 mg) per milliliter.
Tablets: 125, 250, and 500 µg (0.125, 0.25, and 0.5 mg, respectively).
Injection: 100 and 250 µg (0.1 and 0.25 mg) per milliliter.

DOSAGES IN ADULTS AND CHILDREN 10 YEARS OF AGE AND OVER

Oral: Digitalizing dose is 0.75–1.50 mg. For rapid digitalization, 0.50–0.75 mg initially, followed by 0.25–0.50 mg every 6–8 hours until therapeutic effect is achieved or adverse effects intervene. Maintenance dose is 0.125–0.500 mg daily (0.125–0.250 in the elderly). Digitalization (achieving therapeutic blood levels) may be accomplished in 4–6 days by administering maintenance doses only.
IV: Digitalizing dose is 0.5–1.0 mg; 0.25–0.50 mg is given initially, followed by 0.25 mg at 4- to 6-hour intervals until therapeutic effect is achieved. Total dose should not exceed 1 mg.

DOSAGES FOR PREMATURE AND FULL-TERM INFANTS AND CHILDREN UNDER 10 YEARS

Digoxin elixir is usually given to infants and children for oral dosing, and digitalizing doses are divided into two or more portions and administered every 6–8 hours [1].

The oral digitalizing dose (in µg/kg) is as follows:

Premature infants	20–25
Full-term newborn infants	25–35
Infants 1 month to 2 years	25–35
Children 2–5 years	20–30
Children 5–10 years	15–25

Maintenance dose is generally 25–35% of the digitalizing dose. (It is lower, 20–30%, for premature infants.)

Digoxin injection is used for IV dosing, and the digitalizing dose is divided into three or more doses and given every 4–8 hours. The initial dose should be approximately one-half of the total.

The IV digitalizing dose (in µg/kg) is as follows:

Premature infants	15–25
Full-term newborn infants	20–30
Infants 1 month to 2 years	20–30
Children 2–5 years	15–30
Children 5–10 years	15–25

Maintenance dose is generally 25–35% of the digitalizing dose. (It is lower, 20–30%, for premature infants.)

Digitoxin

DOSAGE FORMS AND STRENGTHS AVAILABLE

Tablets: 50, 100, 150, and 200 µg (0.05, 0.10, 0.15 and 0.20 mg, respectively).
Injection: 200 µg (0.2 mg) per milliliter.

DOSAGES IN ADULTS

Oral: For rapid digitalization, administer 0.8 mg initially, followed by 0.2 mg every 6–8 hours for two or three doses. For slower digitalization, 0.1–0.20 mg 1–3 times daily to a total of 1.2–1.8 mg. Maintenance dose is 0.1 mg (0.05–0.20 mg) daily.
IV: Use the same dosages and schedule as indicated for oral administration.

Digitoxin is not recommended in infants and children.

Deslanoside

Deslanoside is administered by IV or IM injection only and is used for rapid digitalization. The patient should be switched to maintenance doses of an orally effective glycoside within 12 hours. Generally, digitalizing doses should be given in divided doses. The alternative, digitalizing in a single dose, is listed below but should only be done in acute emergencies.

DOSAGE FORMS AND STRENGTHS AVAILABLE

Injection: 200 µg (0.2 mg) per milliliter.

DOSAGES IN ADULTS

IV and IM: 0.8 mg initially, followed by 0.4 mg every 2–4 hours to a maximum of 2 mg. Alternatively,
IV: 1.6 mg as a single dose or 0.8 mg initially followed by 0.8 mg in 4 hours.
IM: 0.8 mg given at each of two separate injection sites.

DOSAGES IN INFANTS AND CHILDREN

The following doses are divided into two or three equal portions and administered every 3 or 4 hours (or as a single dose in emergencies).

The IV and IM dose (in μg/kg) is as follows:

Newborn infants to children 3 years old 25
Children over 3 years 20

Plasma Digoxin and Digitoxin Assays

After digoxin- and digitoxin-specific antibodies were reported in 1967–68, a sensitive radioimmunosassay for measuring serum or urine levels of the glycoside became available. However, because of variability in digoxin absorption, skeletal muscle mass and activity, plasma and extracellular volumes, affinity for digitalis receptor, renal function, age, sex, and tissue sensitivity, the question of whether measurements of serum digoxin level improve patient therapy remains unanswered some 20 years later. Nevertheless, serum concentration of digoxin in adults is significantly higher in toxicity than in nontoxic states, even though considerable overlap between the two groups exist.

While the digoxin assay appears to be straightforward, a number of confounding factors reduce the specificity of the reaction. Among the factors is an antibody-reacting substance present in the plasma of infants; in patients with uremia, liver disease (acute viral hepatitis and cirrhosis), hemolyzed serum, and hyperbilirubinemia; and in pregnant women in the last trimester. Receiving ^{125}I isotope within a day or two leads to spurious values. Also, the activity may be increased in patients with hypertension complicating pregnancy. Whether or not a similar cross reactivity exists between digitoxin antibodies and endogenous digitalis-like factors is uncertain.

The major clinical usefulness of the serum digoxin assay is to verify the suspicion of digitalis intoxication. But after acquiring serum levels consistent with digitalis toxicity and discontinuing the drug, one should require evidence that the signs of toxicity (arrhythmia or symptoms) are abolished within the anticipated half-life of the cardiac glycoside. Other indications for serum digoxin measurement are verification of drug compliance, dose regulation with changing renal function, or after cardiac surgery.

Digitalis Toxicity

In experimental animals, radioactive digitalis localizes itself within the T tubule along the myofibrillar sarcomere in the distribution of the Na^+-K^+ ATPase activity. Estimated therapeutic doses of digitalis given to digitalize rapidly, followed by daily maintenance doses, may produce focal degeneration of myocardial fibers, with subsequent fibrosis in the papillary muscles and the free wall of the left ventricle and in the ventricular septum. Histologic changes occur most commonly in the subendocardial region. These morphologic localizations identify the potential sites of digitalis action in therapeutic and toxic ranges.

Identifying digitalis toxicity in humans is made difficult because of the overlap in signs of digitalis toxicity and those of CCHF. Diagnosis of digitalis toxicity requires clinical testing (removal of drug to observe for changes within the half-life of the digitalis preparation), the assessment of ECG and cardiac and extracardiac symptoms, and measurement of digitalis blood levels by RIA.

The most common ECG signs of digoxin intoxication are as follows:

Nonconducted premature atrial complexes
Supraventricular (atrial or AV junctional) tachycardia with block
Nonparoxysmal AV junctional tachycardia with or without exit block
Multifocal ventricular premature beats, bidirectional ventricular rhythm, or tachycardia with exit block
Atrial fibrillation with a slow ventricular response (<50/minute)
Sinus rhythm with second- or third-degree AV block

Because of the steroid (genin or aglycone) element of digitalis, the drug may have hormonal effects and even produce gynecomastia in males. Interesting in this regard is a protective action of other steroid drugs and hormones (estrogen or the aldosterone inhibitor spironolactone) against the toxic effects of digitalis in experimental animals and perhaps in humans as well.

Myocardial sensitivity to digitalis may vary with age, sex, or disease. In an experimental model, sensitivity to digitalis toxicity (arrhythmia) in ischemic hearts may be influenced by local production of prostaglandins PGE_2, PGF_2, PGI_2. Unfortunately, there are no available means for assessing variations in tissue sensitivity to digitalis in humans.

Mechanisms of Cardiac Toxicity

Inhibition of Na^+-K^+ ATPase by digitalis leading to the loss of cellular K^+ underlies most arrhythmias arising in the atria and ventricles and in the Purkinje cells of the conduction system.

Digitalis increases the slope of phase 4 of the action potential, particularly in Purkinje cells, and may induce delayed afterdepolarization in these as well as myocardial cells. Either of these effects can result in digitalis-induced ectopic impulse generation or automaticity. A second mechanism by which digitalis induces arrhythmias is its ability to slow ventricular conduction velocity and increase the ERP in Purkinje cells and, to a lesser extent, in ventricular muscle cells. As a consequence, a nonhomogeneity between myocardial cell types develops, favoring the occurrence of reentry arrhythmias.

Interactions between digitalis and the adrenergic and cholinergic (vagal) influences on the cardiac conduction tissue increase triggered activity and produce many of the ECG manifestations of digitalis toxicity. Dysrhythmias, often multiple, occur in 80–90% of patients with digitalis toxicity. The mechanisms of these dysrhythmias are summarized in Table 1-6.

Electrocardiogram in the Diagnosis of Digitalis Toxicity

In the therapeutic concentration range, digitalis alters the ECG (increased PR interval, ST segment depression, flattened or inverted T waves, and QT interval shortening). In some patients, these changes intensify, and arrhythmias, AV block, or both develop as the digitalis blood concentration moves into the toxic range. However, there is poor correlation between ECG changes and development of toxicity. Moreover, in some cases, extracardiac symptoms of toxicity occur in the absence of

Table 1-6. Dysrhythmias in digitalis toxicity

Site of digitalis action	Toxic effect
SA node	Antiadrenergic (direct drug action)
Atrium	Exit block — first-degree AV block
	Increased atrial cell automaticity
AV node	Direct and cholinergic effect — first-degree AV block
Purkinje fibers	Increased automaticity, delayed after depolarization
Ventricular muscle	Reentry mechanism

Key: SA = sinoatrial; AV = atrioventricular.

major ECG changes. Clearly, while the ECG is a useful diagnostic tool, it cannot be relied on alone to diagnose digitalis toxicity.

The initial ECG changes corresponding to digitalis toxicity may be a further progression of those seen at therapeutic drug levels, namely, an increase of PR interval, troughlike depression of the ST segment, flattening or inversion of the T wave, and shortening of the QT interval. On the other hand, these changes may be absent. Approximately one-third of patients have arrhythmia or AV block as the first ECG sign of toxicity.

There are special circumstances in which identifying digitalis toxicity presents difficulties. Patients with atrial fibrillation may require toxic doses of digitalis to maintain a satisfactory ventricular response. In this setting, clues of digitalis toxicity are excessively slow ventricular response, complete AV block with junctional escape rhythms of 40–50 beats/minute, nonparoxysmal AV junctional tachycardia at a rate of 70–100 beats/minute, accelerated junctional rhythm with variable exit block resulting in a rapid irregular (or regularly irregular) rhythm, and bidirectional tachycardia.

Identifying digitalis toxicity may also be difficult in the patient with a pacemaker rhythm. Retrograde P waves of 70–130 beats/minute may suggest AV junctional tachycardia. Slower rates may suggest AV junctional escape. Premature ventricular complexes and ventricular tachycardia or fibrillation may be manifestations of digitalis toxicity.

Extracardiac Symptoms of Digitalis Toxicity

The most common extracardiac symptoms of digitalis toxicity are anorexia, nausea, fatigue, blurred vision, and chromatopsia (the appearance of everything in specific colors or within halos of color, most commonly yellow and green). Vomiting is also common, especially after the rapid administration of a large dose. Additional frequent symptoms include diarrhea, confusion, and mental depression, the latter seen most commonly in geriatric-

Table 1-7. Extracardiac symptoms of digitalis toxicity

Gastrointestinal system
  Anorexia
  Nausea
  Vomiting
  Lower stomach pain
  Diarrhea
Central nervous system
  Headache
  Fatigue
  Malaise
  Drowsiness
  Dizziness
  Delirium
  Confusion
  Mental depression
  Bad dreams
  Agitation
  Acute psychoses
  Hallucinations
Visual system
  Blurred vision
  White vision (white borders on dark objects)
  Chromatopsia (may be yellow, green, blue, brown, or red)
  Xanthopsia (yellow vision)
Other (rare incidence)
  Skin rash or hives
  Eosinophilia
  Thrombocytopenia (with digitoxin but not digoxin)

age patients. The extracardiac symptoms and signs of digitalis toxicity are listed in Table 1-7.

Factors Influencing Myocardial Tolerance and Digitalis Toxicity

A number of clinical problems affect the action of digitalis on the myocardium as well as the toxicity of digitalis. These factors are listed in Table 1-8.

HYPOKALEMIA. Hypokalemia may occur from several causes, including loss from the gastrointestinal tract (e.g., prolonged vomiting or diarrhea), impaired renal function, and primary aldosteronism. However, the most frequent and important cause in the patient receiving digitalis is concomitant diuretic therapy.

K^+ and digitalis compete for the same or overlapping sites on the myocardial Na^+-K^+ ATPase enzyme. Thus, in low-K^+ states the binding of digitalis to cardiac membranes is greater, leading to greater inhibition of the Na^+ pump at any given

Table 1-8. Factors influencing myocardial tolerance and digitalis toxicity

Electrolyte abnormalities
   Hypokalemia
   Hypomagnesemia
   Hypercalcemia
Endocrinopathy
   Hypothyroidism
   Hyperthyroidism
Myocardial pathology
   Myocarditis
   Myocardial infarction
   Cardiomyopathies
Renal failure
Advanced age
Extracorporeal circulation
Central nervous system disease
   Cerebrovascular accidents
   Spinal cord sections (require high serum digoxin levels)
Concomitant drug administration

---

plasma concentration of digitalis. In the hypokalemic patient, toxicity may occur even when digitalis blood levels are in the normal range.

HYPOMAGNESEMIA. Hypomagnesemia may result from either malabsorption states, alcoholism, or dialysis. However, as with hypokalemia, the most frequent cause in patients with CHF is concomitant use of digitalis and diuretic therapy. Hypomagnesemia sensitizes the heart to digitalis, leading to the dysrhythmias of digitalis toxicity. The hypomagnesemia can be corrected by the administration of either the sulfate or chloride salts of magnesium (Mg^{2+}).

Mg^{2+} is a key cofactor of the Na^+-K^+ ATPase enzyme; the enzyme function is impaired in the presence of low-MG^{2+} states. This impaired enzyme function may account for an increased sensitivity to digitalis.

INTERACTION BETWEEN HYPOMAGNESEMIA AND HYPOKALEMIA. Recently an awareness has developed of Mg^{2+} as well as K^+ depletion with diuretic therapy. K^+ supplementation alone may not correct hypokalemia in the Mg^{2+}-deficient patient. Infusion of K^+ may not correct low cellular K^+ content in patients with hypomagnesemia; Mg^{2+} may be required to increase cellular K^+ content. The effect of Mg^{2+} on intracellular K^+ is not mediated by an action on the Na^+-K^+ ATPase enzyme. Rather, Mg^{2+} prevents cellular K^+ loss, possibly by decreasing K^+ conductance via a specific membrane K^+ channel.

Two options are available for treating hypomagnesemia and hypokalemia associated with diuretic therapy. One is the concomitant supplementation of both ions. Magnesium aspartate is a potentially useful orally effective preparation and is under investigation in the United States. Magnesium sulfate (milk of magnesium, 1 teaspoonful daily) may protect against the depletion of this cation. Numerous oral preparations of K^+ are available. Another option is to add one of the potassium-sparing diuretics (spironolactone, amiloride, triamterene), which appear to spare Mg^{2+} loss, to the therapy regimen (see Chap. 3).

HYPER- OR HYPOCALCEMIA. Ca^{2+} blood levels may be elevated by either disuse atrophy (prolonged bed rest or other long-term immobilization), myeloma, or hyperparathyroidism. Higher extracellular levels of Ca^{2+} increase the concentration gradient for Ca^{2+} to enter the cell. Since digitalis also elevates intracellular Ca^{2+}, the combined effects can lead to toxicity. Higher Ca^{2+}, and therefore positive charge, within the cell displaces intracellular K^+, which in turn contributes to the toxicity. Patients with hypocalcemia secondary to untreated hypoparathyroidism may have depressed left ventricular ejection fractions and may present with CHF. Hypocalcemia is an uncommon but reversible cause of CHF; a prompt reversal of CHF may occur with normalization of the serum Ca^{2+} levels.

HYPO- OR HYPERTHYROIDISM. In hypothyroidism, the elimination of digitalis is reduced, and the heart becomes more sensitive to the glycoside. Consequently, hypothyroid patients require lower digitalis doses. The opposite is true in hyperthyroidism, in which larger than normal doses must be used.

RENAL FUNCTION. Changes in renal function, primarily glomerular filtration, affect blood levels of digoxin but not digitoxin. Lower than normal doses are required in the elderly and in premature infants, while higher than normal doses are required in infants and children, based on age-related differences in renal function.

HEART DISEASE. Any condition that impairs the function of cardiac tissue — for example, ischemic heart disease, myocardial infarction, acute myocarditis, and congestive heart disease — may increase the sensitivity of the heart to digitalis. In part, the increased sensitivity is related to a reduction in myocardial energy stores leading to lowered Na^+-K^+ ATPase activity.

SEVERE PULMONARY DISEASE. Cor pulmonale, emphysema, and other conditions causing chronic hypoxia may also increase cardiac sensitivity to digitalis. Reduced myocardial energy stores and the lowered blood pH that accompanies hypoxia both depress Na^+-K^+ ATPase activity.

HEART BLOCK. Digitalis slows AV conduction. In patients with preexisting partial heart block, digitalis treatment may advance the block to complete AV dissociation.

Treatment of Digitalis Toxicity

Therapy for digitalis toxicity is indicated for hemodynamically important bradyarrhythmias or tachyarrhythmias, for potentially malignant arrhythmias, and in the presence of hyperkalemia. Administration of digitalis should be stopped as the first step in the treatment of toxicity. Mild overdose may be treated simply by withholding one or more digitalis doses until symptoms of toxicity subside.

In the presence of hypokalemia (<3.5 mEq/liter), administration of K^+ may reverse signs of toxicity. IV potassium chloride is usually an initial therapy for ventricular ectopy, ventricular tachycardia, atrial tachycardia with block, and nonparoxysmal AV junctional tachycardia. It is contraindicated in renal failure, hyperkalemia, and depressed AV conduction (greater than first-degree AV block). Potassium chloride should be given in saline rather than a glucose-saline solution.

Acting on the central nervous system by depressing sympathetic outflow, phenytoin is a drug of choice in treating digitalis-induced atrial tachycardia with AV block, ventricular ectopy, ventricular tachycardia, and nonparoxysmal AV junctional tachycardia. The drug suppresses digitalis-induced enhanced automaticity and delayed afterdepolarizations without reversing digitalis-mediated inotropism and reverses digitalis-induced depression of AV and sinus node conductance. Phenytoin does not change or may improve AV conduction. It is administered by intermittent IV injection at a rate of 100 mg every 5 minutes until a desired effect or a total dose of 1000 mg is reached. Then 400–600 mg/day is given until the toxicity is resolved.

Lidocaine suppresses digitalis-induced automaticity and delayed afterdepolarization without depressing AV conduction. Indications are ventricular ectopy or tachycardia.

Intravenous Mg^{2+} can suppress digitalis-induced ventricular arrhythmias. It is contraindicated in renal failure, hypermagnesemia, and advanced AV block and is indicated for ventricular ectopy and tachycardia and AV junctional tachycardia.

Atropine may be used for control of sinus bradycardia, sinoatrial arrest, and second- or third-degree AV block.

Propranolol is used to treat both atrial and ventricular arrhythmias. The drug should not be used in the presence of digitalis-induced AV block.

Either cholestyramine or colestipol may be used as a component of the treatment of digitoxin toxicity. These ion exchange resins bind digitalis glycosides in the intestinal tract, and since digitoxin undergoes enterohepatic circulation, the reabsorption of this glycoside is prevented and the rate of decline of digitoxin blood levels is increased.

Fab fragments of antibody to digoxin are available for the treatment of life-threatening digitalis toxicity. These fragments cause a rapid increase in blood levels of both digoxin and digitoxin but a marked reversal of digitalis effect by reducing tissue binding. Subsequently digoxin clearance increases if renal function is adequate.

Digitalis-Drug Interactions

While many drugs have been reported to interact with digitalis glycosides, only those identified in the drug interaction literature as being clinically important have been included in the following list. When the name of a specific glycoside, such as digoxin, is used, it implies that the interacting drug alters the patient response to this glycoside only. The term *digitalis* is used to indicate that all glycosides participate in the interaction. Since the therapeutic dose of the digitalis glycosides is between 30 and 50% of the toxic dose, any drug that alters the plasma concentration of digitalis has the potential to cause an adverse drug reaction. The addition of a drug that increases digitalis plasma concentration by any mechanism could lead to toxicity, while removal of the same drug from a patient who was digitalized in its presence may lead to loss of therapeutic effect.

Amphotericin B

Amphotericin B can cause hypokalemia, which in turn increases the sensitivity of the heart to digitalis. Under this condition, digitalis toxicity may occur at lower plasma glycoside concentrations, even in the therapeutic range.

Calcium Chloride Injection

Parenteral Ca^{2+} administration increases plasma and extracellular fluid concentrations of Ca^{2+}. Digitalis, on the other hand, increases the movement of Ca^{2+} into cardiac cells and enhances release of Ca^{2+} from intracellular stores. The overall effect of digitalis is to increase the concentration of free intracellular Ca^{2+} responsible for initiating cardiac contraction. Elevation of extracellular Ca^{2+} concentration (by parenteral Ca^{2+} administration) enhances these actions of digitalis and may lead to toxicity.

When it is deemed necessary to administer calcium chloride to the patient receiving digitalis, the Ca^{2+} must be administered slowly with continuous monitoring of the ECG and other variables for signs of toxicity.

Cholestyramine

Cholestyramine is an anionic exchange resin capable of binding drugs in the gastrointestinal tract and preventing their systemic absorption. When cholestyramine or other anionic exchange resins are prescribed for other reasons, plasma levels of digitoxin decline if the drugs are taken concurrently. Digitoxin should be taken at least 1½ hours before cholestyramine to avoid this interaction. Colestipol is another anionic exchange resin and may also reduce the absorption and the enterohepatic circulation of digitoxin.

Potassium-Depleting Diuretics

The following diuretics almost invariably cause hypokalemia: bumetanide, ethacrynic acid, furosemide, and thiazide and thiazide-related diuretics. The clinical importance of the resultant hypokalemia is in debate and, in many patients, probably is nil. Nevertheless, in patients receiving digitalis, extracellular K^+ concentration is an important determinant of cardiac sensitivity to glycoside therapy. Because K^+ and digitalis compete for the same or overlapping sites on the membrane Na^+-K^+ ATPase, the binding of digitalis to cardiac membranes is increased with hypokalemia, and signs of toxicity may appear even when the plasma digitalis concentration is within therapeutic range. Prevention of hypokalemia in the patient receiving digitalis and diuretic concurrently may be accomplished with either K^+ supplementation or the addition of a K^+-sparing diuretic (spironolactone, amiloride, triamterene) to the regimen.

Erythromycin and Tetracycline

In approximately 10% of patients, substantial bacterial metabolism of digoxin occurs in the gastrointestinal tract. Broad-spectrum antibiotics such as erythromycin and tetracycline kill the intestinal bacteria, which in turn decreases the metabolism and causes a marked increase in plasma digoxin concentration.

To avoid toxicity during the concurrent use of erythromycin or tetracycline and digoxin, digoxin serum levels should be monitored and the dose of digoxin reduced as needed.

Hydroxychloroquine Sulfate

Hydroxychloroquine can increase the plasma concentration of digoxin, possibly by decreasing the rate of its renal elimination. The patient should be monitored for signs of toxicity during concurrent therapy, and the digoxin dose should be reduced as needed.

Ibuprofen

Ibuprofen may increase digoxin plasma levels, possibly by decreasing the renal elimination of digoxin. The same appears to be true of indomethacin. Ibuprofen may also unmask the vasoconstricting effect of digoxin on renal and coronary circulation, since endogenous prostaglandin production modulates the vascular effects of digoxin.

The patient should be monitored for signs of toxicity during concurrent therapy, and the digoxin dose should be reduced as needed.

Kaolin-Pectin

Kaolin-pectin preparations may absorb digoxin (and possibly the other glycosides) in the gastrointestinal tract, preventing their systemic absorption. Thus, underdigitalization may occur. Kaolin-pectin should be given at least 2 hours after digoxin to prevent drug interaction.

Magnesium Trisilicate

Magnesium trisilicate, magnesium hydroxide, and aluminum hydroxide antacids may absorb digoxin (and possibly the other glycosides) in the gastrointestinal tract, preventing their systemic absorption. Thus, underdigitalization may occur.

Antacids should be given at least 1–2 hours before or after digoxin to prevent drug interaction.

Metoclopramide Hydrochloride

Metoclopramide increases gastrointestinal motility and decreases gastrointestinal transit time. When digoxin in the form of slow-dissolving tablets is administered concurrently, less glycoside is absorbed and bioavailability decreases, leading to underdigitalization. In these circumstances the digoxin serum levels should be monitored and digoxin dose increased as needed. Alternatively, the use of rapid-dissolving tablets or soft gelatin capsules containing digoxin in liquid form should avoid this drug interaction.

Neomycin Sulfate

Neomycin decreases gastrointestinal absorption of digoxin by an unknown mechanism, even if given 3–6 hours before digoxin is administered. The concurrent use of these drugs leads to a decrease in plasma digoxin levels and to underdigitalization.

To avoid an interaction between neomycin and digoxin, the digoxin plasma concentration should be monitored during both initiation and termination of the neomycin therapy, and the digoxin dose should be adjusted appropriately.

Penicillamine

Penicillamine reduces steady-state digoxin plasma concentrations during concurrent therapy. The mechanism of this interaction is unknown.

The patient receiving both penicillamine and digoxin should be monitored for loss of digoxin cardiotonic effect, and the dose of digoxin should be adjusted appropriately.

Phenobarbital

The following drugs induce hepatic microsomal enzymes: phenobarbital, phenylbutazone, phenytoin, and rifampin. Since digitoxin is eliminated primarily by liver metabolism, coadministration of one or more of the enzyme-inducing drugs increases the rate of metabolism and, therefore, decreases the plasma half-life of this glycoside. Introduction of, for example, phenobarbital into the drug regimen of a patient already stabilized on digitoxin leads to a decline in plasma digitoxin concentration and the possible loss of therapeutic effect. Alternatively, removal of an enzyme-inducing drug from the regimen of a patient whose digitoxin dosage was established in its presence leads to an elevation of plasma glycoside concentration, and possibly toxicity.

The patient must be monitored for under- or overdigitalization, respectively, when an enzyme-inducing drug is either added or removed from the drug regimen. The digitoxin dose must be adjusted as needed.

Propantheline Bromide

Propantheline and other anticholinergic agents slow peristalsis and increase intestinal transit time. Addition of propantheline bromide to therapy with slow-dissolving digoxin tablets increases digoxin absorption and bioavailability, with the possibility of causing toxicity.

The patient should be monitored for toxicity and the digoxin dose appropriately reduced when propantheline is added to the drug regimen. Alternatively, the use of fast-dissolving tablets or soft gelatin capsules containing digoxin in liquid form may avoid changes in bioavailability when coadministered with propantheline.

Quinidine

The opportunity for interaction between quinidine and digoxin is high, given that these drugs are often combined for the treatment of atrial tachyarrhythmias. Quinidine causes a rise of approximately 0.5 ng/ml or more in plasma digoxin concentration in about 90% of patients. The magnitude of serum digoxin rise varies considerably, ranging from none to sixfold. The mechanism of the increase in serum digoxin is apparently by reducing the renal clearance of the glycoside and by displacing it from tissue and albumin binding sites.

It is recommended that the digoxin dose be reduced to half on adding quinidine to the drug regimen and that the patient be monitored and digoxin dose adjusted until the desired therapeutic effect is achieved in the presence of quinidine.

No apparent interaction occurs between quinidine and digitoxin. Other antiarrhythmic drugs may elevate serum digoxin concentration:

Verapamil
Quinine
Amiodarone

Those that **do not** elevate serum digoxin levels are

Procainamide
Mexiletine
Disopyramide

Spironolactone, Amiloride, and Triamterene

Concurrent therapy with any one of these diuretics and digoxin increases the steady-state digoxin plasma concentration, possibly by reducing renal clearance of the glycoside (see Pediatric Considerations, below). Patient response as well as plasma levels of K^+ and digoxin should be monitored to detect signs of toxicity, and the digoxin dose should be reduced appropriately.

Succinylcholine Chloride

Succinylcholine may induce cardiac arrhythmias in patients stabilized on a digoxin regimen. The mechanism of this interaction is unknown.

Succinylcholine should be administered cautiously to the patient taking digoxin, and the ECG and other variables should be monitored to detect signs of toxicity.

Sulfasalazine

Sulfasalazine, but apparently not other sulfonamides, reduces plasma levels of digoxin. The mechanism of this interaction is unknown.

The patient receiving sulfasalazine plus digoxin should be monitored for loss of therapeutic effect of the glycoside. This drug interaction is best avoided by using a different sulfonamide.

Thyroid

Either hyperthyroidism or administration of thyroid hormone increases renal clearance and lowers the plasma concentration of digoxin. Since digoxin has lower cardiotonic activity in the hyperthyroid patient, there may also be a decrease in the sensitivity of cardiac tissue to digitalis glycosides.

The patient receiving thyroid and digitalis glycoside concurrently should be monitored for loss of therapeutic effect, and the glycoside dose adjusted as needed.

Verapamil Hydrochloride

Verapamil decreases both renal and extrarenal clearance of digoxin, leading to an increase in digoxin plasma concentration and to the possibility of toxicity. Diltiazem may have a similar effect.

When verapamil and digoxin are combined, the patient should be monitored for signs of digoxin toxicity. Particular attention should be given to AV block, since both drugs can induce this condition and their combination is additive. Plasma digoxin concentration should also be monitored and the dose of digoxin appropriately adjusted.

Indomethacin

Indomethacin, the drug of choice for pharmacologic closure of a patent ductus arteriosus in preterm infants, may inhibit digoxin elimination. The combination of the two drugs may raise the serum digoxin concentration by 50% and decrease the distribution volume of digoxin. The two drugs may adversely affect coronary blood flow.

Amiodarone Hydrochloride

Amiodarone inhibits the renal tubular uptake of digoxin; consequently, serum digoxin concentrations may rise when the two drugs are administered concurrently. Because amiodarone has a long induction and elimination half-life, digoxin toxicity may take months to manifest. Most distressingly, cardiac asystole may be a fatal manifestation of amiodarone-digoxin interaction.

Pediatric Considerations

Differences in digoxin pharmacokinetics and pharmacodynamics between children and adults do not permit a direct extrapolation from adult to pediatric-age population in considering drug interactions. Digoxin given to pediatric-age patients receiving spironolactone, quinidine, or amiodarone is associated with the same problems of toxicity noted for adult patients.

Nonglycoside Inotropic Agents

The ideal inotropic agent for CCHF should increase myocardial contractility without affecting chronotropy and peripheral vascular resistance. The agent should not induce tachyphylaxis and should have a wide margin of safety.

Intermittent Parenteral Inotropic Therapy

Leier and associates [15] first reported that after 72 hours of continuous dobutamine infusion (10–15 µg/kg/min), left ventricular performance and symptoms and signs of CHF improved. The improvement may be sustained for periods from 2 days to 10 months. Others modified the regimen, giving intermittent DBT infusions, and noted similar responses. While the infusions improved the quality of life, they did not appear to prolong life. In fact, the incidence of sudden death may be increased [14, 16].

Orally Active Sympathomimetic Amines

LEVODOPA. Oral doses of levodopa exert a positively inotropic effect by stimulating cardiac β_1-adrenoceptors. Levodopa is converted to dopamine after oral ingestion, and doses of 1.0–1.5 gm result in cardiac and renal effects similar to those produced by IV dopamine infusion at rates of 2–4 μg/kg/min. Such oral levodopa doses may improve LV performance in patients with severe CHF. Pyridoxine (50 mg/day) appears to be important in converting levodopa to dopamine. Other drugs with similar effects on the myocardium include ibopanine, which is converted to N-methyl dopamine (epinine), and propylbutyl dopamine.

PIRBUTEROL HYDROCHLORIDE (INVESTIGATIONAL). Pirbuterol, a nonselective β-adrenoceptor oral agonist, increases cardiac contractility (β_1) and causes vasodilation (β_2), leading to a decrease in diastolic and mean blood pressure. In general, the heart rate does not increase in response to either the β_1 stimulation or as a reflex response to the reduced blood pressure. Except for its greater vasodilator action, the hemodynamic effects of pirbuterol resemble those of dobutamine. However, tolerance to pirbuterol may develop after several weeks of therapy, and its effect may be lost entirely after 1 or more months. Pirbuterol is used for the management of severe CCHF.

Pirbuterol is available as a 20-mg tablet and is taken 3 times daily. **Adverse effects** include ventricular arrhythmias, tremors, muscle cramps, and the development of tolerance. More clinical experience with pirbuterol is required in order to identify the full range of both its beneficial and its adverse effects.

OTHERS. Other orally administered sympathomimetic drugs that have been tested include terbutaline sulfate and albuterol sulfate (salbutamol), which are relatively selective for β_2-receptors; prenalterol, xansterol, and butopanine, which are relatively selective for β_1-receptors; and ibopamine, propylbutyl dopamine, and dopexamine, which activate dopamine receptors. Although many orally administered sympathomimetic drugs may improve myocardial performance in the short term, the response is extremely variable, and most lose their effectiveness with continuous administration. The reduced effectiveness is apparently due to a desensitization of myocardial β-adrenoceptors resulting from a decrease in β-adrenoceptor numbers and an uncoupling of the receptor from adenylate cyclase.

The desensitization or down-regulation of β-adrenoceptors is a key phenomenon in the positively inotropic response to sympathomimetic drugs. Another important phenomenon is whether a sympathomimetic agent is a full or a partial adrenoceptor agonist. A partial agonist stimulates the receptor to a lesser extent than a full agonist but competes with full agonists for receptor occupancy. This may favorably influence receptor number and coupling in CCHF with elevated endogenous catecholamines. However, even partial agonists will induce a down-regulation in receptor number and efficiency. Therefore, long-term improvement in myocardial inotropy is more likely with intermittent rather than continuous administration of a full agonist. Recent studies have demonstrated myocardial down-regulation of β-adrenoceptors secondary to chronically elevated endogenous catecholamines. This has led to the idea that beta blockers may reduce down-regulation of the β-adrenoceptors by competitively blocking receptor occupancy by endogenous catecholamines. This potential to return myocardial adrenergic reserve is being explored with $β_1$-selective antagonists such as metroprolol.

Phosphodiesterase Inhibitors

Inhibition of phosphodiesterase may increase intracellular concentration of cyclic AMP and cyclic guanosine monophosphate (cyclic GMP) by reducing degradation of cyclic nucleotides. Among inhibitors used clinically, theophylline (1, 3-dimethylxanthine) increases intracellular cyclic AMP levels, directly antagonizes adenosine (a negative myocardial inotrope), inhibits Ca^{2+} by directly affecting troponin, stimulates synthesis and release of endogenous catecholamines, and potentiates β-adrenoceptor agonist effect on myocardial contractility. Theophylline has limited usefulness clinically because of its nonselective effect (not limited to myocardium) and because of adverse systemic and myocardial (arrhythmogenic) effects. The bipyridine derivatives, amrinone and milrinone, on the other hand, appear to be selective for the myocardial cyclic AMP by inhibiting phosphodiesterase.

The phosphodiesterase inhibitors induce vasodilation and a tendency toward tachycardia, thereby aggravating arrhythmias. The drugs act directly on the enzyme and not via a receptor mechanism, and thereby avoid a down-regulation type of tolerance. In addition, the inotropic effect is prominent because of high sympathetically mediated stimulation of cyclic AMP levels via adenylate cyclase.

Bipyridine Derivatives

AMRINONE LACTATE. Amrinone is currently available for short-term management of severe refractory CCHF. Amrinone is effective orally and parenterally, does not cause tachyphylaxis, and has only minimal effects on heart rate.

Amrinone possesses both inotropic and vasodilator actions. The inotropic effects are independent of β-adrenoceptors and Na^+-K^+ ATPase; a positive correlation is reported between a rise in myocardial cyclic AMP and an increased inotropy. Increased inward Ca^{2+} flux appears to be a major pathway for the pharmacologic effect on the myocardium, in addition to other mechanisms for a positive inotropy with amrinone. Amrinone inceases cardiac contractility and output, even in patients who have not responded adequately to digitalis. In contrast to the β-adrenergic agonists, the hemodynamic improvement achieved with amrinone is sustained with continued therapy. Long-term oral therapy, however, may produce adverse effects. Thus, amrinone is available for IV administration only, and is used for the short-term management of severe and chronic CHF.

Amrinone is available as a 5-mg/ml injection. It may be injected undiluted or diluted to a concentration of 1–3 mg/ml in 0.45% or 0.9% sodium chloride solution. Dextrose-containing solutions should not be used.

Amrinone is administered by the IV route. The initial dose is 0.75 mg/kg, followed by a maintenance IV infusion of 5–10 µg/kg/min. An additional dose of 0.75 mg/kg may be given minutes after initiation of the therapy. The total daily dose should not exceed 10 mg/kg.

Amrinone may cause thrombocytopenia, hypotension, and an increased frequency of premature ventricular complexes. Discomfort and tissue necrosis can occur at the injection site. Therefore, caution must be used to avoid extravasation.

MILRINONE. Milrinone is approximately 15 times more potent and has fewer side effects than amrinone on a per-milligram basis and has similar pharmacologic and hemodynamic effects. The drug improves myocardial contractility in patients with severe CHF when given intravenously or orally and may also improve myocardial relaxation. Milrinone improves exercise tolerance and maximal oxygen uptake during long-term administration. As with amrinone, milrinone has not been documented to affect the progression of CHF or patient survival. Of particular concern is the high mortality of patients receiving milrinone, and presently multicenter studies are examining the responses of patients with class III (New York Heart Association) CCHF and ejection fraction of 20–40% treated with milrinone, ACEI plus digitalis, and digitalis alone. The results of these controlled studies should clarify the long-term benefits of milrinone.

Treatment of Chronic Congestive Heart Failure (Left Ventricular Diastolic Dysfunction)

Severe forms of CCHF are due, for the most part, to impaired LV systolic function, as already noted. Less severe CCHF may have normal or near-normal LV systolic function. Such forms of CCHF are seen most commonly with hypertension and are diagnosed by echocardiograms as diastolic dysfunction [9]. Diastolic dysfunction is most severe in hypertensive patients with LV hypertrophy. Perhaps 15–30% of patients with CCHF have diastolic, rather than systolic, dysfunction of the LV.

Another group of patients with diastolic dysfunction of the LV are those with symptomatic or asymptomatic ischemic heart disease. Some of these patients develop high intraventricular pressures, while their LV systolic performance may be normal. Patients with diabetes mellitus may have diastolic dysfunction.

Nothing of note distinguishes the symptoms or signs of diastolic from systolic LV dysfunction. The diagnosis is made by echocardiogram or nuclear studies (Fig. 1-7).

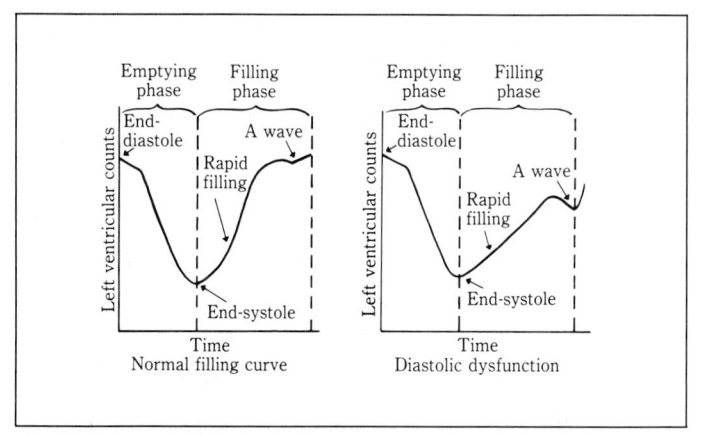

Fig. 1-7. Left ventricular (LV) filling curves (radionuclide ejection fraction) contrasting the slopes of the rapid filling phases of normal subjects (*left*) with those of patients with diastolic dysfunction (*right*). A greater proportion of LV filling occurs during the late diastolic period, coinciding with atrial contraction, in hearts with diastolic dysfunction than in normal hearts. (Modified from B. M. Massie. Congestive heart failure in patients with normal systolic function. *The Complicated Cardiovascular Patient*, p. 7, summer 1987.)

The most effective first-line treatment is similar to the treatment of CCHF secondary to LV systolic dysfunction. Where therapy for the two conditions differ is in the use of diuretics (affecting the preloading of the LV). Patients with CCHF secondary to LV diastolic dysfunction will note fatigability and have markedly reduced blood pressure with excessive diuresis. In general, low doses of thiazides should be carefully titrated.

Vasodilators and ACEI drugs have little or no beneficial effects in patients with CCHF and LV diastolic dysfunction. Ca^{2+} channel blockers, by acting directly on the LV, may be the second-line therapy. The drug of choice appears to be verapamil or diltiazem. Nitrates can also be effective therapy for these patients.

References

1. Artman, M., et al. Congestive heart failure in childhood and adolescence: Recognition and management. *Am. Heart J.* 105:479, 1983.
2. Chadda, K., et al. Effect of propranolol after myocardial infarction in patients with congestive heart failure. *Circulation* 73:503, 1986.
3. Cody, R. J., et al. Atrial natriuretic factor in normal subjects and heart failure patients: Plasma levels and renal, hormonal and hemodynamic responses to peptide infusion. *J. Clin. Invest.* 78:1362, 1986.

4. Cohn, J. N., et al. Effect of short-term infusion of sodium nitroprusside on mortality rate in acute myocardial infarction complicated by left ventricular failure. *N. Engl. J. Med.* 306:1129, 1982.
5. Cohn, J. N., et al. Plasma norepinephrine as a guide to prognosis in patients with chronic congestive heart failure. *N. Engl. J. Med.* 311:819, 1984.
6. Cohn, J. N., et al. Effect of vasodilator therapy on mortality in chronic congestive heart failure. *N. Engl. J. Med.* 314:1547, 1986.
7. The Consensus Trial: A cooperative North Scandinavian enalapril survival study. *N. Engl. J. Med.* 316:1429, 1987.
8. Crozier, I. G., et al. Haemodynamic effects of atrial peptide infusion in heart failure. *Lancet* 2(8518):1242, 1986.
9. Dougherty, A. H., et al. Congestive heart failure with normal systole function. *Am. J. Cardiol.* 54:778, 1984.
10. Fowler, M. B., et al. Assessment of the β-adrenergic pathway in the intact failing human heart: Progressive receptor down-regulation and subsensitivity to agonist response. *Circulation* 74:1290, 1986.
11. Garnett, W. R., and Barr, W. H. *Geriatric Pharmacology.* Upjohn Co., 1984.
12. Grabenkort, W. R. A cardiopulmonary physiologic profile for use with the Swan-Ganz catheter. *Resid. Staff Physician* 29:80, 1983.
13. Killip, T., III, and Kimball, J. T. Treatment of myocardial infarction in a coronary care unit: A 2-year experience with 250 patients. *Am. J. Cardiol.* 20:457, 1967.
14. Krell, M. J., et al. Intermittent, ambulatory dobutamine infusions in patients with severe congestive heart failure. *Am. Heart J.* 112:787, 1986.
15. Leier, C. V., et al. The cardiovascular effects of the continuous infusion of dobutamine in patients with severe cardiac failure. *Circulation* 56:468, 1977.
16. Massie, B. M. Congestive heart failure in patients with normal systolic function. *The Complicated Cardiovascular Patient,* p. 7, summer 1987.
17. Packer, M., et al. Comparison of captopril and enalapril in patients with severe chronic heart failure. *N. Engl. J. Med.* 315:847, 1986.
18. Rouby, J. J., et al. Hemodynamic and metabolic effects of morphine in the critically ill. *Circulation* 64:53, 1981.
19. Weinstein, J. S., and Baim, D. S. The effects of acute dobutamine administration on myocardial metabolism and energetics. *Heart Failure* 2:110, 1986.

Selected Reading

ARTICLES

Aronson, J. L. Digitalis intoxication. *Clin. Sci.* 64:253, 1983.

Bourdarias, J. P., et al. Inotropic agents in the treatment of cardiogenic shock. *Pharmacol. Ther.* 23:53, 1983.

Colucci, W. S., et al. New positive inotropic agents in the treatment of congestive heart failure. *N. Engl. J. Med.* 314:290, 1986.

Lathers, C. M., and Roberts, J. Digitalis cardiotoxicity revisited. *Life Sci.* 27:1713, 1980.

Loffelholz, K., and Pappano, A. J. The parasympathetic neuroeffector junction of the heart. *Pharmacol. Rev.* 37:1, 1985.

BOOKS

Cohn, J. N., (ed.). *Drug Treatment of Heart Failure*. New York: Yorke Medical, 1983.

Ewy, G. A., and Bressler, R. (eds.). *Cardiovascular Drugs and the Management of Heart Disease*. New York: Raven, 1982.

Greef, I. K. (ed.). *Cardiac Glycosides. Part I: Experimental Pharmacology,* Vol. 56, part I. Berlin: Springer, 1981.

Greef, I. K. (ed.). *Cardiac Glycosides. Part II: Pharmacokinetics and Clinical Pharmacology*. Vol. 56, part II. Berlin: Springer, 1981.

Cardiac Arrhythmias

Clinical Guides to Therapy for the Arrhythmias

A most stressful task for many physicians is the rapid diagnosis and identification of appropriate management for cardiac arrhythmias, oftentimes in a high-tension clinical setting in which procedures and drug therapy must be instituted promptly. Presently, there are at least 15 antiarrhythmic drugs from which to choose. Accordingly, this chapter begins with a brief review of the arrhythmias, with tables that provide ready access to first- and second-line drugs in the management of supraventricular, ventricular, and preexcitation syndromes and atrioventricular (AV) blocks, as well as guidelines for electrical procedures. A complete description of the pharmacology of each drug is provided in later sections of this chapter.

SUPRAVENTRICULAR TACHYCARDIA

Table 2-1 presents the first- and second-line therapies for supraventricular tachycardia (SVT).

Vagal maneuvers to interrupt an attack of paroxysmal supraventricular tachycardia (PSVT) include: (1) the Valsalva maneuver, (2) squatting plus Valsalva, (3) gag reflex (finger in throat), (4) upside-down position (legs against wall), and (5) dive reflex (immersion of face in cold water). Electrical cardioversion may be the initial, first-line therapy for PSVT or atrial fibrillation if ventricular function is severely compromised by the rapid heart rate.

VENTRICULAR ECTOPY

Management of ventricular ectopy is a major clinical challenge. A flow pattern designed to provide rapid identification of appropriate therapy is offered in Table 2-2.

LONG QT INTERVAL: PROLONGED REPOLARIZATION

The QT interval is that period of the electrocardiogram (ECG) that begins with the onset of the QRS and terminates with the final deflection of the T wave. A prolonged QT interval may be congenital. Congenital prolonged QT interval has been associated with sudden death in the following syndromes: (1) congenital deafness and syncopal episodes [5], indicating an autosomal recessive inheritance [7]; and (2) similar cardiac findings, but normal hearing, suggesting an autosomal dominant transmission [11].

A prolonged QT interval is a potential contributing factor in sudden death only when it exists concurrently with dispersion of repolarization. The following conditions increase the dispersion of repolarization:

In collaboration with Vilma I. Torres, M.D., Assistant Professor of Medicine and Director, Clinical Electrophysiology Laboratories, Loma Linda University School of Medicine.

Table 2-1. Supraventricular tachycardia therapy

Type of tachycardia	First-line therapy	Second-line therapy
Paroxysmal (140–240 beat/min)	Vagal stimulation, adenosine, electrical cardioversion	Beta blockers
Repetitive (short salvos of ectopic rhythm)	Digitalis, beta blockers	
Sustained (usually in infants and children, lasting months to years)	Verapamil, digitalis; beta blockers, adenosine, adenosine triphosphate	Procainamide
Atrial fibrillation		
Acute	Electrical cardioversion (clinically unstable), IV digitalis, quinidine	Verapamil
Chronic	Anticoagulate, then: Digitalis, propranolol	Anticoagulate, then: Quinidine, procainamide
Atrial flutter	Electrical cardioversion	Digitalis, beta blockers, verapamil

Central nervous system effects. In this situation, beta blockers are first-line therapy.

Myocardial infarction (MI) and prolonged QT interval. This combination indicates a high risk for sudden death (probably related to ischemia-related heterogeneity of repolarization and imbalance in sympathetic activity).

Metabolic and electrolyte disorders: hypokalemia, hypocalcemia, and hypomagnesemia.

Drug-induced. Many drugs can increase the dispersion of repolarization: phenothiazines; probucol; tricyclic antidepressants; lithium; prenylamine; all class Ia antiarrhythmic drugs — quinidine, procainamide hydrochloride, and disopyramide phosphate; class III agents — amiodarone hydrochloride (usually torsades de pointes type of VT).

Drug treatment for arrhythmias associated with a prolonged QT interval is as follows:

First-line: Stop drugs that prolong QT interval; overdrive pacing or phenytoin, or propranolol hydrochloride.
Second-line: Lidocaine or isoproterenol infusion.

These therapies are aimed at decreasing the dispersion of myocardial repolarization.

PREEXCITATION SYNDROME

The preexcitation syndrome is an arrhythmia that "exists if, in relation to atrial events, the whole or some part of the ventricular

Table 2-2. Treatment of ventricular ectopy

Type of ventricular ectopy	First-line therapy	Second-line therapy	Other therapy
Couplets, premature extrasystole	None	Antianxiety drugs	
Nonsustained VT	Reassure	Class I beta-blockers	
Potentially malignant arrhythmias (with organic disease)	Correct causes; use mexiletine, tocainide, procainamide, quinidine		
Parasystole	None		
Accelerated idioventricular rhythm	Cardioversion (if unstable)		
Recurrent sustained VT			
Acute	Lidocaine, procainamide, bretylium, cardioversion	Overdrive pacing	
Chronic	Quinidine, procainamide mexiletine, mexiletine + quinidine	Flecainide, encainide, amiodarone	Endocardial resection, implantable defibrillator, aneurysmectomy
Torsades de pointes	Correct causes, i. e. antiarrhythmics, organophosphates, tricyclic antidepressants; use magnesium sulfate*	Overdrive pacing; isoproterenol	

Key: VT = ventricular tachycardia.
* $MgSo_4$, 2 gm in 25–50% solution given as a bolus. Second bolus given within 5 minutes followed by continuous infusion of 2–3 mg/min for 2 hours [13].

muscle is activated earlier by the impulse originating from the atrium than would be expected if the impulse reached the ventricles by way of the normal specific conduction system only" [4].

There are several pathways by which a part of or the whole ventricle is activated earlier than expected. As shown in Fig. 2-1, sites of prolongation of refractory periods of AV nodal, His, and accessory AV pathways are different for various drugs [12].

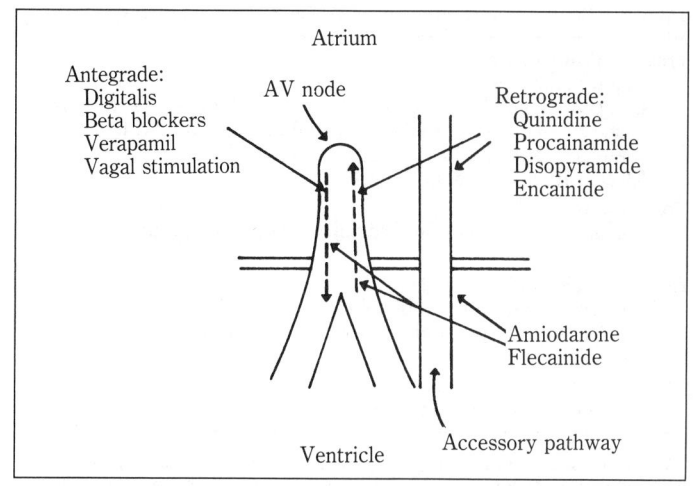

Fig. 2-1. Atrioventricular (AV) conduction system and accessory pathway sites for drug-induced prolongation of the refractory period. Drugs such as quinidine, amiodarone, and flecainide lengthen the refractory period of the retrograde pathway through the AV node and His-Purkinje tract as well as the accessory pathway. (Modified from H. J. J. Wellens et al. The management of preexcitation syndromes. *J.A.M.A.* 257:2325, 1987.)

The two most common arrhythmias, circus-movement tachycardia and atrial fibrillation, may be benign or produce a life-threatening situation in the preexcitation syndrome. The mode of therapy depends on the type of arrhythmia. A guide for drug therapy in circus-movement tachycardia or atrial fibrillation is provided in Table 2-3.

"SICK SINUS NODE" OR THE BRADYCARDIA-TACHYCARDIA SYNDROME

The bradycardia-tachycardia syndrome, consisting of paroxysmal atrial fibrillation, flutter, or tachycardia followed by sinoatrial (SA) block or sinus arrest, may present as Stokes-Adams syncopal attacks. The mechanism, as identified by clinical electrophysiology (EP) studies, includes a depression of pacemaker function or its conduction (exit block) plus depression of AV junctional impulse formation. The proper therapy usually requires electrical pacing plus pharmacologic blockade of the AV node (digitalis or beta blocker or both).

CLINICAL ELECTROPHYSIOLOGY STUDIES: INDICATIONS

The physiologic mechanism or mechanisms underlying many arrhythmias may be identified by invasive EP evaluation. With a sensing and pacing electrode positioned in the high right atrium, His bundle area, and right ventricle, atrial pacing is used to ascertain SA node automaticity, atrial conduction, and AV node refractoriness and to provide data as to whether or not the patient

Table 2-3. Circus-movement tachycardia in the preexcitation syndrome

Treatment during an attack
  Vagal maneuvers
  Drugs: verapamil, 10 mg IV; diltiazem, 0.25 mg/kg IV; adenosine phosphate, 37.5 µg/kg IV, repeated at 1-min intervals; procainamide, 10 mg/kg IV
  Electrical pacing, countershock
Prophylaxis
  Amiodarone hydrochloride, flecainide, encainide, quinidine-like drugs
Atrial fibrillation treatment*
  Hemodynamically intolerable: direct current shock
  Hemodynamically tolerable: procainamide, disopyramide phosphate
Potential cure
  Resection of accessory pathway

* Verapamil and digitalis should not be used for atrial fibrillation in patients with preexcitation ventricular complexes because of potential for ventricular fibrillation.

can develop SVT and, if so, by what mechanism — AV nodal reentry, AV reentry concealed by accessory fibers, or dual AV nodal pathways. Abnormal refractoriness in the His-Purkinje system and the ventricular response (tachycardia) to an induced premature beat are also mechanisms underlying SVT. Finally, the efficacy of drugs in exaggerating or abolishing arrhythmias may be tested. A list of indications for EP testing is given in Table 2-4.

Combined use of ambulatory (Holter) monitoring and EP studies can reliably predict drug efficacy in patients with ventricular tachyarrhythmia or fibrillation.

BRADYARRHYTHMIA; PERMANENT PACEMAKER

Patients with symptomatic bradyarrhythmia should be considered for permanent cardiac pacemaker therapy. It is essential, however, to ensure that the arrhythmia is not due to a drug, an electrolyte imbalance, or an acute inflammatory or ischemic process. Drugs that may reduce SA node discharge, AV nodal conduction, and carotid sinus sensitivity include methyldopa, clonidine, reserpine, verapamil, diltiazem, digitalis, quinidine, procainamide, beta blockers, and amitriptyline. When the bradyarrhythmia is not reversible, the implantation of a permanent cardiac pacemaker is indicated. The causes of bradyarrhythmias requiring a permanent pacemaker are summarized in Table 2-5.

ANTIARRHYTHMIC DRUGS

Table 2-6 provides ready access to the four classes of antiarrhythmic drugs.

Table 2-4. Indications for clinical electrophysiologic testing

Problem	Study objective
1. Syncope or near syncope	Evaluate sinus and AV node function and detect covert atrial tachycardia or VT
2. Suspected sinus node dysfunction	Ascertain need for pacemaker therapy
3. AV conduction defect	Ascertain need for pacemaker therapy
4. Recurrent sustained SVT or nonsustained VT with coronary artery disease	Evaluate mechanism; define therapy
5. Survival after cardiac arrest	Test for inducible VT; define therapy
6. Preexcitation syndrome	Evaluate induced SVT and determine location of accessory pathway
7. Mitral valve prolapse with involvement of SA or AV nodal tissue	Search for sinus node disease, anomalous AV connections, inducible VT; define therapy
8. Safety of drugs in patients with disease of SA node or AV node or both	Search for adverse drug effects in a controlled environment

Key: AV = atrioventricular; VT = ventricular tachycardia; SVT = supraventricular tachycardia; SA = sinoatrial.

Overview of Electrical and Mechanical Properties of the Heart

Electrical and mechanical properties of the heart are integrally linked: Electrical depolarization of cardiac cells elevates free intracellular calcium (Ca^{2+}), which in turn activates mechanisms responsible for contraction. A coordinated depolarization wave, initiated in the SA node, moves across the atrium and activates

Table 2-5. Indications for permanent cardiac pacemaker

Sinus node dysfunction (symptomatic)
    Sinus bradyarrhythmias (severe)
    Bradycardia-tachycardia syndrome: for severe and symptomatic bradycardia or to facilitate drug use for tachycardia
Atrioventricular (AV) block
    Complete (third-degree)
    Incomplete (second-degree)
        Mobitz type I (Wenckebach's disease: rare condition)
        Mobitz type II
        Incomplete with 2 : 1 or 3 : 1 AV response (widened QRS complex) (AV block localized in the bundle branches)

Table 2-6. A ready access to prototypes of the four classes of antiarrhythmic drugs

Class	Drug	Parenteral dose	Oral dose	Half-life (hr)	Therapeutic serum level (µg/ml)
Ia	Quinidine	Up to 800 mg slow IV	200 mg q6h	6	2–6
	Procainamide (Pronestyl)	100 mg q3–5 min IV; total dose 1.0 gm	250–500 mg q3–6h	1½–3	4–8
	Disopyramide (Norpace)		100–200 mg q6h	5–7	2–4
Ib	Lidocaine	30–100 mg IV bolus, 1–6 mg/min drip	None	½–2	1.2–6.0
	Tocainide (Tonocard)	750 mg IV over 15-min period	200–800 mg q8h	12–14	4–10 µg/ml
	Mexiletine	150–250 mg IV over 5–10-min period; 0.5–1.5 mg/min	400–600 mg q8h	8–12	0.7–2.0 >3.0 toxic
	Phenytoin (Dilantin)	100–500 mg slow IV	1.0-gm loading dose; 300 mg/day	6–24	10–18
Ic	Flecainide (Tambocor)		100–300 mg bid	14	300–900 ng/ml; >1000 ng/ml toxic
	Encainide		75–200 mg	Variable with metabolism; 2½–11	Serum level not helpful clinically because of active metabolites; PR should be <280 msec; QRS, <160–170 msec

II	Propranolol (Inderal)	0.1–1.0 mg q3min; maximum, 10 mg	10–40 mg q6h	3.5–6	30–50 ng/ml
	Pindolol (Visken)		5–20 mg bid	3–4	1.0–2.5 ng/ml
III	Bretylium	5–10 mg/kg over 15-min period	None	8–12; variable	
	Amiodarone (Cordarone)	5 mg/kg slow IV	200–600 mg/day loading dose; variable; usually 800–1200 mg/day for 7–14 days	13–>100 days at equilibrium	
IV	Verapamil	5–10 mg IV	240–360 mg/day	3–7	
	Diltiazem	None	240–480 mg/day	3–5	

the AV node. After a pause in the AV node, the wave spreads along the Purkinje tracts (right and left bundles and their branches) to depolarize specific regions of ventricular muscle and leads to sequential contractions of heart muscle segments. Arrhythmias occur when the electrical properties of the heart become uncoordinated, that is, when sites other than the SA node generate the depolarization wave or when marked regional differences in conduction velocity or duration of refractoriness occur. In either case, the resulting arrhythmias range from occasional extra beats or intermittent tachycardia to fibrillation. Cardiac pump function may be inconsequentially impaired or lost completely with the arrhythmia.

The actions of the antiarrhythmic drugs are best understood in terms of their effects on the electrical properties of the heart. Certain of these agents slow the rate of spontaneous depolarization generation by ectopic pacemakers. Others alter either conduction velocity or the duration of refractoriness. The objective of these agents is to move the heart toward more homogeneous electrical behavior and, thus, reduce or eliminate arrhythmias.

In this chapter, the physiologic and pathologic electrical activities of the heart, as well as the mechanisms of the antiarrhythmic agents, are described in terms of the cardiac action potential (AP). But first an overview of the AP in the different regions of the heart is presented, followed by a review of current concepts of mechanisms underlying ectopic impulse formation and reentrant arrhythmias. The four categories of antiarrhythmic agents according to mechanism of action are then reviewed, and the pharmacologic, pharmacokinetic, and therapeutic properties of individual agents are discussed. The chapter concludes with a guide to antiarrhythmic drug interactions.

Cardiac Electrical Activation and the Myocardial Contractile Response

The heart is activated (depolarized) in a coordinated manner that assures the greatest efficiency for myocardial contraction. Depolarization is initiated in the SA nodal cells (P cells) as an AP that spreads rapidly over the atria and triggers contraction of the atria and subsequent delivery of blood during the diastolic interval of the ventricles. The slowness of conduction of the depolarization front through the AV node is essential to allow a complete emptying of the atria before the ventricles contract. After passing through the AV node, the depolarization front travels rapidly down the right and left bundle branches of the Purkinje system, ultimately to reach the endocardial surface of the ventricles. Sequential depolarization of the ventricular muscle is necessary to accommodate an initial contraction of the inflow and the subsequent contraction of the outflow myocardial components of the two chambers.

Several properties of the heart are essential for coordinated pump function. First, the atria and ventricles behave as syncytia, since the cells are linked by low-resistance junctions (intercalated disks). Thus, an AP occurring in one cell spreads rapidly to the adjacent cells of the structure, either atria or ventricles. A second essential property of P cells located in the SA and selected cells of the AV nodes and the Purkinje system is the capacity to generate APs spontaneously. However, cells of the SA node have the most rapid inherent rate of AP generation and therefore serve as pacemaker cells. The third and fourth essential properties of cardiac cells are the rates of conduction from cell to cell and the duration of refractoriness after excitation. For example, the time required for an AP to conduct through the Purkinje system and ventricular muscle mass is approximately 0.06 seconds. However, the duration of refractoriness is 0.3 seconds. Thus, the whole of the ventricles is refractory during systole, and the possibility for reexcitation of one portion of ventricle by another is eliminated by the combination of rapid conduction plus prolonged refractory period.

A myocardial ischemic episode, mechanical stretching, intense nerve stimulation, or infection may alter one or more of the essential properties of cardiac cells and lead to arrhythmic activity. For example, an ischemic site in the atrium or ventricle may generate impulses at a rate greater than that of the SA node and become the predominant pacemaker for tachycardia, or multiple ectopic pacemakers may cause high-frequency tachyarrhythmias such as flutter or fibrillation. Ectopic pacemakers develop most commonly in the AV node, the bundle of His, or the Purkinje system; however, modified cells of the atria or ventricles may become aberrant pacemakers. Alterations of either conduction velocity or the duration of refractoriness may also lead to arrhythmias by creating a nonhomogeneity of either or both of these characteristics. For example, the refractory period may be shortened in a damaged region of heart muscle, leading to a more rapid recovery there than in the surrounding tissue. In this situation, the depolarization wave reenters and excites the damaged region and cycles back and forth between the damaged and normal tissue, generating reentry tachycardia or higher frequencies of tachyarrhythmias. The mechanisms underlying reentrant arrhythmias are discussed in detail below.

Cardiac Action Potential

The depolarization phase of cardiac APs in fast-response tissues is carried by sodium (Na^+) inward current. Such tissues include the atria, bundle of His, Purkinje fiber system, and the ventricles. Depolarization of the slow-response tissues, the SA and AV nodes, is carried by calcium (Ca^{2+}) inward current. Injury to fast-response tissues can impair Na^+ channel function, converting these to Ca^{2+}-dependent depolarization.

The normal fast-response tissues have an average resting potential of -90 mV. The voltage-dependent Na^+ channel is in a resting state at this potential but becomes activated as the potential decreases to a threshold of about -60 mV. Na^+ cascades into the cell via the Na^+ channel and carries the membrane potential to approximately $+20$ mV. This constitutes the 0 phase of the AP (Fig. 2-2). The Na^+ channel inactivates

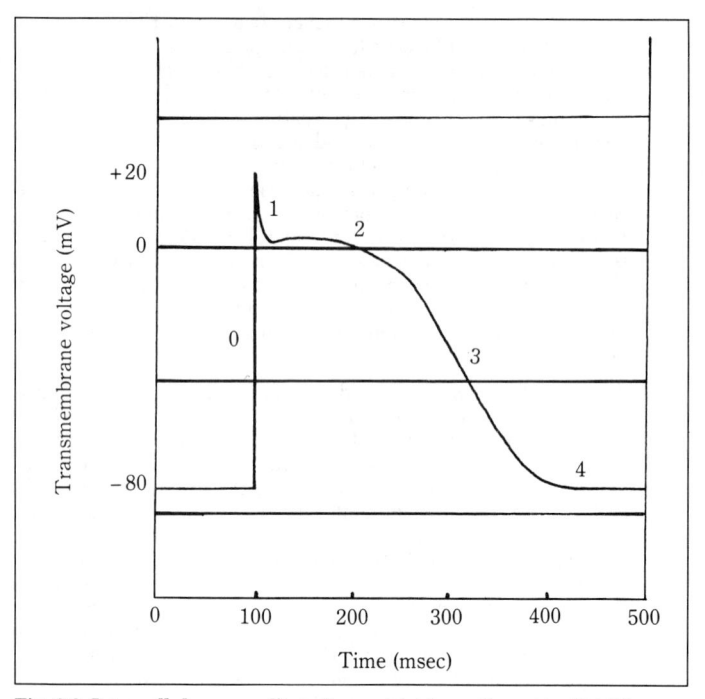

Fig. 2-2. Intracellular recording of a ventricular action potential. The ionic basis for each phase is described in the text.

within 1–2 msec, and a passive inward movement of chloride ion (Cl$^-$) occurs as the AP returns rapidly to 0 mV. These events are responsible for phase 1 of the AP.

During phase 2, the potential is maintained at a plateau near 0 mV for approximately 100–200 msec. Three factors account for this. The Ca^{2+} channel, which is also voltage dependent, is activated during 0 phase as the membrane potential becomes more positive than −40 mV. Thus, inward Ca^{2+} current contributes to the phase 2 plateau. Outward potassium (K$^+$) conductance is also reduced during phase 2 and becomes rectified in that K$^+$ enters the cell more easily than it leaves. Phase 2 is terminated when (1) the Ca^{2+} channel inactivates, stopping the inward flow of positive current, and (2) the K$^+$ channel opens, leading to the outward positive current that repolarizes the cell during phase 3, returning the cell to resting potential. The period between the APs, when the membrane potential remains stable in atrial and ventricular muscle, or depolarizes slowly in the SA and AV nodes, the bundle of His, and the Purkinje fiber system, is called phase 4. The slow diastolic depolarization of the SA nodal cells carries the membrane potential to threshold and spontaneously initiates an AP.

Several currents are primarily responsible for maintaining the resting potential. The Na$^+$ pump is electrogenic since it exchanges three sodium ions for two K$^+$ ions. It represents positive

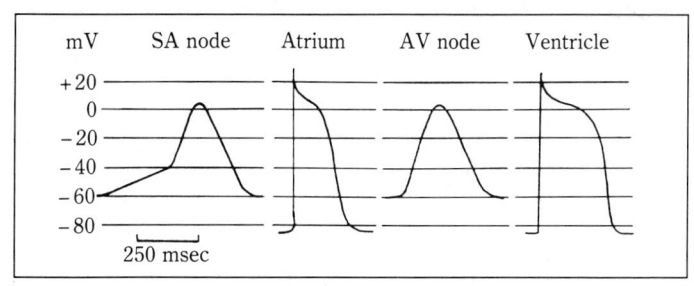

Fig. 2-3. Intracellular recordings of action potentials at different sites in the heart. (SA = sinoatrial; AV = atrioventricular.)

current out. Background K$^+$ current also contributes to positive current out. These are opposed by background Na$^+$ and Ca^{2+} currents moving into the cell. (The term **background** refers to the general leakiness of the membrane. The background currents are active during all five phases of the AP.) The diastolic depolarization that occurs most predominantly in the SA node is carried by "pacemaker" currents that are active only during phase 4. These include both outward K$^+$ and inward Na$^+$ flux. Presently, it is thought that depolarization is carried by increased Na$^+$ current in while outward K$^+$ current remains constant.

The AP in the SA and AV nodes (Fig. 2-3) differs from that of the fast-response tissues in that the resting potential of the former is approximately -60 mV. Moreover, the 0 phase depolarization is carried by Ca^{2+} current. As described below, this accounts for marked differences in conduction velocity between the fast-response and slow-response tissues.

REFRACTORY PERIOD

Na$^+$ channel reactivation occurs during phase 3 repolarization, beginning at approximately -60 mV. The cardiac cell becomes absolutely refractory beginning with 0 phase depolarization and remains so until the cell has repolarized to approximately -55 to -60 mV. The cell remains relatively refractory — refractory to all but a superintense second AP — during the remainder of phase 3 as the potential moves from -60 to -90 mV. The relative refractoriness is due to the lack of Na$^+$ channels available for activation. Since Na$^+$ channel recovery occurs between -60 and -90 mV, the degree of refractoriness steadily declines over this voltage range. In all subsequent discussion, the term **effective refractory period** (ERP) is used to refer to the absolute plus the relative refractory periods.

THE 0 PHASE AND THE RATE OF CONDUCTION

The rate of rise of the 0 phase is a function of the availability of activatible Na$^+$ channels. This can be demonstrated experimentally by applying an electrical stimulus to a cardiac cell at several points during phase 3 recovery. If the intensity of stimulation is sufficient to elicit a second AP, the rate of rise of the 0 phase of that potential will be slowest when the stimulus is applied at

A

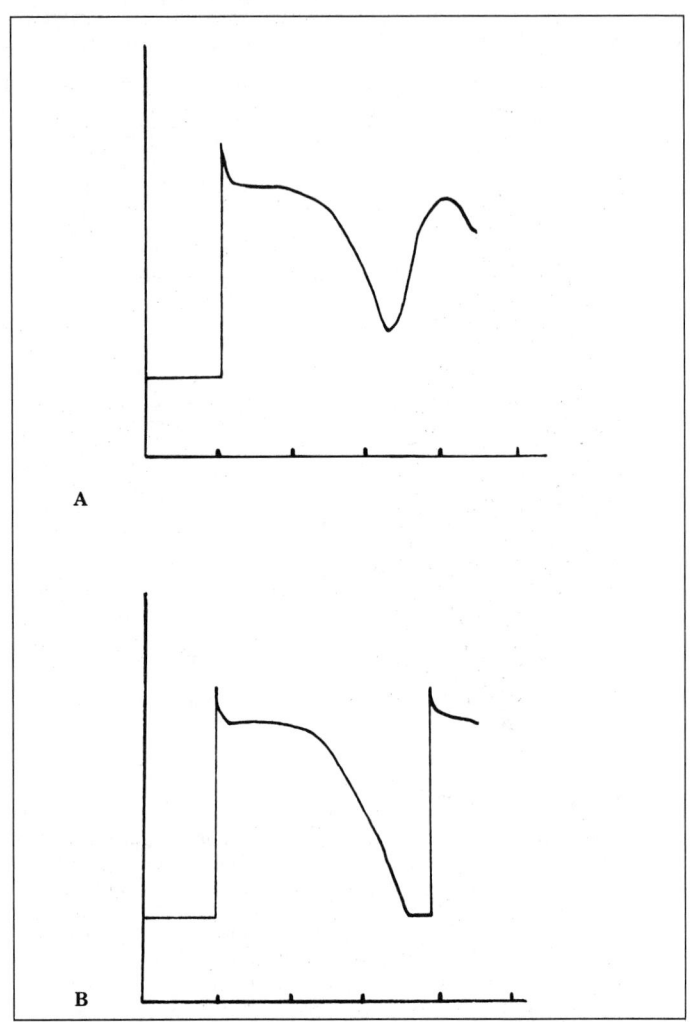

B

Fig. 2-4. Action potentials showing stimulation during phase 3 and resultant depolarization (A), and during phase 4 (B). Stimulation before full repolarization results in a slower rate of rise of the 0 phase.

-55 to -60 mV. The rate of rise will increase as the stimulus is applied at more negative potentials and will be greatest when the cell has recovered to -90 mV at the time of stimulus (Fig. 2-4).

The rate of conduction between cardiac cells is a function of the rate of rise of the 0 phase in each cell. A finite period of time is required for each cell to depolarize to the point that the wave of excitation is passed to the next cell. Thus, rate of conduction through cardiac tissue is the cumulative reflection of the 0 phase rates of rise of the constituent cells.

Therefore, the availability of activatible Na^+ channels determines the rate of rise of the 0 phase as well as the conduction velocity and is the definitive concept underlying changes in conduction velocity brought about by diseases and by the antiarrhythmic drugs. Ischemic assault, hyperkalemia, infection, and other pathologic processes can make the resting potential of fast-response tissues less negative. Full recovery of Na^+ channel function requires a return to normal resting potential (-90 mV), while limited recovery of the resting potential in cells of diseased tissue reduces the conduction velocity through the region. Healthy myocardial tissues conduct at 0.5–5.0 m/sec, while impaired tissue may conduct at a rate of less than 0.1 m/sec. Certain antiarrhythmic drugs act by binding to and inactivating the Na^+ channels to reduce the number of Na^+ channels available during the 0 phase and thereby slow conduction velocity through the tissue.

The availability of Na^+ channels influences not only the rate of rise but also the amplitude of the 0 phase. In normal cells undergoing repolarization to a resting potential of -90 mV, the AP amplitude ranges between 90 and 135 mV. In contrast, impaired fast-response tissues and slow-response tissues exhibit an amplitude of 40–70 mV. The AP amplitude determines the conductivity rate of the depolarization wave through the myocardium. When the amplitude is less than approximately 55 mV, conduction becomes decremental rather than all-or-none. The amplitude of the AP progressively declines, and conduction failure may occur before the wave of depolarization can emerge from the region of impaired fast-response tissue.

AUTONOMIC CONTROL OF THE HEART RATE

The vulnerability of the heart to arrhythmias is altered by changes in the vagal and sympathetic neural input into the conduction tissues. Depolarization waves from the SA node and conduction delay through the AV node are particularly sensitive to sympathetic and parasympathetic (vagal) impulses.

During sinus rhythm, heart rate is determined by the intrinsic frequency of discharge of the P cells in the SA node and the tonic influence of the autonomic nervous system. An antagonism and an interaction between sympathetic and vagal influences on heart rate is shown by vagally mediated presynaptic inhibition of norepinephrine release from cardiac sympathetic nerve endings, summarized as follows:

Inhibitory vagal effects are mediated in part by a direct effect of acetylcholine on muscarinic receptors on P cells plus an indirect effect of muscarinic receptor-mediated inhibition of norepinephrine release at the sympathetic nerve endings.

Sympathetic tone, partly attenuated by presynaptic inhibition (indirect muscarinic effect) is mediated by a fraction of the total β-adrenoceptor activity to determine the resting tone.

The presynaptic interaction between vagal and sympathetic nerve endings on the P cell of the SA node is shown in Fig. 2-5.

In an infrequently cited but important report, Rossi [8], of the University of Milan, identified the pathologic changes in the

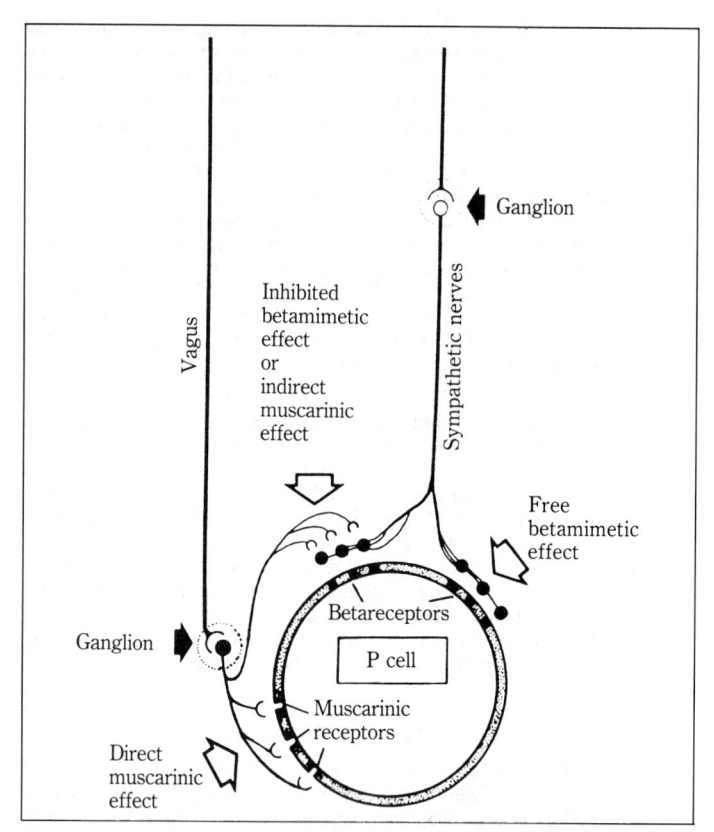

Fig. 2-5. Interactions between vagal and sympathetic nerve endings at the pacemaker (P cell) in the sinoatrial node. Vagal impulses affect P cell function by direct activation of muscarinic receptors and indirectly by inhibiting transmitter release from sympathetic nerve endings. The remaining sympathetic tone comes from stimulation of the free betamimetic receptors. (From V. S. Murthy and T. F. Hwang. Antiarrhythmic drugs and the modulation of autonomic control of heart rate in rabbits. *Fed. Proc.* 45:2186, 1986.)

cardiac autonomic nerve plexus among 32 human hearts from individuals with precocious atrial arrhythmias. In many instances, the nervous tissue lesions were independent of myocardial or connective tissue lesions. A summary of his findings is presented below.

1. Atrial fibrillation (AF) (20 cases). There were 3 hearts with normal nerves from patients with chronic AF (>2 years); 4 cases had normal myocardial and connective tissue components but pathologic changes of the nervous tissue. Severe pathology in the SA node innervation was present in 7 cases; moderate pathology, in 4 other cases. SA node fibrosis was present in 5 cases, and severe sclerosis in only 2 cases. Inflammation or hemorrhage in and around the SA node was seen in more than 50% of the cases.

2. Paroxysmal supraventricular tachycardia (2 cases). In both cases, severe nerve changes (interrupted axons with extensive degeneration and abnormal proliferations) and ganglia changes in and around the SA node were present.

3. AV nodal rhythms (7 cases). Damage to nerves and ganglia was seen in 6 cases. Lesions in and around the nodes of Keith-Flack and of Tawara were present in all cases.

Mechanisms of Arrhythmia: Automaticity and Abnormalities of Conduction and Refractoriness

INCREASED RATE OF DIASTOLIC DEPOLARIZATION

Spontaneous impulse generation results from a depolarization during diastole — that is, an increased slope of phase 4 — that carries the membrane potential to threshold for activation. Such diastolic depolarization characterizes the P cells of the SA node, which has an inherent rate of approximately 70–80 beats/min. The AV node and the Purkinje fibers also exhibit an increased phase 4 slope and have inherent rates of impulse generation of 40–60 and 15–40 beats/min, respectively. Atrial and ventricular muscle do not exhibit diastolic depolarization; however, when the resting membrane potential is reduced by disease or experimentally, an increase in phase 4 slope may develop to accelerate the inherent rate of impulse generation to levels that exceed the intrinsic rates of the P cells of the SA node. Ischemia, hyperkalemia, and other pathologic processes produce less-negative resting potentials in fast-response tissues and may increase the slope of phase 4. Diseased atrial and ventricular tissue from human hearts with membrane potentials in the range of -50 to -60 mV exhibits phase 4 depolarization and spontaneous impulse generation.

TRIGGERED BEATS

Early and delayed afterdepolarizations (see below) are linked to and "triggered" by a prior AP. Each can result in a single extra beat, referred to as a coupled beat, or to a series of extra beats, all originating from the initial AP. In contrast, the ectopic impulse generation described above is not linked to a prior AP, and its rate is determined exclusively by the steepness of the phase 4 depolarization.

EARLY AFTERDEPOLARIZATIONS

Early afterdepolarizations are initiated during phase 3 of the AP. The rate of repolarization is slower than normal, allowing the potential to remain momentarily at a stable point in the range of -30 to -50 mV. However, this potential is above threshold for initiating an AP, and the membrane depolarizes once again (Fig. 2-6A). Multiple APs can also be generated by this mechanism as the potential oscillates between approximately -30 to -50 mV and 0 mV. While the mechanisms underlying early afterdepola-

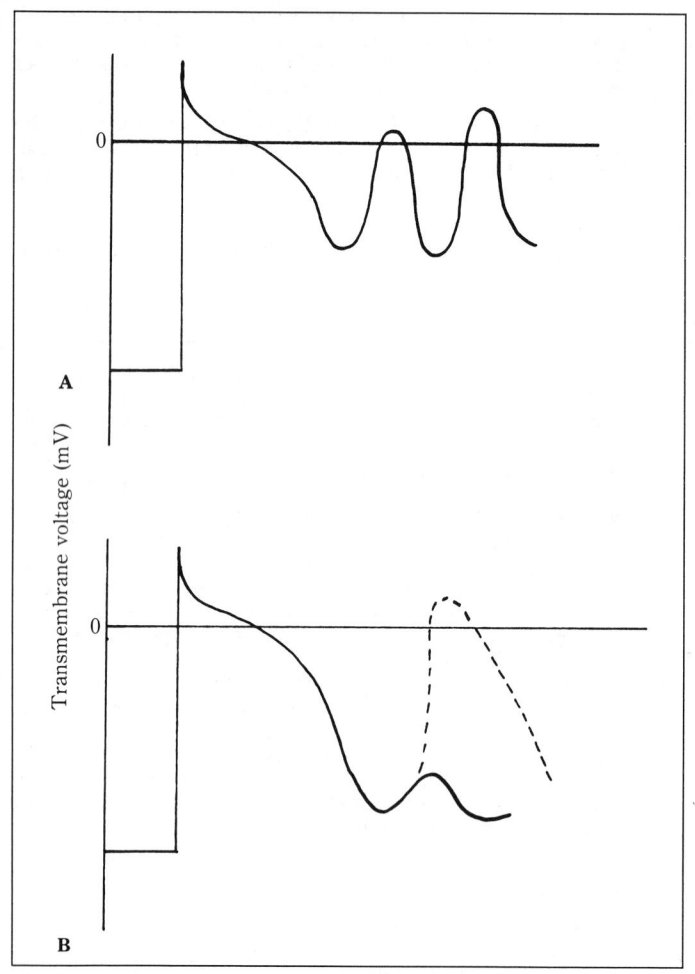

Fig. 2-6. Action potentials followed by early (A) and delayed (B) afterdepolarizations. Ionic mechanisms underlying these events are given in the text.

rizations are not fully understood, two requirements are recognized: (1) The rate of repolarization during phase 3 must be slowed. Either decreased background outward current (K^+) or increased background inward current (Na^+ or Ca^{2+} or both) could account for this. (2) Cardiac fibers must possess the capacity to "rest" at -30 and -50 mV as well as at the normal resting potential of approximately -90 mV. Evidence for two such stable resting potentials was obtained in Purkinje fibers [3].

Clinical conditions associated with early afterdepolarizations include high concentrations of catecholamines, hypoxia, elevated pCO_2, and mechanical stretching. One or more of these conditions may exist in cardiac tissue damaged by ischemia or other pathologic assaults.

DELAYED AFTERDEPOLARIZATIONS

Delayed afterdepolarizations are oscillations of the membrane potential during phase 4 (Fig. 2-6B). Such oscillations can result in premature APs when the magnitude of the upstroke is sufficient to carry the membrane potential to threshold for activation. Moreover, delayed afterdepolarizations may result in a single coupled beat or in a series, as shown in Fig. 2-6.

Delayed afterdepolarizations generally occur under conditions of elevated intracellular Ca^{2+} concentrations and are most commonly associated with toxic levels of the digitalis glycosides. They may also be associated with elevated catecholamines. It has been proposed that an elevated intracellular Ca^{2+} may fluctuate due to alternating uptake and release of Ca^{2+} from the sarcoplasmic reticulum. Since Ca^{2+} can influence the permeability of Na^+ ion, the Ca^{2+} fluctuation results in the transient inward current of Na^+ during phase 4 and leads to oscillatory changes in membrane potential that characterize delayed afterdepolarizations.

REENTRY

Reentry requires a nonhomogeneity of both conduction velocity and refractory period. Using the ventricles as the example, reentry cannot occur when conduction throughout this tissue is complete within 0.06 seconds and the entire muscle mass remains refractory for 0.3 seconds. However, regional, pathologic alterations such as ischemia may reduce the resting potential (make it less negative) by impairing Na^+ channel function and thereby dramatically reduce conduction velocity from perhaps 5 m/sec to 0.01–0.10 m/sec. Under these conditions, a wave of depolarization could travel slowly through a damaged region of cardiac tissue and emerge to reexcite recovered normal tissue.

Mechanisms underlying reentry are complex and beyond the scope of this text. Only the original model of Schmitt and Erlanger [9] will be described, since it clearly illustrates requirements for reentry and provides a basis for understanding how antiarrhythmic agents might interrupt this form of arrhythmia. Accessory pathways such as Kent fibers in Wolf-Parkinson-White (WPW) syndrome provide the only anatomic model of reentry in humans (see Fig. 2-1).

Reentry implies that a wave of depolarization traverses an abnormal circuit repetitively and also passes away from this circuit to depolarize the remainder of the heart. This process generates coupled extra beats and higher frequencies of tachyarrhythmias that are uninfluenced by and independent of the pacemaker activity of the SA node. The abnormal circuit may be defined by an anatomic object such as the circumference of a discrete region of ischemic tissue. Alternatively, it may continuously change its size and location with time.

The requirements for reentry are (1) a long pathway of conduction or (2) a reduced rate of conduction or both, (3) unidirectional

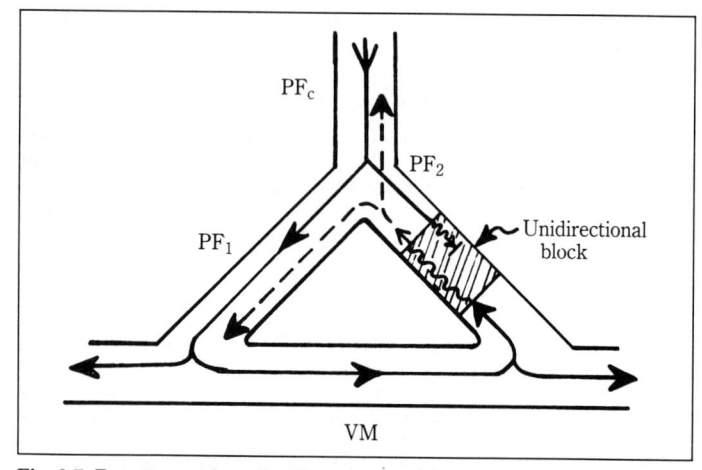

Fig. 2-7. Reentry, as described by Schmitt and Erlanger [9]. The anterograde impulse travels down the common Purkinje fiber (PF_c) and its two branches (PF_1, PF_2); however, ischemic damage in PF_2 creates a block in the anterograde direction. The wave of excitation travels down PF_1 through ventricular muscle (VM) and excites the terminal end of PF_2, leading to retrograde conduction through the damaged area (unidirectional block) and up the PF_c. The depolarization wave may also cycle down PF_1 repeatedly, creating a reentrant circuit. (From M. F. Arnsdorf. Basic understanding of the electrophysiologic actions of antiarrhythmic drugs. Sources, sinks and matrices of information. *Med. Clin. North Am.* 68: 1247, 1984.)

block, and (4) a reduced effective refractory period. Reentry is illustrated in Fig. 2-7, using a branching Purkinje fiber. The shaded area on the right branch denotes an area of injury where conduction in the normal direction is blocked. However, conduction in the retrograde direction can occur at a greatly reduced rate. Thus, the area of injury provides both the reduced rate of conduction and the unidirectional block. A depolarization front is conducted down one Purkinje fiber but is blocked in the other. The wave front traveling down the healthy left branch emerges into the ventricular muscle, reaches the distal tip of the diseased right branch, and conducts in the retrograde direction. A portion of the right branch proximal to the shaded area is depolarized by the normally conducted AP. However, if retrograde conduction through the shaded area is sufficiently slow, the proximal portion of the right branch recovers and the conduction continues up the Purkinje fiber, generating a coupled extra beat. A series of extra beats would be generated if the wave of depolarization cycled repeatedly down the left branch and retrogradely up the right branch. In this example, slow conduction through the area of injury would provide the time needed for recovery of the depolarized proximal portion of the right branch. A reduced effective refractory period in that portion would decrease the time requirement and, thus, work in concert with the slow rate of conduction to ensure the survival of the reentrant circuit.

Arrhythmogenic Properties of Digitalis

ELECTROPHYSIOLOGIC EFFECTS OF DIGITALIS

While stimulating myocardial contractility, a digitalis-mediated increase in vagal function serves as a first-line treatment of SVT, including paroxysmal tachycardia, flutter, and fibrillation. The goal of the therapy is to induce AV block in order to maintain ventricular rate in the normal range. Using atrial flutter as an example, impulses are generated in the atria at an average rate of 300/minute. Given the characteristically long ERP of the AV node, many of these impulses are extinguished within the node, resulting in a 2 : 1 or greater AV block. By increasing the ERP, digitalis can increase the block to 4 : 1, providing an ideal ventricular rate of 75. The effect of digitalis on the atrial rate is unpredictable, however. The flutter may either convert to normal sinus rhythm or to fibrillation, or may not change. The degree of conduction block is dependent on the atrial rate. Thus, in paroxysmal atrial tachycardia, AV node conduction may be 2 : 1 or 3 : 1 with digitalis, and thereby provide protection to the ventricles. The digitalis-mediated AV block may be reduced by increased sympathetic stimulation, and the dose of digitalis must be sufficiently high to prevent loss of AV block during exercise or stress.

DIGITALIS EFFECTS ON VENTRICULAR ACTION POTENTIAL AND THE ELECTROCARDIOGRAM

The ECG reflects the different stages of the ventricular AP and, thus, ionic events at the level of the cardiac cell membrane. Since both therapeutic and toxic effects of digitalis are related to drug-induced alterations in ionic membrane events, the ECG becomes an important clinical means for assessing drug effects throughout digitalis therapy. In this section, relationships between different phases of the AP and ECG are summarized. Changes in these variables brought about by digitalis are then reviewed. It will be seen that these changes account for the following characteristic effects of digitalis on ventricular muscle and Purkinje cells: reduced conduction velocity, decreased AP duration (APd) and ERP, and increased automaticity. These same changes occur in atrial muscle whenever the direct effects of digitalis predominate in this tissue; however, this usually occurs only in the toxic concentration range.

In Fig. 2-8 the atrial and ventricular APs are shown together with an ECG on the same time scale. The atrial AP corresponds to the P wave of the ECG and represents the depolarization of atrial muscle cells. Atrial cell repolarization (T wave) is buried in the QRS complex. The 0 phase of the ventricular AP corresponds to the QRS complex and represents depolarization of ventricular muscle mass. Phase 2 corresponds to the ST segment. Since phase 2 is nearly isoelectric in the normal heart, the ST segment of the ECG is also isoelectric. Repolarization during phase 3 corresponds to the T wave.

The major changes that occur in the AP elicited by digitalis are also shown in Fig. 2-8. Digitalis decreases the rate of rise of the 0

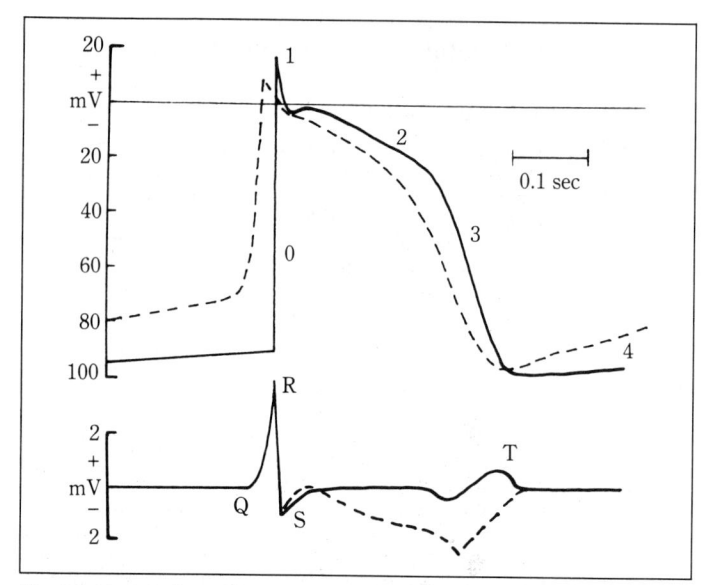

Fig. 2-8. Ventricular action potential (top) and consequent ECG (bottom) in the absence (solid line) and presence (dashed line) of digitalis. Note the digitalis-induced changes in QT interval, ST segment, and T wave.

phase, increases the slope of phase 2, decreases the slope of phase 3, and may increase the slope of phase 4 in the Purkinje but not the ventricular muscle cells. While the decreased rate of the 0 phase is not generally revealed in the ECG, it is nonetheless an important event. The 0 phase determines conduction velocity between cells, and the reduced rate of rise accounts for the reduced conduction velocity throughout the ventricles and the Purkinje cells with digitalis. The increased slope of phase 2 is responsible for a depressed ST segment on the ECG. The increase in slope of phase 3 causes the T wave of the ECG to be diminished, isoelectric, or inverted. As shown in Fig. 2-8, the combined changes in phases 2 and 3, a reduced APd, and therefore ERP, result in a decreased QT interval on the ECG. Finally, digitalis increases the time between atrial and ventricular APs, which is manifested as an increase in the PR interval. The PR interval is a measure of the rate of conduction of impulses between the atria and the ventricles. The AV node is the rate-limiting structure along the conduction path between the SA node and the ventricles, and digitalis decreases the AV nodal conduction velocity.

The digitalis-mediated increase in the PR interval of the ECG in therapeutic concentrations allows clinical recognition of the drug effect, and results from a prolongation of AV nodal conduction velocity. Digitalis may also induce AV block, which, of course, represents a toxic manifestation in patients with normal sinus rhythm. The induction of AV block, however, is a therapeutic goal in patients with atrial flutter or fibrillation or other atrial tachyarrhythmias. The digitalis effects on the ECG are summarized in Table 2-7.

Table 2-7. Effects of digitalis on the electrocardiogram

PR interval increased
QRS unchanged
QT interval decreased
ST segment depressed
T wave diminished, isoelectric, or inverted

INCREASED AUTOMATICITY

Digitalis reduces AP duration in therapeutic concentrations but increases automaticity in toxic concentrations. Increased automaticity can occur within therapeutic plasma digoxin concentrations and is among the earliest signs of digitalis toxicity. This accounts for many of the arrhythmias seen during digitalis excess.

Digitalis enhances phase 4 depolarization of Purkinje cells (see Fig. 2-8) and increases automaticity in these cells. As digitalis increases the diastolic depolarization rate within the Purkinje system beyond that of the SA node, one or more Purkinje cells may take over as a site of repetitive ectopic impulse formation.

Development of delayed afterdepolarizations is a second mechanism by which digitalis increases potential for ventricular automaticity. As shown in Fig. 2-8, delayed afterdepolarization is the result of membrane potential oscillatory behavior during phase 4. The upward stroke of an oscillation may bring membrane potential to threshold, resulting in an ectopic impulse or tachycardia. The complete ionic mechanisms of delayed afterdepolarizations are uncertain; however, the oscillatory behavior during phase 4 is due to transient influxes of Na^+. This appears to be related to Ca^{2+} mechanisms, since digitalis-induced delayed afterdepolarizations can be blocked by the Ca^{2+} channel antagonist verapamil hydrochloride.

Classification of Antiarrhythmic Agents

Antiarrhythmic drugs are currently divided into four categories according to the major electrophysiologic or pharmacologic properties considered to underlie beneficial drug action. Class I agents are generally local anesthetics on nerve and myocardial membranes that slow conduction velocity by decreasing the maximal rate of depolarization (AP) without changing the resting potential. The prototype class I agent is quinidine. Class II agents are beta-adrenoceptor blockers (beta blockers), which depress the adrenergically enhanced phase 4 depolarization. The prototype drug is propranolol hydrochloride. Class III agents homogeneously prolong the AP duration, thereby increasing the ERP. Bretylium tosylate is a prototype drug. Class IV agents inhibit the slow Ca^{2+} channel and thereby increase both AP and ERP, particularly in the SA and AV nodes and atria. Verapamil hydrochloride is the prototype drug. While the above classification facilitates an understanding of the most important properties of the antiarrhythmic agents, from a therapeutic point of view it is an oversimplification. For example, many of the drugs in a given class possess actions characteristic of one or more of the other classes or may fall outside the four categories. In addition, marked differences in the effect of the class I drugs on conduction velocity have necessitated a subdivision into three subcategories, classes Ia, Ib, and Ic. Furthermore, the digitalis glycosides and adenosine triphosphate (ATP) or adenosine do not fit into this scheme even though they are clearly indicated in the treatment of certain supraventricular arrhythmias. Table 2-6 lists the four classes of antiarrhythmic drugs that are considered below.

Drug Actions Responsible for Opposing Arrhythmias

REVERSAL OF AUTOMATICITY

The three subclasses of class I agents have little or no effect on the rate of SA nodal impulse generation but can slow the rate of impulse generation in an ectopic pacemaker by decreasing the slope of the phase 4 depolarization. The mechanism underlying this action is unknown for the Ia and Ic agents. However, the class Ib agents accomplish this by increasing background outward K^+ current and decreasing inward pacemaker current carried by Na^+.

Two additional drug actions also contribute to the reversal of ectopic pacemaker activity. The class Ia agents make the threshold potential less negative without changing the resting potential. This results from the action of these agents on the Na^+ channel. The class Ib agents have been shown to increase the maximum resting potential, probably by increasing background outward K^+ current.

The consequences of the drug-induced changes in phase 4 slope, threshold potential, and maximum resting potential are shown in Fig. 2-9. The steep phase 4 slope of the ectopic pacemaker rapidly carries the membrane potential to threshold, thereby generating an AP. It can be seen that reducing the slope of phase 4 increases the time required for the membrane to move from maximum resting potential to threshold for activation. Making the threshold less negative (Ia agents) or making the maximum resting potential more negative (Ib agents) further increases that time and, when the drug therapy is successful, reduces the rate of ectopic impulse generation below that of the SA node. The SA node once again becomes the predominant pacemaker, and the arrhythmia is terminated.

A number of class I drugs have arrhythmogenic properties. Pharmacologic actions with high arrhythmogenic potential are associated with drugs that directly or indirectly enhance the nonhomogeneity of electrical properties, enhance a depressed contractility, or alter autonomic function. The incidence of exacerbations of rhythm disturbances or arrhythmogenicity for class I drugs is estimated to be 10–15%.

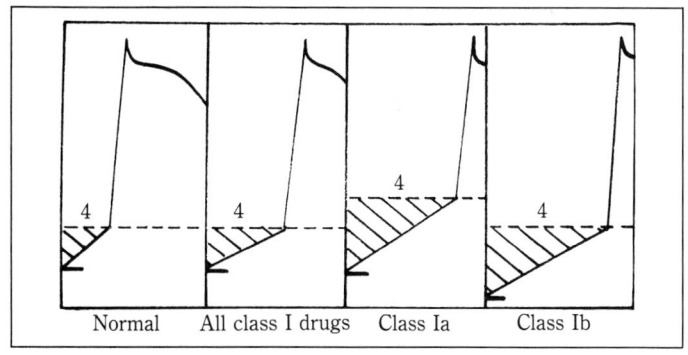

Fig. 2-9. Effects of antiarrhythmic agents on phase 4 of the cardiac action potential. All class I agents decrease the slope (slow diastolic depolarization). Class Ia agents make threshold potential (dashed line) less negative; class Ib agents hyperpolarize or make the maximum resting potential more negative (short solid line).

REVERSAL OF REENTRANT ARRHYTHMIAS

All class I agents decrease conduction velocity in the myocardium. The class Ia and Ic agents do this in all cardiac tissue, while the class Ib agents slow conduction velocity only in impaired fast-response tissue characterized by a markedly less negative resting potential, such as ischemic myocardium. Class Ib agents do not alter conduction in normal fast-response tissues.

Reduction in conduction velocity may interrupt reentrant circuits by converting the one-way conduction block in damaged tissue to two-way block. In one-way block (see Fig. 2-7), conduction in the normal direction along the Purkinje fiber branch is blocked at the site of damage; however, retrograde conduction can occur. The key issue is that the rate of retrograde conduction is dramatically reduced in the damaged tissue because of impairment of Na^+ channel function. This implies that the AP amplitude is low, perhaps less than -70 mV. Since AP amplitude determines success or failure to propagate a depolarization wave, when a class I agent further reduces the AP amplitude and rate of conduction, conduction becomes decremental and may fail before the wave of depolarization emerges from the damaged tissue. In this case, the one-way block is converted to two-way block and the reentrant circuit is broken, terminating the arrhythmia.

Increasing the ERP may also terminate reentrant arrhythmias. Retrograde conduction reentry depends on recovery of the Purkinje fiber and its branch proximal to the damaged tissue (see Fig. 2-7). The retrograde conduction wave may then emerge from the damaged tissue to reexcite Purkinje fiber and the remainder of the heart. However, if the ERP of the Purkinje fiber and its branches can be prolonged, the tissues may remain refractory when the retrograde conduction wave arrives. In this case, the wave is extinguished and the re-entrant circuit broken. The class III agents cause a marked prolongation of the AP duration and the ERP. It seems likely that this action accounts for the ability of these agents to interrupt reentrant arrhythmias.

Table 2-8. Major effects of class I agents on cardiac action potential (AP)

Drug	Action potential duration	Effective refractory period (ERP)[a]	Conduction velocity[b]	Phase 4 slope[c]
Ia (e.g., quinidine)	↑	↑↑	↓	↓↓
Ib (e.g., lidocaine)	↓→	↓→	[d]	↓↓
Ic (e.g., flecainide acetate)	↓→	↑→	↓↓	↓

Key: ↑ = moderate increase; ↓ = moderate decrease; ↑↑ = marked increase; ↓↓ = marked decrease; ↑→ = no change or a slight increase; ↓→ = no change or a slight decrease.
[a] Increasing ERP can terminate reentrant arrhythmias.
[b] The major action shared by all class I agents in terminating reentrant arrhythmias is reduction of conduction velocity, thereby converting one-way to two-way block in reentrant circuit.
[c] Phase 4 slope, i.e., diastolic depolarization rate, is reduced by all class I agents to terminate ectopic arrhythmias.
[d] Class Ib agents reduce conduction velocity primarily in ischemic tissue.

Effects of Class I Antiarrhythmic Agents on Cardiac Action Potential

The major effects of the class I antiarrhythmic agents on the cardiac AP are listed in Table 2-8.

Certain differences between the subcategories should be emphasized. For example, class Ia and Ic agents reduce the rate of rise of the 0 phase in all cardiac tissue, while the Ib agents do this only in impaired fast-response tissue exhibiting less-negative resting potential. In addition, class Ia agents increase AP duration while class Ib agents reduce it. The ERP normally terminates at the point of full repolarization, that is, on completion of phase 3 of the AP. However, class Ia and Ib agents extend refractoriness well into phase 4, a "postrepolarization refractoriness." In contrast, class Ic agents have little or no effect on either AP duration or ERP.

Many of the important differences between the effects of the antiarrhythmic agents on the AP are due to their interactions with the Na^+ channel. All class I agents bind to the Na^+ channel in a use-dependent manner. However, the three subcategories differ in their rates of association and dissociation with the channel. The concept of use dependence and the consequences of the different kinetic properties of class I agents are reviewed in the following discussion.

STATES OF THE SODIUM CHANNEL

The Na^+ channel is modulated by both voltage and time. During diastole, it exists in a resting or closed state, R, in which no Na^+ current is conducted but the channel is capable of being activated (Fig. 2-10A). As the membrane potential moves from -90 to -60 mV, progressively more Na^+ channels convert to an activated or open state, A, and are capable of conducting Na^+ current. Threshold for activation is between -60 and -75 mV. When threshold is reached, all available Na^+ channels are in the activated state, and Na^+ cascades into the cell, giving rise to the 0 phase of the AP. The time constant for inactivation of the Na^+ channel is short, 0.5 msec, after which time most of the channels convert to an inactivated state, I, within 1–2 msec after completion of the 0 phase. Na^+ channels in the I state can convert only to the R, not the A, state, and this conversion is also voltage dependent. Thus, the channels return progressively to the R state during phase 3 as the membrane potential moves from -60 to -90 mV.

USE DEPENDENCE OF THE ANTIARRHYTHMIC AGENTS

The class I agents bind reversibly to the Na^+ channel, rendering it incapable of conducting Na^+ current (Fig. 2-10B). The term *use dependence* means that the antiarrhythmic agents bind only to channels undergoing use, that is, cycling through the R, A, and I states that accompany repetitive stimulation. The evidence for use dependence comes from experiments using isolated cardiac muscle preparations and measuring the ability of the antiarrhythmic agents to reduce the rate of rise and the amplitude of the 0 phase of the AP. Reductions in these parameters imply a reduction in the number of available Na^+ channels. If an unstimulated preparation is exposed to drug for an appropriate period of time and then stimulated once, little or no change is seen in the 0 phase of the AP. However, if the preparation is stimulated repetitively over the exposure time, both the rate of rise and the amplitude of the 0 phase decline steadily. Moreover, the rate of decline increases with an increase in the frequency of stimulation. The Na^+ channel is almost exclusively in the R state in the unstimulated preparation. Since no drug effect is seen in this case, it implies the drug has very low affinity for the R state. In contrast, the Na^+ channel cycles repetitively between R, A, and I states in the stimulated preparation, and then a frequency-dependent binding of drug to either the A or I states of the Na^+ channel occurs with high affinity. Since the channels are in these states more often at higher frequencies of stimulation, the opportunity for drug binding is also greater with fast heart rates, thereby explaining the frequency dependence of the drug effect.

KINETICS OF DRUG ASSOCIATION AND DISSOCIATION WITH NA^+ CHANNEL

It is accepted that the class I antiarrhythmic drugs bind to the A or I state of the Na^+ channel, resulting in a complex that is incapable of conducting Na^+ current. In order to facilitate the

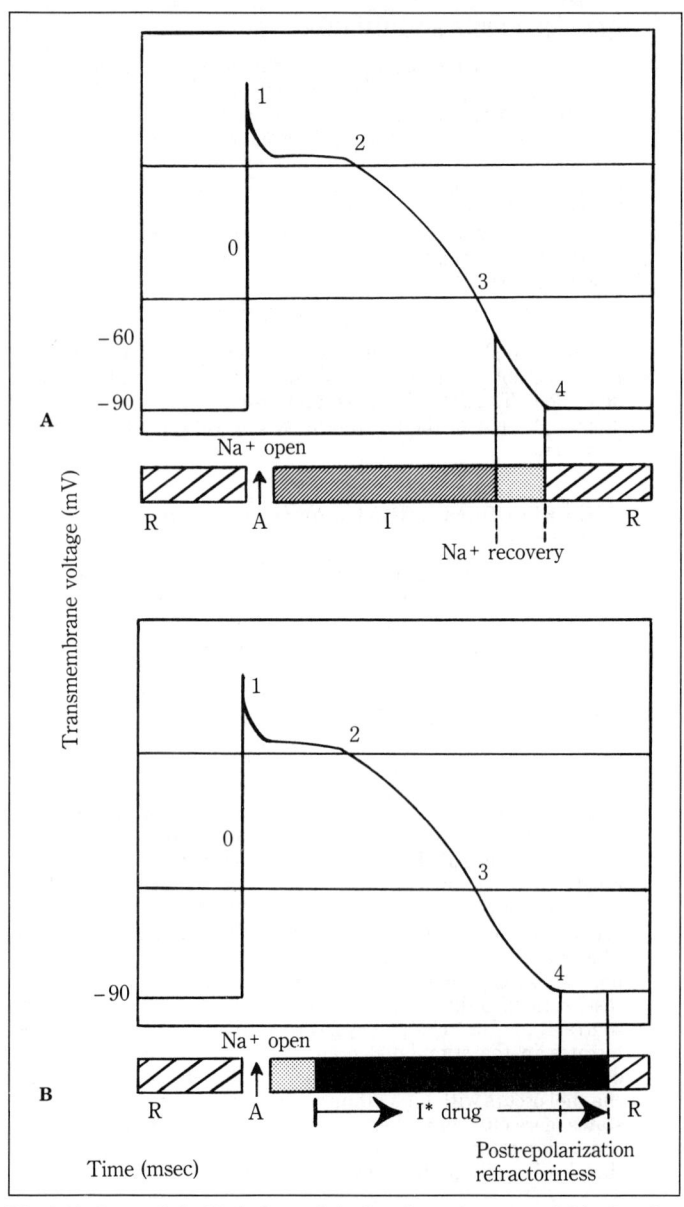

Fig. 2-10. State of the Na⁺ channel during the action potential in the absence (A) and presence (B) of class I agents. (R = resting; A = activated; I = inactivated; I* drug = channel held in the inactivated state by being bound to class I agent.) The Na⁺ channel can return to the R state only after dissociation from the class I agent.

following discussion, two simplifying assumptions are made that are consistent with these observations, namely, that it is the I state that is bound (I* drug) and that I* drug must dissociate to I before I can convert to R.

Studies using isolated cardiac muscle preparations indicate that the class Ib agents dissociate from the Na^+ channel with a time constant of approximately 0.5 seconds. The Ic agents have a much longer time constant of 15–20 seconds, while the Ia agents are intermediate. Considering the Ib agents first, no drug is bound to Na^+ channels during diastole since all of the channels are in the R state. However, on initiation of an AP, all channels convert first to the A and then to the I state, allowing drug binding to occur. Subsequently, more than half the drug will dissociate from the channel within 0.5 seconds. However, since the AP duration is approximately 0.3 seconds, many Na^+ channels will remain in I* drug state, and therefore inactivated, well into the diastolic period. This underlies the drug-induced extension of the ERP beyond the completion of the AP. In the case of Ib drugs, dissociation from the channel, which allows a return to the R state, is essentially complete by the time the next AP arrives. However, if the heart rate is markedly increased, the period of diastole is reduced and APs may arrive while the cell is still relatively refractory. This, in turn, reduces conduction velocity as discussed below in relation to the Ia agents. The relationship among Ib agent association and dissociation with the Na^+ channel, duration of ERP, and the phases of the AP is shown in Fig. 2-10B.

The Ia agents bind to and inactivate the Na^+ channel in the same manner as the Ib agents. However, Ia drugs behave as though they have a somewhat longer time constant for dissociation. Thus, they remain bound to Na^+ channels not only into the diastolic period but also during at least the initiation of the next AP. Like the Ib agents, the Ia agents extend the ERP beyond the completion of the AP. Unlike the Ib agents, the Ia agents slow the rate of rise of the 0 phase of all subsequent APs and thereby reduce conduction velocity throughout the heart at normal heart rates.

Drug dissociation from the Na^+ channel is time dependent. Consequently, the effect of Ia and Ib agents on conduction velocity increases with heart rate; that is, the shorter the period between APs, the greater the fraction of drug-bound, inactivated channels at the initiation of each AP. However, with Ib drugs essentially all Na^+ channels are available at normal heart rates. Higher heart rates may reduce the diastolic time sufficiently that APs arrive before complete drug dissociation and Na^+ channel recovery. Under these conditions, Ib agents may also reduce conduction velocity throughout the heart.

The class Ic agents have little or no effect on the ERP and do not extend refractoriness beyond phase 3 of the AP. These agents dissociate from the Na^+ channel with a time constant of 15–20 seconds. Thus, bound channels are inactivated over many heartbeats, which resemble the irreversible inactivation of the Na^+ channel. Thus, the AP is dependent on the remaining, unbound channels whose kinetics are unaltered. These channels are in the

R state during diastole and activate during 0 phase. Subsequently, they rapidly inactivate during phase 1 and recover during phase 3 as illustrated in Fig. 2-10A for non-drug-exposed cardiac tissue.

The Ic agents can have a more profound effect on conduction velocity than the Ia or Ib agents. This reflects their greater capacity to reduce the fraction of functional Na^+ channels. As reviewed above (see Cardiac Action Potential), reduction of the number of Na^+ channels decreases the rate of rise of the 0 phase of the AP and, thus, cell-to-cell conduction.

Basis for the Antiarrhythmic Action of Class II Drugs—Beta Blockers

Beta blockers inhibit beta-adrenergic receptors in the heart and, thus, depend on the preexistence of sympathetic tone to exert an effect. Such tone does exist, since most patients experience a decrease in both heart rate and cardiac output on receiving beta blocker therapy. Beta blockers exhibit the greatest antiarrhythmic efficacy under conditions of either increased sympathetic tone or increased cardiac sensitivity to sympathetic stimulation. Such conditions include exercise, pheochromocytoma, thyrotoxicosis, myocardial ischemia, congestive heart failure, digitalis toxicity, anesthesia with halothane and other gaseous anesthetics, and administration of exogenous catecholamines. Other actions by certain beta blockers, such as membrane stabilization, appear to contribute little to the antiarrhythmic action of these agents. (An important exception to this may be the prolongation of AP duration and ERP that results from long-term beta blocker therapy.)

Increased sympathetic tone changes several important electrical properties of the heart. The slope of phase 4 is increased both in the SA node and in ectopic pacemakers. In addition, conduction velocity is increased and ERP shortened throughout the heart. Therapy with beta blockers is understood in terms of reversing these effects. For example, these agents decrease the phase 4 slope and are effective in reducing ectopic arrhythmias, particularly in the atria. Atrial tachyarrhythmias ranging from extra beats to fibrillation may respond to beta blocker therapy. The beta blockers also reduce conduction velocity and prolong ERP in the AV node. This protects the ventricles during atrial flutter and fibrillation. Many ectopic atrial impulses fail to conduct through the AV node, allowing the ventricular rate to remain in or near the normal range. In many cases, paroxysmal atrial tachycardia involves a reentrant pathway that includes the AV node. Beta blockers are often effective in terminating this arrhythmia, probably by increasing AV nodal ERP or by slowing conduction further in the slow antegrade alpha pathway. Beta blockers may also terminate ventricular ectopic beats. However, these agents are not considered to be first-line therapy for higher grades of ventricular tachyarrhythmia.

Recent clinical trials have shown that beta blocker therapy, instituted after a myocardial infarction, provides significant protection against a second infarction and sudden death. The mechanism underlying this beneficial effect is unknown. It may be due to beta blockade, which reduces cardiac work and oxygen demand and the subsequent ischemic episodes. Alternatively, the prolongation of the AP duration that accompanies long-term beta blocker therapy could also account for the protective effect. This latter action appears to be due to an adaptive change in the heart in response to beta blocker therapy rather than to some property of the drugs. In contrast, the experimental beta blocker sotalol and the class III antiarrhythmic agents possess the capacity to increase AP duration and ERP directly.

Basis for the Antiarrhythmic Action of Class III and IV Drugs

While the class III agents, amiodarone hydrochloride and bretylium, possess a number of pharmacologic actions, their main antiarrhythmic action is a prolongation of the AP duration and ERP. This interrupts reentrant arrhythmias and may be understood in terms of the idealized model for reentrant circuits given above. The requirements for reentry include a long conduction pathway or a slow rate of conduction, a one-way conduction block, and a short ERP. This combination ensures that recovery from depolarization along the circuit occurs at the same rate or more rapidly than conduction of the next AP. On the other hand, prolongation of the ERP allows the conducted potential to "catch up" to refractory tissue along the circuit and thus to be extinguished.

The class III agents have a greater efficacy than other antiarrhythmic agents and are often held in reserve for cases that are unresponsive to other therapy. This may reflect the benefit of changing only one of the determinants of the reentrant circuit. For example, the class Ia agents not only prolong ERP but also slow conduction velocity. Because of the requirements for reentrant circuits, these changes actually may cancel each other out; that is, even though ERP is prolonged, the slower conduction may still allow sufficient time for recovery of the tissue in front of the reentrant AP.

Prolongation of the ERP always affects the relationship between recovery and conduction along a reentrant circuit. On the other hand, slowing conduction velocity, the hallmark effect of the Ia agents, may not. According to the idealized model for reentry, the most likely mechanism by which Ia agents interrupt a reentrant circuit is to convert the one-way block to a two-way block. The lesser efficacy of these drugs compared to the class III agents implies that slowing conduction velocity does not automatically cause retrograde conduction failure and, thus, conversion of one-way to two-way conduction block.

The class IV agents exert their antiarrhythmic action by reducing Ca^{2+} current during the AP. Verapamil and diltiazem do this in a use-dependent manner; that is, blockade occurs only in cardiac tissue undergoing repetitive depolarization and increases with the rate of depolarization. In contrast, blockade by nifedipine and the other dihydropyridine Ca^{2+} antagonists is not use dependent.

The contribution of Ca^{2+} current to the AP differs among the regions of the heart and determines the sites of action of the Ca^{2+} channel blockers. In Purkinje fibers and cardiac muscle cells, the 0 phase of the AP is mediated by Na^+ entering through its own channel. The Ca^{2+} channel is voltage dependent and is activated as the cell depolarizes over the range of -40 to $+10$ mV. The Ca^{2+} channel blockers have little effect on Purkinje fibers and cardiac muscle cells. Phase 2 plateau may be lower (more negative) and the AP may be slightly reduced in these tissues.

The AP of the SA and AV nodes is carried entirely by Ca^{2+} current and these structures are highly sensitive to the Ca^{2+} channel blockers. Ca^{2+} channel blockers decrease (1) the rate of diastolic depolarization, (2) the threshold potential (it becomes less negative), and (3) the rate of rise and amplitude of the 0 phase. They also prolong AP duration and ERP. Thus, the main effects of the Ca^{2+} channel blockers are to decrease heart rate and slow conduction through the AV node. In atrial tachyarrhythmias, Ca^{2+} channel blockers may induce 2 : 1 or higher grades of AV block.

The Ca^{2+} channel blockers have little benefit in treatment of ventricular arrhythmias, which probably reflects the relative lack of electrophysiologic effect in Purkinje fibers and cardiac muscle. In contrast, they are very useful in treating supraventricular arrhythmias. They can rapidly terminate PSVT, an arrhythmia most often involving a reentrant circuit that includes the AV node. The circuit may be limited to the atria (intraatrial reentry) or may traverse between the atria and ventricles via the AV node and an accessory AV pathway (AV reentry tachycardia as in WPW syndrome). In either case, the reentrant circuit depends on a balance between conduction and refractoriness. The Ca^{2+} channel blockers disrupt this balance and terminate the arrhythmia by slowing conduction and prolonging ERP in the AV node.

The Ca^{2+} channel blockers may be used to induce AV block and reduce the ventricular rate in the treatment of atrial fibrillation and flutter, but the drugs usually do not terminate the arrhythmia.

Antiarrhythmic Properties of Adenosine Triphosphate and Adenosine

It has been known for more than 50 years that ATP and adenosine exert pronounced electrophysiologic effects on the mammalian heart. Administration of adenosine compounds results in a slowing of discharge from the SA node and delayed conduction through the AV node. Both ATP and adenosine administered to humans as well as animal models exert transient negative chronotropic and dromotropic effects. ATP, when given as acute therapy, will reverse PSVT.

A 15- to 30-mg dose of ATP given as an IV bolus produces sinus bradycardia and a first- or second-degree AV block, and the effect is mimicked by adenosine. Dose-dependent negative chronotropic and dromotropic effects occur within seconds after an IV dose of adenosine.

MECHANISM OF ACTION

The action of ATP [6] appears to be in part due to its degradation to adenosine. In experimental preparations, adenosine depresses the automaticity of the SA node and Purkinje fibers, hyperpolarizes the membrane, shortens the plateau phase of the AP of atrial myocytes, and depresses AV nodal conduction. Adenosine depresses the Ca^{2+}-mediated slow-channel conduction, increases K^+ conductance, and may have antiadrenergic effects by a mechanism involving specific membrane P_1-purinoreceptors, which are different from muscarinic cholinergic receptors.

CLINICAL EFFICACY

Clinical studies show that ATP (20 mg) administered by a rapid IV infusion (central vein) will terminate tachycardias within half a minute. The ATP may cause a transient cardiac standstill followed by atrial and ventricular extrasystoles.

Two types of tachycardias are amenable to ATP (10–20 mg):

Supraventricular (3–25 mg in paroxysmal atrial tachycardia in pediatric-age patients)
AV junctional

ATP has no effect on ventricular tachycardias.

EFFECTS ON CLINICAL ELECTROPHYSIOLOGY DURING PAROXYSMAL ATRIAL TACHYCARDIA

Termination of AV reentrant tachycardia by ATP (20 mg IV) results from a block in the slow antegrade AV nodal pathway without affecting the retrograde conduction through the fast AV nodal pathway or the accessory pathway. The effect is not altered by atropine but is suppressed by aminophylline. Inosine and dipyridamole potentiate the ATP effect.

AV reentrant tachycardia can be terminated within seconds with adenosine. (Adults: inject 6 mg IV over 2 seconds. If the arrhythmia is not terminated, two minutes later inject 12 mg IV over 2 seconds. Infants and children: inject 0.05–0.25 mg/kg IV. Arrhythmia is terminated within 20 seconds.)

SIDE EFFECTS

There is a high incidence of cardiac and noncardiac side effects that occur within a few seconds and last less than 1 minute. Cardiac effects, including sinus bradycardia, sinus arrest, and various degrees of AV block and sinus tachycardia, are transient and require no intervention. Noncardiac effects include malaise, hyperpnea, flushing, headache, and, less commonly, cough and retching. Side effects may be less frequent with adenosine than with ATP.

Properties of Individual Class Ia Antiarrhythmic Drugs

Quinidine

Quinidine, historically the first antiarrhythmic agent, is the dextrostereoisomer of quinine derived from the bark of the *Cinchona* tree. Both quinine and quinidine were used for the treatment of malaria, and the antiarrhythmic action of quinidine was first noted several decades ago during the treatment of patients with malaria who also had arrhythmias.

PHARMACOLOGY

Antiarrhythmic Action

The antiarrhythmic actions of quinidine depend on its direct electrophysiologic effects on cardiac membranes. It slows the rate of diastolic depolarization, decreases the rate of rise of the 0 phase, increases the AP duration, and extends refractoriness into the diastolic period. The effect on refractoriness in the diastolic period is responsible for the quinidine-induced increase in the ratio of ERP/APd. Identified in individual cells, these events translate to the following changes throughout the heart: reduced conduction velocity, increased ERP, and reduced automaticity (spontaneous ectopic impulse generation).

Effects on the Electrocardiogram

Quinidine increases the QT interval by effects on its two components, the QRS complex and the ST interval. In the following discussion, these changes are related to the underlying effects of quinidine on the cardiac AP.

The QRS complex of the ECG represents ventricular depolarization. Quinidine slows the rate of depolarization (reduced rate of rise of the 0 phase) and results in a widening of the QRS complex. Widening occurs at therapeutic concentrations, is dose-related, and is a useful diagnostic tool for monitoring drug effect. A 25% widening may be seen at therapeutic blood levels, while a 50% widening may indicate toxicity and a need to reduce the dosage.

The ST interval represents the period between the end of the QRS complex and the T wave (full repolarization of the ventricles) and corresponds to phases 1, 2, and 3 of the AP. The ST interval is prolonged by quinidine. Since quinidine directly decreases conduction velocity in the AV node, His bundle, and Purkinje fibers at therapeutic doses, prolongation of the PR interval will also be seen.

Autonomic Effects

Quinidine exerts an antivagal (atropinelike) action on the heart, which is inconsequential in most patients. However, under conditions of elevated vagal stimulation, quinidine reduces vagal activity in the SA and AV nodes to increase the sinus rate and improve AV conduction. Such increases in heart rate are a special risk for quinidine therapy in patients with atrial flutter or fibrillation. A certain level of AV block exists in these patients, allowing the ventricles to follow the atria at a slower rate. In past decades, quinidine was administered by itself to convert the arrhythmia to normal sinus rhythm. However, some patients experienced a sudden, marked increase in the ventricular rate before conversion to sinus rhythm occurred. The atropinelike action of quinidine increases AV conduction, allowing the ventricles to receive a much higher frequency of impulses from the atria. Current practice dictates the establishment of a stable level of AV block by digitalis before quinidine is administered to such patients.

It should be noted that at higher therapeutic and toxic concentrations the direct effects of quinidine predominate and conduction through the AV node is reduced. Indeed, AV block is a manifestation of quinidine toxicity.

Quinidine is a weak α-adrenergic receptor antagonist. This action can lead to vasodilation and hypotension by reducing the α-mediated vasoconstrictor response to sympathetic tone while leaving the β-mediated vasodilator response unopposed. However, quinidine-induced vasodilation is only seen after large doses of intravenous administration of the drug.

THERAPEUTIC USE

Quinidine is used to treat supraventricular tachyarrhythmias including extrasystoles, paroxysmal atrial and AV nodal reentry tachycardia, flutter, and fibrillation. Quinidine may be used for conversion as well as prevention of recurrent tachyarrhythmias. However, conversion of hemodynamically important AV nodal or AV reentry tachycardia, flutter, and fibrillation is more effectively and safely achieved with electrical cardioversion.

Quinidine is also useful for treatment of ventricular premature complexes and tachycardia. However, the drug is not useful in the acute treatment of serious ventricular arrhythmias. Quinidine in combination with class Ib agents has synergistic therapeutic effects in the treatment of simple and complex ventricular arrhythmias. Such a synergism allows for a reduction in the dosage of either or both agents, thereby reducing the potential for toxic side effects.

PHARMACOKINETICS

Absorption and Distribution

The time to peak plasma concentration after oral administration is 1–1½ hours with quinidine sulfate and 3–4 hours with quinidine gluconate. Bioavailability is 80 and 70%, respectively, for the sulfate and gluconate salts. Quinidine is 70–95% plasma protein bound and has a volume of distribution of 2.0–3.5 liters/kg. The half-life of quinidine is 6 hours and may be prolonged in the elderly and in those with cirrhosis.

Elimination

Quinidine consists of quinoline and quinuclidine rings, and is extensively metabolized. It is first oxidized in the liver to form 3-hydroxyquinidine, 2'-oxoquinidine, and O-desmethylquinidine. These products are subsequently conjugated and eliminated via the kidneys as glucuronides.

3-Hydroxyquinidine and 2'-oxoquinidine are cardioactive and have been reported to be equipotent with quinidine. However, their contribution to the antiarrhythmic action of quinidine may be slight since they show little accumulation in most patients.

ADVERSE EFFECTS

Cinchonism

Quinidine (and quinine) can cause a series of central nervous system and gastrointestinal symptoms characteristic of the syndrome called **cinchonism.** In mild form, these include tinnitus, loss of hearing, blurred vision, and gastrointestinal upset. More severe forms of cinchonism include headache, diplopia, photophobia, altered color perception, confusion, delirium, psychosis, nausea, vomiting, and diarrhea. The development of hot and flushed skin with pruritus may also accompany these more serious symptoms.

Cardiovascular Symptoms

Without preexisting impairment of cardiac function, the incidence of quinidine-induced cardiovascular toxicity is relatively low, and the symptoms listed below are observed mainly at toxic drug concentrations. However, toxicity — impairment of SA and AV nodal function or contractility or both — can occur at therapeutic blood levels. Quinidine can slow heart rate or cause sinus arrest, induce either partial or total AV block, and cause myocardial depression.

Quinidine syncope, which may occur at subtherapeutic or therapeutic drug levels, is due to transient ventricular tachycardia or polymorphic ventricular tachycardia (torsades de pointes). In a small fraction of patients this arrhythmia is irreversible and results in sudden cardiac death. The phenomenon results from the prolongation of the QT interval, which is an inherent action of the drug. This, in turn, can lead to ventricular stimulation occurring in the vulnerable period, the so-called R-on-T phenomenon. Many of the ventricular cells still recovering are in phase 3 of the AP at the time the next SA nodal impulse is conducted to the ventricles. Thus, some cells are fully recovered, others are relatively refractory, and still others are absolutely refractory to the impulse. This produces a dispersion of activation throughout the ventricles, generating multiple ectopic foci and ventricular fibrillation. Patients who are most susceptible to quinidine syncope are those who have a prolonged QT interval or who show a marked prolongation of the QT interval on receiving quinidine. Such patients should not be treated with this drug.

Hypersensitivity Reactions

Some patients develop an immediate (i.e., within a few days) idiosyncratic reaction characterized by cutaneous flushing, pruritus, skin rashes, fever, respiratory distress, anaphylactic reactions, vascular collapse, thrombocytopenia, or hemolytic anemia. In general, these reactions are rare. However, some of them, such as thrombocytopenia and acute hepatitis, may be life-threatening. Isolated fever with minimal organ system involvement has been reported to occur months after quinidine administration, and it is important to include this in the differential diagnosis of fever of unknown origin.

The hypersensitivity reaction may take the form of systemic lupus erythematosus (SLE). Quinidine-induced SLE may cause dermatitis, lymphadenopathy, hepatosplenomegaly, polyarthritis, hemolytic anemia, leukopenia, thrombocytopenia, and positive antinuclear antibody (ANA) and direct Coombs' test results. Even a quinidine-induced nephropathy is reported. Some develop coagulation abnormalities — thrombocytopenia, prolonged prothrombin time, and a factor IX (Christmas factor) deficiency. The mechanism underlying the quinidine-induced SLE is uncertain, but the ANA is of the IgM and IgG classes and directed mainly to nuclear histones. Resolution of the quinidine-SLE is slow (months) and may require prednisone therapy.

PATIENT MONITORING

Careful monitoring of the patient can greatly reduce the likelihood of adverse reactions. ECG recordings should be taken before and periodically during quinidine therapy. Blood platelet count after a test dose is a valuable means of identifying a rapid or idiosyncratic reaction. Renal and hepatic function tests provide an initial basis for predicting changes in quinidine plasma half-life and concentration. These tests, plus confirmation with a serum quinidine determination, provide a basis for appropriate dosage adjustment. Levels should be maintained in the therapeutic range (2–6 µg/ml). Periodic blood cell and platelet counts should also be performed to detect thrombocytopenia or hemolytic reactions. When an SLE-like reaction is considered, a blood ANA determination should be made.

PREPARATIONS AND DOSAGES

The patient should receive a single oral dose (200 mg) initially as a test for idiosyncratic reactions. Oral doses should be taken with a full glass of water 1 hour before or two hours after meals for better absorption. However, quinidine may be taken with food to reduce gastric irritation.

Quinidine Polygalacturonate

Tablets: 275 mg.
Oral: *Adults* — initial doses of 275–825 mg every 3–4 hours for three or four doses with subsequent doses being increased by 137.5–275.0 mg every third or fourth dose until rhythm is restored or toxic effects occur. Maintenance dose — 275 mg 2 or

3 times daily. *Pediatric* — 8.25 mg/kg body weight or 247.5 mg/m² of body surface 5 times a day.

Quinidine Gluconate

Extended-release tablets: 324 and 330 mg.
Injection: 80 mg/ml.
Oral: *Adults* — maintenance doses of 324–660 mg every 6–12 hours.
IM: *Adults* — 600 mg initially followed by 400 mg every 4–6 hours or every 2 hours in emergencies. Absorption of intramuscularly administered quinidine is erratic and incomplete.
IV: *Adults* — 200–800 mg in a dilute solution given at a slow rate (10–20 mg/min). IV route is rarely indicated. ECG and blood pressure must be continuously monitored. *Adult infusion* — 800 mg in 40 ml of 5% dextrose injection administered at a rate of 1 ml/min.

Quinidine Sulfate

Tablets: 100, 200, and 300 mg.
Capsules: 200 and 300 mg.
Extended-release tablets: 300 mg.
Injection: 200 mg/ml.
Oral: *Adults* — initial doses for premature atrial and ventricular contractions, 200–300 mg 3–4 times daily. Maintenance doses of 200–400 mg every 6 hours, tablets or capsules, or 600 mg every 8–12 hours, extended-release tablets. *Pediatric* — 6 mg/kg body weight or 180 mg/m² of body surface 5 times a day.
IV: *Adult infusion* — 600 mg in 40 ml of 5% dextrose injection administered at a rate of 1 ml/min with continuous monitoring of ECG and blood pressure.

Procainamide Hydrochloride

The antiarrhythmic actions of procaine were recognized many decades ago. However, this compound has a very short duration of action and is not effective by the oral route. Thus, numerous congeners of procaine were investigated, leading to the introduction of procainamide into clinical practice in 1950.

PHARMACOLOGY

Antiarrhythmic Action

The electrophysiologic effects of procainamide closely resemble those of quinidine. Procainamide slows the rate of diastolic depolarization, decreases the rate of rise of the 0 phase, increases the AP duration, extends refractoriness into the diastolic period, and increases the ERP/APd ratio. Thus, conduction velocity and automaticity are reduced, and ERP is increased throughout the heart.

Effects on the Electrocardiogram

Procainamide increases the QT interval by increasing the duration of its two components, the QRS complex and the ST interval.

The widening of the base of the QRS occurs in the therapeutic range and is a useful indicator of drug effect. PR prolongation also occurs because of prolongation of AV, His bundle, and Purkinje conductions in a fashion similar to that seen with quinidine.

Autonomic Effects

Procainamide exerts a much weaker atropinelike action than that of quinidine. Nevertheless, the same precautions are required for both drugs in the treatment of rapid atrial tachycardias, flutter, and fibrillation; that is, a stable AV block must be established using, for example, digitalis or Ca^{2+} channel blockers such as verapamil before initiating procainamide therapy. Procainamide has no other autonomic effects.

THERAPEUTIC USE

The therapeutic use of procainamide resembles that of quinidine in the treatment of atrial arrhythmias. Procainamide is effective against extrasystoles, paroxysmal atrial and AV nodal reentry tachycardia, flutter, and fibrillation. The drug may be used for conversion as well as prevention of lower-frequency tachyarrhythmias. However, conversion of higher-frequency tachycardia, flutter, and fibrillation is more effectively and safely achieved with electrical cardioversion.

Procainamide is effective against chronic ventricular arrhythmias ranging from extrasystoles to tachycardia and is an important alternative to lidocaine in the treatment and prevention of acute, hemodynamically important ventricular tachycardia. The treatment of ventricular flutter and fibrillation may require cardioversion, the use of lidocaine or bretylium tosylate, or both (see below). Procainamide is not usually the first choice of therapy for these arrhythmias but may be effective in preventing reversion once they have been controlled.

Procainamide is chosen over quinidine when parenteral injection or infusion of a class Ia agent is required. On the other hand, quinidine is often selected over procainamide for a long-term oral therapy in order to avoid procainamide-induced SLE. Procainamide-induced SLE is more commonly seen than quinidine-induced SLE.

PHARMACOKINETICS

Absorption and Distribution

Procainamide is rapidly absorbed with an oral availability of 75–95%. The time to peak effect is 60–90 minutes after oral administration and 15–60 minutes after IM injection. Drug effect is immediate after IV injection. Procainamide is only slightly bound to plasma proteins and has a volume of distribution of 2 liters/kg.

Elimination

Approximately 50–60% of procainamide is excreted unchanged, while the remainder undergoes acetylation in the liver to form the main metabolite, N-acetylprocainamide (NAPA). NAPA is cardioactive, with one-third the potency of procainamide. Whether or not NAPA accumulates sufficiently to contribute to the antiarrhythmic action depends on two factors: the acetylation status and kidney function of the patient. Rapid acetylators convert more procainamide to NAPA than do slow acetylators. However, if renal function is normal, it is likely that NAPA accumulation is low even in fast acetylators. On the other hand, NAPA accumulates extensively if renal function is impaired and may contribute to both antiarrhythmic and toxic effects of procainamide. The half-life of procainamide is 3 hours in patients with normal renal function and 11–20 hours with renal impairment. The half-life of NAPA, 6 hours, increases to 21 hours with renal impairment.

ADVERSE EFFECTS

Myocardial Reactions

The toxic effects of procainamide on the heart resemble those of quinidine. Procainamide can cause partial or total AV block, myocardial depression, hypotension, and ventricular tachyarrhythmias including polymorphic ventricular tachycardia (torsades de pointes); however, prolongation of the QT interval and the potential for R-on-T-induced ventricular arrhythmias is less frequently seen than with quinidine. Perhaps this is due to the fact that quinidine is one of the most widely used antiarrhythmics.

SLE-like Syndrome

From 50–80% of patients receiving procainamide will have elevated serum ANA levels, and 10–15% will develop SLE-like symptoms. Most antibodies in procainamide-induced SLE are formed to denatured single-stranded deoxyribonucleic acid (DNA). These patients develop a fine specificity of IgG antibodies to the nucleoside guanosine (G). Patients with procainamide-induced SLE will have high levels of anti-G antibodies in the serum, and there is evidence of a sympathomimetic action of the antibodies on the myocardium. Serum anti-G antibody levels correlate positively with the presence of arthritis, pleuritis, and pericarditis.

Agranulocytosis and Pancytopenia

Agranulocytosis and pancytopenia occur rarely but can be fatal. Fever or sore mouth, gums, or throat, usually innocuous, require immediate attention in the patient receiving procainamide.

Other Adverse Effects

Oral administration of procainamide can cause anorexia, nausea, and vomiting. Central nervous system effects including depression, hallucinations, and psychoses are rare.

PATIENT MONITORING

Continuous ECG and blood pressure monitoring is required during parenteral procainamide therapy and should also be performed before and occasionally during long-term oral therapy. ANA testing should also be performed intermittently during oral therapy and procainamide withdrawn if ANA titer steadily increases or if lupuslike symptoms appear. Complete blood cell counts should be performed every 2–3 weeks during the first 3 months of procainamide therapy and intermittently during the remainder of therapy. A reduction of leukocytes requires withdrawal of procainamide. Renal and hepatic function tests must be performed periodically since decreased function will increase both half-life and concentration of the drug in the plasma.

PREPARATIONS AND DOSAGES

Capsules: 250, 375, and 500 mg.
Tablets: 250, 375, and 500 mg.
Extended-release tablets: 250, 500, and 750 mg.
Injection: 100 and 500 mg/ml.
Oral: *Adults* — initially, 1.25 gm, followed in 1 hour by 750 mg as needed; then 500–1000 mg every 2–3 hours as needed and tolerated (capsules or tablets). Maintenance doses of 250–1000 mg every 3–6 hours around the clock (capsules or tablets). Extended-release tablets — maintenance doses of 500–1000 mg every 6 hours. (Doses up to 2 gm every 6 hours have been used, with monitoring of serum levels.) Prophylaxis of ventricular arrhythmias: 50 mg/kg body weight per day in 8 divided doses; every 3 hours around the clock (capsules and tablets).
Pediatric — 12.5 mg/kg of body weight or 375 mg/m^2 of body surface 4 times daily.
IM: *Adults* — 500–1000 mg every 4–8 hours.
IV: *Adults* — initially, inject 100 mg (diluted in 5% dextrose injection) at a rate no greater than 50 mg/min, repeating every 5 minutes until arrhythmia is controlled (maximum, 1 gm). Alternatively, infuse 500–600 mg at a constant rate over 25–30 minutes. Maintenance — infuse at a rate of 2–6 mg/min with monitoring of serum levels. Recommended therapeutic levels: 4.0–10.0 μg/ml; toxic levels, more than 12.0 μg/ml.

p-Amino-*N*-(2-diethylamino ethyl) Benzamide

The *N*-acetyl metabolite of procainamide, *p*-amino-*N*-(2-diethylamino ethyl) benzamide (NAPA) is an investigational antiarrhythmic agent currently undergoing clinical trials in the United States. NAPA has been shown to have antiarrhythmic efficacy by suppressing chloroform-induced ventricular fibrillation in mice and reversing aconitine-induced atrial fibrillation in dogs. It has been shown to be effective in clinical trials and in the electrophysiology laboratory in preventing ventricular tachycardia. NAPA and procainamide have been shown to be distinctively different from a pharmacodynamic point of view. Electrophysiologically, NAPA does not suppress the rate of phase 4 depolarization of Purkinje fibers, does not change resting membrane potential, and does not change AP amplitude or maximum upstroke velocity (all of which are effects of procainamide).

NAPA exerts a marked effect on AP duration and repolarization. NAPA, like its parent compound procainamide, may depress automaticity and prolong repolarization time at every high dosages. NAPA increases atrial effective refractory and atrial functional refractory periods in a dose-dependent fashion. It has no effect on AV nodal conduction. It causes prolongation of both ventricular function and ERP. During clinical studies, NAPA has not been found to alter sinus node recovery time or atrial-His (AH) or His-ventricle (HV) intervals significantly. Based on this information, the antiarrhythmic action of NAPA is felt to be due to a prolongation of repolarization, possibly in a uniform manner, which places this agent in the class III category. The hemodynamic effects of NAPA are complex and are felt to be secondary, in part, to its effect on sympathetic tone. Unlike procainamide, NAPA has been shown to raise myocardial contractility slightly.

PHARMACOKINETICS

Absorption and Distribution

Studies have shown that NAPA has a high degree of bioavailability. It is well absorbed orally and reaches peak levels in 1½ hours in normal subjects and approximately 2½–3½ hours in patients with congestive cardiomyopathies.

Elimination

Eighty percent of NAPA is eliminated in the urine unchanged, 2% is deacytylated to procainamide, 0.2% is metabolized to p-acetamido-N-benzamide, and for the approximately remaining 18%, the metabolism is unknown. The renal clearance of NAPA in some studies has been reported to exceed the patient's creatinine clearance, which suggests secretion by the renal tube. The mean half-life of NAPA is 6.1 hours for an IV dose and 8–10 hours following an oral dose after chronic administration. NAPA is eliminated by hemodialysis, and its half-life in anephric patients not undergoing dialysis has been reported to be approximately 42 hours. It is recommended that in patients with impaired renal function, plasma drug levels should be carefully monitored to avoid toxic side effects.

THERAPEUTIC USE

NAPA has been shown to have modest antiarrhythmic properties, producing reduction in both premature ventricular depolarizations and control of ventricular tachycardia. This drug is not superior to any other available antiarrhythmic, but an addition to the inventory of drugs for patients with ventricular arrhythmias, especially those with abnormal left ventricular (LV) function. Although the antiarrhythmic properties of NAPA and procainamide are different, NAPA has been found to be useful in patients whose arrhythmias have been controlled by procainamide who developed side effects such as systemic lupus erythematosus (SLE) from the latter.

ADVERSE EFFECTS

The major systemic adverse effects of NAPA are severe nausea and vomiting, blurred vision, headaches, constipation, fatigue, possible sexual dysfunction, and insomnia. Isolated cases of moderately positive results of Coombs' test for hemolytic anemia have also been reported. Bone marrow suppression and renal or hepatic dysfunction have not been reported with the use of NAPA.

SLE-like Syndrome

The major proposed advantage of *N*-acetyl procainamide over procainamide is that NAPA does not induce the lupuslike syndrome that is frequently seen with procainamide. A possible mechanism for the development of the lupuslike syndrome is that procainamide forms an active metabolite that combines with nuclear macromolecules to yield a hapten, which stimulates the production of antibody to single-stranded DNA. There have been isolated reports of patients who have developed positive ANA results and arthralgia with development of de novo NAPA-induced lupus syndrome. This can probably be explained by the reverse conversion of NAPA to small amounts of procainamide.

Electrocardiographic Changes

NAPA does not change the duration of the PR or QRS interval; however, there is prolongation of the QT interval, because of NAPA's effects on repolarization and AP duration.

DOSAGE AND ADMINISTRATION

NAPA can be administered both intravenously and orally. Caution should be used during rapid IV infusion, since hypotension similar to that experienced with procainamide can occur.

IV: 18 mg/kg over a 30-minute period by constant infusion.

Tablets: 500 mg. Recommended dose is 1000–1500 mg orally every 8 hours, not to exceed a dose of 3000 mg every 8 hours. Recommended therapeutic levels: 15–30 µg/liter although in some clinical studies levels up to 40 µg/liter have been recommended to be therapeutic. Toxicity has been reported at levels greater than 40 µg/liter.

Disopyramide Phosphate

PHARMACOLOGY

Antiarrhythmic Action

The electrophysiologic effects of disopyramide closely resemble those of quinidine. Disopyramide slows the rate of diastolic depolarization, decreases the rate of rise of the 0 phase, increases the AP duration, extends refractoriness into the diastolic period, and increases the ERP/APd ratio. Thus, conduction velocity and automaticity are reduced, and ERP is increased throughout the heart.

Effects on the Electrocardiogram

Disopyramide increases the QT interval by increasing the duration of its two components, the QRS complex and the ST interval. The widening of the base of the QRS is not as marked as that seen with quinidine but does occur in the therapeutic concentration range. PR prolongation may also occur at higher doses.

Autonomic Effects

Disopyramide exerts a marked anticholinergic (atropinelike) action. In patients exhibiting vagal tone, this action reduces sinus rate, improving conduction through the AV node. As with quinidine, initiation of disopyramide in treatment of rapid atrial tachyarrhythmias requires AV blockade with digitalis. The atropinelike action also can cause a number of adverse extracardiac effects, which may be due to an accumulation of a disopyramide metabolite.

THERAPEUTIC USE

Disopyramide is effective against supraventricular arrhythmias and is an alternative to quinidine and procainamide for this purpose. However, it is used primarily for the suppression and prevention of ventricular arrhythmias, including extrasystoles, coupled beats, and paroxysmal tachycardia.

PHARMACOKINETICS

Absorption and Distribution

Disopyramide is rapidly absorbed, with an oral availability of 80–90%. The time to peak effect is 30 minutes to 3 hours. Disopyramide is 50% plasma protein bound; however, it may range between 35 and 95% plasma protein bound, varying inversely with serum concentration. The volume of distribution is 0.8 liters/kg. The drug saturates plasma binding in some patients with the usual dose ranges. Consequently, small supplemental doses (100 or 150 mg) cause a major rise in the unbound and active form of the drug.

Elimination

Fifty percent of disopyramide is excreted unchanged in the urine. The remainder is metabolized, primarily to mono-*N*-dealkyldisopyramide. This metabolite has approximately 25% of the antiarrhythmic potency of the parent compound, but is 24 times more potent as an anticholinergic. The major effect of the metabolite is to limit the usefulness of disopyramide by causing atropinelike side effects. The plasma half-life of disopyramide is 8 hours but may increase to 18 hours with impaired renal function.

ADVERSE EFFECTS

Cardiovascular Symptoms

Disopyramide has a more marked adverse effect on hemodynamics than either quinidine or procainamide because of marked myocardial depression plus arteriolar vasoconstriction. Disopyramide may cause congestive heart failure, particularly with previously impaired myocardial function or in the presence of beta blockers (e.g., propranolol). In patients with congestive heart failure or left ventricular ejection fractions of less than 30%, disopyramide must be used with caution or avoided entirely to avoid cardiac decompensation and hypotension. AV block and ventricular arrhythmias including polymorphic tachycardia (torsades de pointes) are additional side effects.

Atropinelike Symptoms

Dry mouth and urinary hesitancy or retention are common anticholinergic symptoms associated with disopyramide therapy. The latter side effect is usually more common in men, especially if prostatic hypertrophy is present. Other less common symptoms include nausea, vomiting, constipation, abdominal pain, diarrhea, urinary retention, blurred vision, and, rarely, acute angle-closure glaucoma.

PATIENT MONITORING

ECG monitoring should be performed intermittently throughout disopyramide therapy, with particular attention focused on widening of the QRS complex and prolongation of the QT interval. Increases of more than 25% in either variable may require dose reduction or discontinuation of therapy. Blood pressure should be monitored to detect possible hypotension. Other features to be monitored include blood glucose level to detect hypoglycemia and renal and hepatic function.

PREPARATIONS AND DOSAGES

Capsules: 100 and 150 mg.
Extended-release capsules: 100 and 150 mg.
Oral: *Adults* — initially, 300 mg (for body weight ≥50 kg; 200 mg for body weight <50 kg). Maintenance dose (capsule) — 100–150 mg every 6 hours. The lower dose should be used in patients with body weight less than 50 kg or with suspected cardiomyopathy or history of cardiac compensation. Maintenance dose (extended-release capsules) — 300 mg every 12 hours for body weight less than 50 kg.

The maintenance dose (capsules) interval should be increased in patients with renal insufficiency in accordance with creatinine clearance rates, as follows:

Creatinine clearance (ml/min)	Approximate maintenance dosing intervals
30–40	Every 8 hr
15–30	Every 12 hr
<15	Every 24 hr

Recommended therapeutic levels are 2–5 µg/ml, with toxic levels not yet established.

Pediatric

Children should be hospitalized and monitored until the maintenance dose is established. The following doses should be divided and given every 6 hours:

Age	Daily dose (mg/kg body weight)
Up to 1 year	10–30
1–4 years	10–20
4–12 years	10–15
12–18 years	6–15

Properties of Individual Class Ib Antiarrhythmic Drugs

Lidocaine Hydrochloride

Lidocaine is a particularly useful drug in the coronary care unit because of its rapid onset and offset of action which, allow continuous control of drug effect. It is effective against many forms of ventricular arrhythmia and has few adverse effects in therapeutic concentrations.

PHARMACOLOGY

Antiarrhythmic Action

Lidocaine decreases the rate of diastolic depolarization. It has little or no effect on the rate of rise of the 0 phase, except in damaged cardiac tissue exhibiting impaired sodium channel function. Lidocaine decreases the maximum AP duration and extends refractoriness into the diastolic period more in depressed, partially depolarized cardiac fibers than in normal cardiac fibers. Lidocaine prolongs the time required to attain maximum AP (and conduction) to recover steady-state value after a preceding response. Therefore, lidocaine causes the maximum AP (and conduction) of an early premature response to be slower than anticipated from the membrane potential level. Lidocaine influences the rapid (Na^+) inward current while not affecting the slow (Ca^{2+}) inward current responsible for the APs whose resting potential is in the -40 mV range. Such APs characterize the sinus and AV nodal fibers and ischemic or depolarized fibers. Lidocaine shortens AP duration. Thus, while ERP does not change at therapeutic concentrations, the ERP/APd ratio increases. These cellular electrophysiologic effects result in decreased automaticity (ectopic activity) and slowed conduction or conduction failure in damaged tissue. This latter action is responsible for the termination of reentrant arrhythmias.

In therapeutic concentrations, lidocaine, while having a limited effect on conduction, does not depress contractility in normal cardiac tissue. In addition, it has little or no effect on the ECG and lacks both atropinelike and α-adrenergic blocking actions.

THERAPEUTIC USE

Lidocaine is a drug of choice for the suppression and short-term prophylaxis of ventricular arrhythmias from a variety of causes including acute myocardial infarction, digitalis toxicity, cardiac surgery, or cardiac catheterization. It has little or no therapeutic benefit in atrial arrhythmias.

PHARMACOKINETICS

Absorption and Distribution

Lidocaine undergoes extensive first-pass metabolism after oral administration and is not used by this route. It is rapidly and completely absorbed after IM injection and has an onset of action of 5–15 minutes. Lidocaine is 70% plasma protein bound and has a volume of distribution of 1 liter/kg.

Elimination

Only 10% of lidocaine is excreted unchanged in the urine; the remainder is metabolized. The half-life is approximately 100 minutes and tends to increase with continuous infusion for more than 24 hours. The rapid distribution of an initial loading dose causes a much shorter apparent half-life after a single injection than after several doses or continuous infusion.

The two major metabolites of lidocaine are formed by the removal of one or both ethyl groups to produce monoethylglycinexylidide (MEGX) and glycinexylidide (GX), respectively. Both compounds are cardioactive. However, MEGX is 85% as potent as lidocaine and has approximately the same half-life, while GX is one-tenth as potent and has a half-life of 9–10 hours. GX probably contributes little to the overall antiarrhythmic action of lidocaine because of its low potency. On the other hand, MEGX accumulates in the plasma to the same extent as or more than lidocaine and may exert a considerable cardiac effect.

ADVERSE EFFECTS

Cardiovascular

Adverse effects are rare at therapeutic concentrations of lidocaine. However, large doses may depress cardiac contractility or cause conduction block, especially in the case of preexisting cardiac dysfunction.

Central Nervous System

Toxicity caused by overdose can cause a series of concentration-related symptoms including drowsiness, blurred vision, ringing in the ears, dizziness, convulsions, respiratory depression, and coma.

PATIENT MONITORING

ECG and blood pressure should be monitored throughout therapy. Serum lidocaine measurements should be performed during long-term infusion.

PREPARATIONS AND DOSAGES

Direct IV: 10 and 20 mg/ml.
Continuous IV: 40, 100, and 200 mg/ml. Infusion solution preparation: Add 1 gm of lidocaine hydrochloride to 1 liter of 5% dextrose solution (final concentration: 1 mg/ml).
IM injection: 100 mg/ml.
In 5% dextrose for continuous IV infusion: 2, 4, and 8 mg/ml.

The following dosages should be reduced in patients with congestive heart failure, cardiogenic shock, or hepatic disease and in elderly patients:

IM: *Adults* — 300 mg (4.3 mg/kg body weight) injected into the deltoid muscle every 60–90 minutes as needed.
IV: *Adults* — initially, 50–100 mg/kg injected over a period of 2–3 minutes. Dose may be repeated after 5 minutes, followed by IV infusion (see below). Give no more than 300 mg in any 1-hour period.
IV: *Pediatric* — initially, 1 mg/kg body weight injected at a rate of 25–50 mg/min. Repeat this dose after 5 minutes, giving no more than 3 mg/kg body weight total. Follow with IV infusion (see below).
IV: *Adult infusion* — 20–50 µg (0.02–0.05 mg) per kilogram body weight at a rate of 1–4 mg/min. Do not exceed 300 mg (4.5 mg/kg body weight) in any 1-hour period.
IV: *Pediatric infusion* — 20–50 µg (0.02–0.05 mg) per kilogram body weight at a rate of 1–4 mg/min.

Recommended therapeutic levels: 1.2–6.0 µg/ml; toxic levels, 9.0 µg/ml.

Phenytoin Sodium (Dilantin, Diphenylan)

Phenytoin is a drug of first choice in the treatment of digitalis-induced atrial and ventricular arrhythmias. Thus, the duration of its use is, at most, a few days. Phenytoin is generally not used for the treatment of arrhythmias from other causes. It has proven to be useful for ventricular tachycardia in children when other class I agents are ineffective or not tolerated.

PHARMACOLOGY

Antiarrhythmic Action

The electrophysiologic effects of phenytoin closely resemble those of lidocaine. Phenytoin decreases the diastolic depolarization rate but has little or no effect on the rate of rise of the 0 phase except in damaged cardiac tissue exhibiting impaired Na^+ channel function. Phenytoin decreases the AP duration because of abbreviation of all phases of repolarization and extends refractoriness into the diastolic period. Thus, while ERP does not change at therapeutic concentrations, the ERP/APd ratio increases. These cellular electrophysiologic effects result in decreased automaticity (ectopic activity) and slowed conduction or conduction failure in damaged tissue. The latter action is responsible for termination of reentrant arrhythmias. Phenytoin tends to hyperpolarize the cardiac cell (make the maximum resting potential more negative), which also contributes to antiarrhythmic action by making the cells less responsive to stimuli. Finally, phenytoin may actually increase conduction velocity in the AV node. In therapeutic concentrations it has little or no effect on conduction and does not depress contractility in normal cardiac tissue. In addition, it has little or no effect on the ECG and lacks both atropinelike and α-adrenergic blocking actions.

THERAPEUTIC USE

The therapeutic use of phenytoin is limited to the treatment of atrial and ventricular arrhythmias induced by digitalis excess. The drug is particularly effective against supraventricular tachycardia (SVT) with AV block and complex ventricular premature depolarizations and ventricular tachycardia.

PHARMACOKINETICS

Absorption and Distribution

Absorption of phenytoin by the oral route is slow and variable. Time to peak effect is 1½–3 hours (prompt capsule; see below) or 4–12 hours (extended capsules). Absorption by the IM route is erratic and unreliable, and this route of administration is not used. Phenytoin is 90% plasma protein bound and has a volume of distribution of 0.6 liter/kg.

Elimination

Phenytoin is eliminated primarily by hepatic metabolism. It is first hydroxylated to the parahydroxyphenyl derivative and subsequently conjugated to form the glucuronide. The metabolite is not cardioactive. The half-life of phenytoin ranges between 6 and 24 hours and is dose dependent at higher therapeutic concentrations. This means phenytoin may unexpectedly accumulate to toxic concentrations.

ADVERSE EFFECTS

The adverse effects related to phenytoin therapy for digitalis-induced arrhythmias are those that would occur over the course of a few days. They are referable to the central nervous system, are dose related, and may reflect phenytoin overdose. The early symptoms include drowsiness, nystagmus, vertigo, ataxia, and nausea. More serious symptoms include blurred or double vision, confusion, hallucinations, and convulsions.

PATIENT MONITORING

ECG and blood pressure should be monitored before and throughout phenytoin therapy. Measurement of phenytoin serum concentrations may be required to predict possible overdose.

PREPARATIONS AND DOSAGES

The preparations listed here are the ones most commonly used in the treatment of arrhythmias. Other available preparations are used in longer-term anticonvulsant therapy.

IV administration of phenytoin should be by intermittent injection. Continuous infusion is usually not recommended, because the high pH (12) of the injection solution may cause phlebitis at the infusion site.

Prompt capsules: 30 and 100 mg.
Extended capsules: 30 and 100 mg.
Injection: 50 mg/ml.
Oral: *Adults* — on the first day, 15 mg/kg body weight given in two or three divided doses over a period of approximately 6 hours. On the second day, 7.5 mg/kg body weight given in two or three divided doses. Maintenance dosage — 4–6 mg/kg body weight given in two divided doses (prompt capsules) or as one dose (extended capsules).
IV: *Adults* — 100 mg injected over a 2-minute period and repeated every 5 minutes until arrhythmia is controlled or adverse effects occur.

Mexiletine Hydrochloride

Mexiletine is an active congener of lidocaine and is a primary amine with local anesthetic, anticonvulsant, and antiarrhythmic properties.

PHARMACOLOGY

The chemical structure of mexiletine closely resembles that of lidocaine, and the two drugs share a spectrum of antiarrhythmic activity. The two drugs are not pharmacologically identical, since some cases are refractory to one of the drugs but respond to the other. Mexiletine has no autonomic or other indirect effects; the antiarrhythmic action is mediated by the membrane effects discussed below. Mexiletine has minimal or no effects on arterial blood pressure.

Antiarrhythmic Action

Mexiletine exhibits many of the same electrophysiologic effects as lidocaine. It slows the maximal rate of the AP depolarization and reduces the rate of rise of the 0 phase in damaged cardiac tissue with impaired Na^+ channel function. Mexiletine decreases the AP duration in Purkinje fibers but extends refractoriness into the diastolic period. Thus, while ERP does not change at therapeutic concentrations, the ratio of ERP/APd increases. Unlike lidocaine, mexiletine makes the threshold potential for activation less negative. These cellular electrophysiologic effects result in decreased automaticity (ectopic activity) and slowed or failed conduction in damaged tissue. This latter action is responsible for termination of reentrant arrhythmias. Rapid onset of rate-dependent blocking of the Na^+ channel by mexiletine suggests a greater drug effect against fast than slow ventricular tachyarrhythmias.

In humans, mexiletine has no consistent effect on sinus node discharge rate and atrial refractoriness but prolongs sinus node recovery times in the presence of preexisting disease. Similarly, it does not effect His-Purkinje conduction time unless preexisting disease exists. Mexiletine also does not affect AV conduction without preexisting disease. Electrophysiologic effects in children are similar to those seen in adults with the exception of a consistent increase in heart rate in children.

THERAPEUTIC USE

Mexiletine can be as effective as Ia agents in the control of simple ventricular arrhythmias such as premature ventricular depolarizations or ventricular couplets. Mexiletine has limited efficacy in suppressing or preventing drug-refractory ventricular arrhythmias and is ineffective in managing atrial arrhythmias. When combined with other Ia agents, specifically quinidine or procainamide, or class II beta blockers, a considerable synergistic effect in controlling simple and complex ventricular arrhythmias occurs. This synergism allows for reduction in the dosage of either or both agents, reducing the potential for toxic side effects. Alternatively, mexiletine can be used for prophylaxis after the arrhythmia has been controlled by lidocaine or other therapy.

Since mexiletine has minimal or no effects on cardiac contractility, patients with impaired myocardial performance (after myocardial infarction or because of dilated cardiomyopathy) can benefit the most from this agent. This is the group of patients usually at high risk for serious ventricular arrhythmias and in whom other antiarrhythmic drugs are contraindicated because of their negative inotropic effects. Patients with renal dysfunction requiring antiarrhythmic therapy can be treated with this drug, since minor adjustments are required in patients with severely impaired renal function. The relatively high incidence of minor but distressing side effects, however, limits the widespread use of this effective drug.

PHARMACOKINETICS

Absorption and Distribution

Mexiletine is rapidly absorbed after oral administration and has a 90% bioavailability. However, absorption is delayed and incomplete in patients with acute myocardial infarction, particularly if they have received narcotic analgesics. Mexiletine is 70% plasma protein bound and has a volume of distribution of 5.5 liters/kg.

Elimination

Only 10% of mexiletine appears in the urine unchanged. The remainder is metabolized, primarily to parahydroxymexiletine, hydroxymethylmexiletine, and their corresponding alcohols. These metabolites lack antiarrhythmic activity. The half-life is 8–12 hours and may increase in patients with acute MI.

ADVERSE EFFECTS

Thirty to eighty percent of patients experience adverse effects from mexiletine, in some cases requiring dosage reduction or discontinuation of the drug. The most common symptoms are referable to the central nervous system and gastrointestinal tract: tremors (usually resting tremors), nystagmus, blurred vision, diplopia, dizziness, ataxia, confusion, and nausea. Thrombocytopenia is a rare but reported side effect, and an elevated ANA titer may occur. Hepatitis is also a rare complication.

Cardiovascular Symptoms

The following cardiovascular symptoms may signal overdose but could also occur at therapeutic drug concentrations in the presence of underlying cardiac disease: sinus bradycardia, tachycardia, atrial fibrillation, AV block, hypotension, and ventricular tachycardia. The incidence of arrhythmia aggravation has been reported to be lower than with other forms of therapy; it is more likely to occur in patients with drug-resistant arrhythmias who have received or are currently receiving other antiarrhythmic therapy.

PATIENT MONITORING

ECG and blood pressure should be monitored before and during stabilization of mexiletine dose and intermittently thereafter.

PREPARATIONS AND DOSAGES

Capsules: 150, 200, and 250 mg.
Injection: 25 mg/ml.
Oral: *Adults* — 200–300 mg every 8 hours.
IV: *Adults* — initially infuse 300 mg over a 30-minute period, followed by 250 mg over a 30-minute period, 250 mg over a 2½-hour period, and finally 500 mg over an 8-hour period.

Recommended therapeutic levels: 0.7–2.0 µg/ml; toxic levels, more than 3.0 µg/ml.

Tocainide Hydrochloride

Tocainide is a second structural analog of lidocaine that shares nearly an identical profile of pharmacologic action and therapeutic use. It is effective against ventricular premature complexes, tachycardia, and other ventricular arrhythmias and has the advantage over lidocaine of being effective by the oral route and thus suitable for long-term therapy.

PHARMACOLOGY

Antiarrhythmic Action

Tocainide produces dose-dependent decreases in Na^+ and K^+ conductance, reduces the rate of rise of the AP, and decreases the rate of diastolic depolarization. The effect on the rate of rise of the 0 phase is most striking in damaged cardiac tissue exhibiting impaired Na^+ channel function. The drug decreases the AP duration but extends refractoriness into the diastolic period. Thus, while ERP does not change at therapeutic concentrations, the ERP/APd ratio increases. These cellular electrophysiologic effects result in decreased automaticity (ectopic activity) and slowed conduction or conduction failure in damaged tissue, thus favoring the termination of reentrant arrhythmias.

Tocainide, in therapeutic concentrations, has little or no effect on conduction and does not depress contractility in normal cardiac tissue. In addition, it has little or no effect on the ECG (although the QT interval may be slightly shortened) and lacks both atropinelike and α-adrenergic blocking actions. Tocainide appears to have minimal or no hemodynamic effects.

THERAPEUTIC USE

Tocainide has the same spectrum of antiarrhythmic activity as lidocaine. Its main use is in the suppression of and prophylaxis against drug-resistant ventricular arrhythmias. It is not effective against atrial arrhythmias. It is given initially in loading doses for arrhythmia suppression followed by long-term maintenance therapy. Alternatively, tocainide may be used for long-term prophylaxis after initial arrhythmia suppression by lidocaine or other antiarrhythmic agent. Therapeutic plasma levels (measured by a 50–80% reduction in premature ventricular contractions) are 4–10 µg/ml.

The QT interval is not affected. There is no major negative inotropy or adverse drug interactions with warfarin sodium, digitalis, or beta blockers. Tocainide can be administered on a 2- or 3-times-a-day basis.

PHARMACOKINETICS

Absorption and Distribution

Tocainide is readily absorbed and has an oral bioavailability of 90%. It has low plasma protein binding (10%) and a volume of distribution of 3 liters/kg.

Elimination

Approximately 40–50% of tocainamide is excreted in the urine unchanged; the remainder undergoes hepatic glucuronidation and subsequent renal excretion. Two major metabolites are glucuronide derivatives, neither of which is cardioactive. The plasma half-life of tocainamide is 12–14 hours but may increase to 17–43 hours in patients with either renal or hepatic disease.

ADVERSE EFFECTS

One-third to two-thirds of patients receiving tocainide experience adverse effects. Approximately 20% have side effects referable to the central nervous system: lightheadedness and vertigo; paresthesias, tremor, and altered mood; ataxia and confusion. A fraction of these patients must reduce the dose or discontinue tocainide therapy. Additional symptoms include nausea (approximately 14%), vomiting (about 5%), anorexia (about 2%), and miscellaneous problems including rash, nightmares, fever, diarrhea, and nystagmus (about 4%).

Sinus bradycardia, tachycardia, atrial fibrillation, AV block, hypotension, and ventricular tachyarrhythmias may signal overdose but may also occur at therapeutic drug concentrations in the presence of underlying cardiac disease.

Rarely, interstitial pneumonitis and pulmonary fibrosis may occur, and fatalities have been reported. In addition, tocainide may cause bone marrow depression leading to leukopenia and agranulocytosis.

PATIENT MONITORING

ECG and blood pressure should be monitored before and during stabilization of tocainide dose and intermittently thereafter. Renal and hepatic function tests should be performed periodically to detect changes leading to tocainide accumulation and toxicity. The patient should be instructed to report any difficulty in breathing, cough, or wheezing. Blood cell counts should be performed periodically to detect possible bone marrow depression.

PREPARATIONS AND DOSAGES

Tablets: 400 and 600 mg.
Oral: *Adults* — initially, 400 mg every 8 hours. Maintenance — 1.2–1.8 gm daily in three divided doses.

Properties of Individual Class Ic Antiarrhythmic Drugs

Encainide

PHARMACOLOGY

Encainide is one of the newly released Ic antiarrhythmic agents. It dramatically affects conduction velocity but has only small effects on the refractory period and does not cause postrepolarization refractoriness. Encainide has no autonomic or other indirect effect and mediates its antiarrhythmic action via its direct membrane effects.

Antiarrhythmic Action

Encainide binds to and inactivates the Na^+ channel with a half-life of 15–20 seconds, thus behaving as an irreversible blocker of the Na^+ channel. As a consequence, it dramatically slows conduction throughout the heart, although the slowing is greater in the Purkinje fiber system and accessory pathways, especially in the retrograde direction, in which conduction may be completely abolished. Encainide decreases the diastolic depolarization rate, an action underlying its effectiveness against ectopic arrhythmias, and increases ERP of atrial and Purkinje fibers and ventricular muscle.

Effects on the Electrocardiogram

Encainide increases the PR interval, markedly widens the base of the QRS complex, and modestly prolongs the QT interval. This last change is due only to the effect of encainide on the QRS complex; no prolongation of the ST interval is observed.

THERAPEUTIC USE

Encainide's greatest use is in treatment of ventricular arrhythmias. It has particular efficacy against ventricular ectopy, causing a reduction of more than 75% in 70–80% of patients, and has been reported to suppress ventricular tachycardia or fibrillation in 30–60% of cases refractory to other drugs. Encainide is also effective against reentrant arrhythmias caused by accessory pathways. Encainide has been shown to be useful against refractory supraventricular arrhythmias.

PHARMACOKINETICS

Absorption and Distribution

Oral encainide is rapidly absorbed with a bioavailability of approximately 40%; 70–80% of the drug is bound to plasma protein. Effective plasma concentration is wide, 1.3–5.6 ng/ml. Plasma concentrations associated with transient side effects range from 135–570 ng/ml.

Elimination

Encainide is eliminated primarily by metabolism to O-dimethyl encainide (ODE) and 3-methoxy-O-dimethyl encainide (MODE). With long-term use, these metabolites contribute substantially to the antiarrhythmic action of encainide. They are both more potent than encainide and accumulate to concentrations more than 5 times that of encainide. The half-life of encainide is 2½–4 hours, while those of ODE and MODE are 11–12 hours and more than 24 hours, respectively. Because of the number of active metabolites, plasma encainide levels are not useful in guiding encainide therapy.

ADVERSE EFFECTS

The most important adverse effect of encainide is its potential to worsen arrhythmias. For example, patients treated for premature ventricular contractions (PVCs) may develop sustained ventricular tachycardia or fibrillation, although the latter complication is usually seen in patients with sustained arrhythmia or low ejection fractions. Other adverse effects include lightheadedness, dizziness, headache, ataxia, tremor, nausea, vomiting, and constipation. These are rarely serious enough to require discontinuation of the drug. In patients with preexisting severe cardiac dysfunction, encainide has the potential to cause hemodynamic deterioration, although in general the drug can usually be administered in patients with depressed left ventricular function. Overall, encainide is fairly well tolerated during long-term therapy.

PATIENT MONITORING

ECG should be monitored before and after initiation of therapy, and ECG recordings obtained intermittently throughout the remainder of therapy. Because of the potential for arrhythmogenicity in patients with sustained VT, the manufacturer recommends hospitalizing patients when encainide therapy is to be initiated in high-risk patients or for increases in dosage to greater than 200 mg a day. Rapid dose adjustments are not recommended.

PREPARATIONS AND DOSAGES

Capsules: 25, 35, and 50 mg.
Oral: *Adults* — recommended dose is 25 mg 3 times a day with increase of dosage in increments of 2–3 days to a maximum dose of 200–250 mg/day. In heart failure, initial dose starts at 25 mg three times a day with weekly dose titrations.

Flecainide Acetate

PHARMACOLOGY

Flecainide, while not exhibiting autonomic or other indirect actions, exerts antiarrhythmic actions by directly affecting cardiac membranes.

Antiarrhythmic Action

Flecainide behaves as an irreversible antagonist of the Na^+ channel, binding to the Na^+ channel with a half-time for dissociation of approximately 15–20 seconds. This property classifies it as a class Ic agent. In addition, flecainide prolongs the AP duration and slows the rate of diastolic depolarization, resulting in a prolongation of conduction and an increase in refractoriness in the atrium, His-Purkinje system, and ventricles. Flecainide also increases retrograde refractoriness and slows conduction in accessory AV pathways and is particularly effective in controlling dangerously rapid tachyarrhythmias in the WPW syndrome.

Effects on the Electrocardiogram

Flecainide increases the PR interval, can markedly widen the QRS complex at the base, and modestly increases the QT interval, largely by widening the QRS complex. There is a minimal prolongation of the ST interval.

THERAPEUTIC USE

Flecainide's principal use is in the treatment of ventricular arrhythmias. It is extremely effective in abolishing PVCs, suppressing more than 90% in 80% of patients. Therefore, drugs of this class, flecainide and encainide, have been dubbed "PVC killers." Flecainide is also effective in controlling serious recurrent ventricular tachycardia refractory to other antiarrhythmic drugs. The overall efficacy in this group of high-risk patients is 30–40%, similar to that of encainide, but better than that of Ia agents. Flecainide is also very effective in suppressing reentrant supraventricular arrhythmias involving accessory pathways and the AV node and in the conversion of atrial flutter and fibrillation.

PHARMACOKINETICS

Absorption and Distribution

Flecainide acetate is rapidly absorbed after oral administration with peak plasma levels at 3 hours and a bioavailability of 95%. Peak plasma concentrations are not affected by food or antacid. Flecainide is 40% plasma protein bound.

Elimination

Approximately 30% of flecainide is eliminated unchanged by urinary excretion. The remainder is metabolized in the liver, and the metabolites, with no recognized antiarrhythmic properties, are excreted in the urine. The drug's plasma half-life of 14 hours may be increased in patients with either congestive heart failure, renal failure, or arrhythmias. Steady state for plasma drug concentration is 3–5 days after multiple dosage.

ADVERSE EFFECTS

Flecainide has little effect on hemodynamics in patients with normal cardiac function. However, where cardiac reserve is reduced, flecainide may cause hemodynamic deterioration, including newly developed congestive heart failure. In patients with abnormal sinus function, flecainide may produce a marked depression of sinus node activity with sinus arrest requiring pacing. The drug also possesses arrhythmogenic potential, converting simple arrhythmias such as PVCs to sustained tachycardia or fibrillation. As with encainide, this occurs in patients with a history of sustained arrhythmias, associated with lowered LV function and during rapid drug titrations.

The most common adverse effects are neurologic, including dizziness, headache, paresthesias, fatigue, nervousness, tremor, and blurred vision. Nausea may also occur. The adverse effects are generally not severe enough to warrant discontinuation of the drug, and this agent is fairly well tolerated during long-term therapy.

PATIENT MONITORING

The ECG should be monitored before and after initiation of flecainide therapy, and ECG should be recorded intermittently thereafter, specifically monitoring the QRS duration.

PREPARATIONS AND DOSAGES

Tablets: 100 mg.

Oral: *Adults* — administer 100–200 mg every 12 hours. Initial recommended dose is 100 mg every 12 hours. In elderly patients, 50 mg every 12 hours has resulted in satisfactory control of arrhythmias. Flecainide levels should be monitored during therapy and maintained between 200 and 1000 ng/ml. They should not exceed 1000 ng/ml.

Lorcainide Hydrochloride (Investigational)

Lorcainide lacks autonomic and other indirect effects. Its antiarrhythmic action is mediated by its direct effects on cardiac membranes.

PHARMACOLOGY

Antiarrhythmic Action

Lorcainide binds to Na^+ channels with a dissociation time of about 15–20 seconds, producing an apparently irreversible blockade of the Na^+ channel. Lorcainide also slows the diastolic depolarization rate. These electrophysiologic effects result in a slowing of conduction in the atria, AV node, His-Purkinje system, ventricles, and accessory AV pathways. Lorcainide has only modest effects on cardiac refractoriness.

Effects on the Electrocardiogram

Lorcainide prolongs the PR interval and widens the QRS complex at the base, which increases the QT interval. The drug has little or no effect on the ST interval.

THERAPEUTIC USE

Lorcainide is effective against ventricular ectopy and arrhythmias that are refractory to other drugs. It may also abolish tachycardia involving accessory pathways. However, it is ineffective against atrial flutter and fibrillation.

PHARMACOKINETICS

Absorption and Distribution

Lorcainide undergoes substantial first-pass metabolism after oral administration. Only 4% of a single dose of 100 mg becomes available systemically. Fifty percent becomes available after a 300-mg dose. Bioavailability increases after multiple doses, possibly because of either saturation or metabolite-induced negative feedback inhibition of the metabolic pathway. Lorcainide is 80–95% plasma protein bound and has a volume of distribution of between 6 and 7 liters/kg.

Elimination

Lorcainide is eliminated primarily by metabolism to the N-dealkylated compound, norlorcainide. The half-life of lorcainide is 6–10 hours initially, but may increase to 10–14 hours with long-term maintenance of therapy. Norlorcainide is nearly equipotent to lorcainide in antiarrhythmic activity. This metabolite accumulates to substantially higher concentrations in the plasma than lorcainide on long-term therapy and has a half-life of 24–30 hours. Thus, it contributes substantially to the antiarrhythmic action of lorcainide.

ADVERSE EFFECTS

Lorcainide may reduce sinus node function in patients with preexisting sinus nodal disease. The drug has little effect on hemodynamics in patients with normal cardiac function. However, hemodynamics may deteriorate and hypotension may occur in patients with congestive heart disease. Like the other class Ic agents, lorcainide has arrhythmogenic potential, converting PVCs to sustained tachycardia or fibrillation.

The most common adverse effects are sleep disturbances characterized by frequent awakening, vivid dreams, and night sweats. Most patients are not unusually tired in the mornings after such frequent awakening. Hypnotics can be effective in reducing insomnia. This side effect results in a high discontinuance rate, thereby limiting lorcainide's usefulness. Other adverse effects include anxiety, headache, paresthesias, nausea, vomiting, and a metallic taste.

PATIENT MONITORING

ECG must be monitored continuously during the first 2–3 days of therapy and intermittently thereafter.

PREPARATIONS AND DOSAGES

Tablets: 100 mg.
Injection: 10 mg/ml.
Oral: *Adults* — administer 100 mg twice daily up to 400 mg. Dosage should not be increased more frequently than at weekly intervals because of slow accumulation. (In some studies,

lorcainide hydrochloride has been shown to be effective during once-a-day dosing.)

IV: *Adult* — 2 mg/min, or 100 mg infused over a 1-hour period.

Properties of Individual Class II Antiarrhythmic Drugs

The physiologist Ahlquist in 1948 [1] observed differences in the relative ability of a series of sympathomimetic amines to affect organs and systems and concluded that there were two distinct types of adrenergic receptors, α and β. Some 10 years later, β-adrenergic receptor antagonists (beta blockers) were discovered, initiating one of the greatest advances in cardiovascular pharmacotherapy. Beta blockers are class II antiarrhythmic drugs.

Beta blockers are defined as drugs with the property of competitive inhibition of isoproterenol, a catecholamine with exclusive β-adrenoceptor agonist properties. Properties common to all beta blockers are (1) structural similarities, (2) ability to slow the heart rate and reduce myocardial oxygen consumption, (3) negatively inotropic effect, and (4) ability to reduce the AV conduction velocity.

MECHANISMS UNDERLYING ANTIARRHYTHMIC EFFECTS

Beta blockers reduce the rate of impulse formation in automatic cells, reduce the conduction velocity in the AV node, and reduce the amplitude of delayed afterdepolarization. They increase the duration of the AP, decrease its upstroke velocity, and decrease phase 4 depolarization.

MECHANISMS UNDERLYING SIDE EFFECTS

Other actions play a primary role in determining the side effects of the different beta blockers. For example, highly lipid soluble drugs will enter the central nervous system to cause a variety of side effects that are absent when beta blockers of low lipid solubility are used. Certain of the beta blockers have a membrane-stabilizing effect, also known as local anesthetic or quinidinelike effect. However, the membrane-stabilizing effect does not relate to the antiarrhythmic action of the drugs because at concentrations that effectively block β-adrenoceptors, the drugs do not stabilize membranes.

Certain beta blockers possess intrinsic sympathomimetic activity and behave as partial agonists of the β-receptor. Others are cardioselective, blocking the β_1-receptor in the heart at low concentrations and the β_2-receptor, located in other sites, as the concentration is increased. Activation of β_2-receptors relaxes bronchiolar smooth muscle in the lung, induces glycogenolysis and lipolysis, and mediates vasodilation in blood vessels. There are metabolic differences between cardioselective and nonselective agents. Hypoglycemia induced by insulin is dependent on beta stimulation in response to circulating catecholamines, which in turn increase glycogen breakdown in the liver (glycogenolysis) and reverse hypoglycemia. Beta blockade reduces glycogenolysis and causes prolonged hypoglycemia. The effect is less with cardioselective (metoprolol and atenolol) than with nonselective drugs (propranolol). Thus, cardioselective agents are preferred in patients with insulin-dependent diabetes mellitus.

Both cardioselective and nonselective beta blockers may equally exhibit lipolysis and affect plasma lipids. High-density lipoprotein (HDL) cholesterol concentration is reduced, HDL_3 is increased, and there are no significant changes in low-density lipoprotein (LDL) cholesterol. Long-term treatment (12 weeks) reduces total cholesterol mainly by lowering HDL. Serum triglyceride concentrations may be increased by short-term beta blocking (6 weeks). Cardioselective drugs (atenolol and metoprolol) have less effect on triglyceride and very-low-density lipoprotein (VLDL) than nonselective beta blockers (propranolol).

Asthma and Bronchospasm

Some cardioselective drugs may induce asthma or bronchospasm. For example, atenolol has less effect on bronchial smooth muscle than metoprolol.

Beta blockers impair extrarenal disposal of an acute potassium load. Patients with impaired potassium disposal may be at increased risk of hyperkalemia with beta blockers.

Beta blockers may have gastrointestinal side effects in the following order of frequency: diarrhea, dyspepsia, nausea, flatulence, abdominal pain, and constipation. Sclerosing peritonitis, which includes abdominal pain, vomiting, and weight loss, has been reported in patients receiving propranolol or metoprolol. Sclerosing peritonitis may develop months after cessation of the beta blocker therapy.

Pregnancy

There are no reports of fetal malformation or retardation of fetal growth resulting from beta blockers, and in fact beta blockers for treatment of hypertension appear to improve the likelihood that the fetus will be normal.

THERAPEUTIC USES

The therapeutic indication for all beta blockers in managing arrhythmias is the treatment of SVT, atrial flutter, and fibrillation. While conversion to normal sinus rhythm occurs in some cases, the major action of the beta blockers is to protect the ventricles by increasing the refractory period and slowing conduction through the AV node. Thus, they produce AV block or increase the degree of existing block. AV block is a key action of the beta blockers when used alone or in combination with digitalis. The beta blockers also have some antiarrhythmic activity against ventricular arrhythmias, particularly those associated with excessive catecholamines, myocardial ischemia, mitral valve prolapse, and digitalis toxicity, and in the prevention and treatment of syncope and ventricular arrhythmias associated with the long QT syndrome. Because of the negatively inotropic effects of beta blockers, they are also useful against PVCs associated with hypertrophic cardiomyopathy. Beta blockers may also provide considerable protection against reinfarction after an acute MI.

Atenolol

PHARMACOLOGY

Atenolol is a cardioselective beta blocker. It lacks both membrane-stabilizing and partial agonist activity. Because of low lipid solubility, it does not accumulate in high concentrations in the brain, thereby reducing the likelihood of centrally mediated side effects. Cardioselectivity may reduce the severity and incidence of bronchospasm, hypoglycemia, and aggravation of peripheral vascular disease.

PHARMACOKINETICS

Absorption and Distribution

Atenolol has an oral availability of 40% and an apparent volume of distribution of 0.7 liter/kg. Atenolol undergoes little or no plasma protein binding.

Elimination

Approximately 85% of atenolol appears in the urine unchanged. The remainder is metabolized. The plasma half-life of atenolol is 6–7 hours and increases in patients with impairment of renal function.

ADVERSE EFFECTS

The most serious adverse effects occur in patients with preexisting cardiac disease. For example, when cardiac output in the congestive heart failure patient is maintained by sympathetic drive, the use of a beta blocker removes this drive and decreases cardiac output, exacerbating cardiac decompensation. Beta blockers may convert preexisting heart block to a higher degree or to total AV block.

Abrupt withdrawal of large doses of beta blocker may result in angina, ventricular tachyarrhythmia, myocardial infarction, sudden death, or a combination of these. The dosage must be withdrawn slowly over a period of 1–2 weeks. Because atenolol is cardioselective and has a low lipid solubility, it has less of a tendency to cause fatigue, lethargy, and other central nervous system side effects or to induce asthma in the asthmatic, hypoglycemia in the diabetic, or peripheral vasoconstriction in the patient suffering from peripheral vascular disease.

PREPARATIONS AND DOSAGES

Tablets: 50 and 100 mg.
Oral: *Adults* — initially, 12.5–25.0 mg once a day. (Dosage may be increased to 50–100 mg/day after 2 weeks, if necessary and tolerated.) In severe renal dysfunction the dose should be adjusted according to creatinine clearance: 50 mg daily if creatinine is 15–35 ml/min/1.73 m^2; 50 mg every other day if creatinine clearance is less than 15 ml/min/1.73 m^2.

Pindolol

PHARMACOLOGY

Pindolol is a nonselective beta blocker that possesses partial agonist activity and slight membrane-stabilizing activity. It is moderately lipid soluble and, therefore, gains access to the central nervous system.

PHARMACOKINETICS

Absorption and Distribution

Pindolol is rapidly absorbed after oral administration with a bioavailability of 90%. Peak plasma concentrations are achieved in 1–2 hours. Pindolol has very low plasma protein binding, 10%, and a volume distribution of 0.9 liter/kg.

Elimination

Thirty to forty percent of pindolol appears unchanged in the urine, while the remainder is metabolized. The half-life of pindolol, 3–4 hours, may increase to 11–12 hours in renal failure and to more than 30 hours in patients with hepatic dysfunction.

ADVERSE EFFECTS

Pindolol may cause fatigue, lethargy, depression, and other central nervous system side effects. Theoretically, its capacity to cause asthma, heart failure, hypoglycemia, or peripheral vasoconstriction in the respective susceptible patients may be reduced because of the partial agonist activity of this beta blocker. Nevertheless, pindolol must be used with great caution in patients with markedly reduced cardiac reserve or preexisting AV block. Pindolol may also cause bradycardia in patients with preexisting sinus nodal impairment. However, in patients with normal SA node function, resting bradycardia is not a major problem but rather an advantage of this type of beta blocker. Paradoxical increases in blood pressure have occurred in some patients and are thought to be due to the partial agonist activity of this drug. Sudden withdrawal of high doses of pindolol may result in unstable angina, ventricular tachyarrhythmias, myocardial infarction, sudden death, or a combination of these. Discontinuation of the drug must be carried out gradually over a 1- to 2-week period.

PREPARATIONS AND DOSAGES

Tablets: 5 and 10 mg.

Oral: *Adults* — initially 5 mg 2 times a day, increased by increments of 10 mg daily at 2–3 week intervals as needed and tolerated. Dosage may have to be decreased in either renal or hepatic dysfunction.

Propranolol Hydrochloride

PHARMACOLOGY

Propranolol is a nonselective beta blocker that lacks partial agonist activity. It is highly lipid soluble and has easy access to the central nervous system. It also possesses marked membrane-stabilizing activity. However, the doses eliciting this effect are above those required to achieve beta blockade.

PHARMACOKINETICS

Absorption and Distribution

Propranolol is rapidly and completely absorbed from the gastrointestinal tract and has an oral bioavailability of 30–50% because of extensive first-pass metabolism. Peak plasma concentrations are achieved within 1–1½ hours. Propranolol is 90–95% plasma protein bound and has an apparent volume of distribution of 3.9 liters/kg.

Elimination

Propranolol is eliminated almost exclusively by liver metabolism. Its metabolite, 4-hydroxypropranolol, is cardioactive; however, it has a shorter half-life than propranolol and probably contributes little to the therapeutic effect. Propranolol's half-life is 3½–6 hours; the therapeutic effect lasts longer, which suggests that plasma concentration is not a useful indicator of duration of drug action. The half-life increases in patients with cirrhosis and is minimally affected by renal insufficiency.

ADVERSE EFFECTS

Propranolol can cause the full range of adverse effects attributable to beta blockers. The central nervous system effects include fatigue, lethargy, vivid dreams, insomnia, and depression. Propranolol may also cause asthma, peripheral vascular constriction, or hypoglycemia in the respective susceptible patient populations. The most serious adverse effects are attributable to the heart, where the drug may induce bradycardia, heart failure, and AV conduction disturbances. Sudden withdrawal of large doses of propranolol may be followed by unstable angina, ventricular tachyarrhythmias, MI, sudden death, or a combination of these. Discontinuation of propranolol therapy should be carried out gradually over a 1- to 2-week period. Other adverse effects include nausea, vomiting, gastric discomfort, diarrhea, constipation, and flatulence.

PREPARATIONS AND DOSAGES

Tablets: 10, 20, 40, 60, 80, 90, and 120 mg.
Extended-release capsules: 60, 80, 120, and 160 mg.
Injection: 1 mg/ml.
Oral: *Adult* (tablets) — initially 10–20 mg 3 or 4 times daily. The dosage may be increased gradually every 3–7 days up to a total of 320 mg/day, if needed. *Adult* (extended-release capsules) — 80, 120, or 160 mg administered once a day for maintenance. *Pediatric* (tablets) — 0.5–4.0 mg/kg daily in four divided doses. (Up to 16 mg/kg daily has been used.)
IV: *Adult* — 0.10–0.15 mg/kg administered in increments of 0.50–0.75 mg every 1–2 minutes with continuous monitoring of ECG and blood pressure. *Pediatric* — 0.01–0.15 mg/kg over a 3- to 5-minute period with continuous monitoring of ECG and blood pressure.

Timolol Maleate

Timolol is a nonselective beta blocker with no membrane-stabilizing or partial agonist activity. Its lipid solubility is low, which suggests that it does not achieve high concentrations in the brain. Otherwise, timolol appears to resemble propranolol closely in its pharmacologic profile.

PHARMACOKINETICS

Absorption and Distribution

Timolol is rapidly absorbed from the gastrointestinal tract but has a 50% oral bioavailability because of marked first-pass metabolism. The time to peak effect is 1–2 hours. Timolol is only 10% plasma bound and has an apparent volume of distribution of 1.8 liters/kg.

Elimination

Timolol is eliminated almost exclusively by hepatic metabolism. The drug has a half-life of 4 hours, but its therapeutic effect lasts longer, which suggests that plasma concentrations do not indicate the duration of therapeutic effect.

ADVERSE EFFECTS

While timolol may cause fatigue, lethargy, and other central nervous system side effects, these are likely to be less frequent and severe than with other, more lipid-soluble beta blockers. Timolol may cause asthma, hypoglycemia, and peripheral vasoconstriction in the respective susceptible patient populations. The most serious adverse effects are related to the heart and are most likely to occur when there is preexisting cardiac dysfunction. These adverse effects include heart failure, AV conduction disturbances, bradycardia, and hypotension. Sudden withdrawal of large doses of timolol may result in unstable angina, ventricular tachyarrhythmias, myocardial infarction, sudden death, or a combination of these.

PREPARATIONS AND DOSAGES

Tablets: 5, 10, and 20 mg.

Oral: *Adult* — initially, 10 mg 2 times daily. Dosage may be increased at 1-week intervals, as needed and tolerated (up to 30 mg twice daily). Myocardial reinfarction prophylaxis: 10 mg twice daily (to be initiated 4 weeks after infarction).

Esmolol

Esmolol is an IV administered drug that is particularly useful in treating supraventricular arrhythmias in patients with myocardial ischemia in whom rapid titration of beta blockade is desirable [2].

PHARMACOLOGY

Esmolol is a cardioselective beta blocker that lacks intrinsic sympathomimetic and membrane-stabilizing properties.

PHARMACOKINETICS

Esmolol has an ultrashort action and an elimination half-life of about 9 minutes. It is metabolized by ester hydrolysis in the blood stream, and the half-life is not appreciably affected by renal or hepatic disease.

ADVERSE EFFECTS

The limiting side effect of hypotension, occurring in over one-third of patients, is dose related and controlled by reducing or discontinuing the infusion. Other side effects are nausea (7%), peripheral ischemia (rare), and bronchospasm (>1%). Precipitation of heart failure and heart block is rare (1% of patients). Depression of LV function, even with ejection fractions of 27 ± 2%, is minimal with doses of 50–100 µg/kg/min (which effectively blocks beta receptors). Doses higher than 110 µg/kg/min may have a slight depressing effect on the LV.

PREPARATIONS AND DOSAGES

The drug is prepared by removing 20 ml from a 500-ml volume of commonly used IV fluids (5% D/W, saline, lactated Ringer's; it is **incompatible with sodium bicarbonate**) and adding the contents of two 2.5-gm ampules of esmolol. It is administered by continuous IV infusion, 10 mg/ml. Give a loading dose infusion of 500 µg/kg/min for 1 min, followed by a 4-min maintenance infusion of 50 µg/kg/min. Wait 5 min. If therapeutic effect is not achieved within 5 min, repeat the loading dose followed by a maintenance infusion increased to 100 µg/kg/min. Continue this titration procedure, increasing the maintenance dose (4 min) by 50 µg/kg/min each time. When desired heart rate or blood pressure effect is approached, omit the loading dose and reduce the increment in maintenance dose from 50 to 25 µg/kg/min. The interval between titration steps may also be increased from 5 to 10 min.

Properties of Individual Class III Antiarrhythmic Drugs

Amiodarone Hydrochloride

PHARMACOLOGY

Amiodarone [10] was first introduced in the early 1970s as an antianginal coronary vasodilator because of its smooth-muscle-relaxing properties. After extensive clinical experience outside the United States, the drug was found to possess marked antiarrhythmic properties.

The molecular structure of amiodarone consists of a procainamide-lidocaine-like element, a diethyl amino radical probably responsible for some of the electrophysiologic properties as a local membrane anesthetic, and a ringed iodine-containing portion responsible for the drug's interaction with the thyroid gland. Some investigators contend that at times the antithyroid properties are responsible for the drug's antianginal and even for some of its electrophysiologic properties. That amiodarone exerts a complex and time-dependent effect on the heart and the circulation is suggested by the slow onset of action, requiring days or weeks, and a plateau effect between 5 and 7 weeks.

Antiarrhythmic Action

Because amiodarone causes a marked prolongation of the AP and the refractoriness of cardiac tissue, it is categorized as a class III antiarrhythmic agent. Amiodarone slows the rate of rise of the 0 phase of the AP in all tissues dependent on the Na^+ fast channel and decreases the rate of rise of the 0 phase in the SA and AV nodes, which suggests an action on the Ca^{2+} entry channel. The drug does not affect the AP amplitude, the overshoot, or resting membrane potential. Amiodarone does not affect electrophysiologic characteristics of the transmembrane APs when isolated cardiac muscles are perfused with homologous plasma containing the drug. It is noteworthy that changes in the cardiac muscle secondary to amiodarone closely resemble those produced by thyroid gland ablation, and in experimental animals the drug's effect on repolarization is prevented by the concomitant administration of the daily requirements of triiodothyronine (T_3). These electrophysiologic effects result in a slowing of the heart rate, a reduction in conduction velocity, and an increase in the duration of the ERP in all cardiac tissues including accessory pathways that participate in the preexcitation syndromes. Clinical electrophysiologic studies identify a prolongation of the AH, PR, and HV intervals and ERP of all tissues.

Effects on the Electrocardiogram

Sinus bradycardia is very common during long-term therapy. Amiodarone increases the PR interval and markedly prolongs the

QT interval. This latter effect is due primarily to a prolongation of the ST interval, since the drug has only minimal effects on the QRS complex.

Autonomic Nervous Tissue Effects

Amiodarone causes a noncompetitive blockade of β-adrenergic receptors in both animals and humans as demonstrated by reduction in the cardiac response to isoproterenol. Amiodarone has also been shown in animal experiments to inhibit the α-adrenergic receptor noncompetitively.

The pharmacologic properties of amiodarone may be summarized as follows:

Long-term administration (>3–6 weeks) (1) lengthens AP duration in all cardiac tissues and (2) depresses phase 4 depolarization.
Coronary artery and systemic artery dilatation.
α- and β-Adrenoceptor antagonism.
No recognized vagolytic or vagomimetic activity.
Negligible negatively inotropic activity.
Hypothyroidism.

THERAPEUTIC USE

Amiodarone is generally reserved for serious atrial and ventricular tachyarrhythmias that are refractory to other drug therapy. Amiodarone is effective against atrial fibrillation, converting many cases to normal sinus rhythm and slowing the ventricular rate via the induction of AV block in the remainder. Amiodarone is also effective against PSVT whether it is due to AV reentry via accessory pathways, AV nodal reentry, or ectopic activity. Amiodarone has been found to be particularly effective against reentry arrhythmias involving accessory pathways, such as the WPW syndrome. The drug is also effective against the bradycardia-tachycardia syndrome, controlling the tachycardia component. However, in many instances a pacemaker may be required to control severe bradycardia. Most forms of ventricular tachyarrhythmias are responsive to amiodarone, which has been called "the drug of last resort." Amiodarone has an efficacy of 40–60% in refractory ventricular arrhythmias, compared to the 20% success rate seen with Ia drugs and the 30% observed with the newer Ic drugs.

PHARMACOKINETICS

Absorption and Distribution

The absorption of amiodarone is variable and incomplete. There is a lag time of ½–3 hours for onset of absorption. Peak plasma concentrations occur between 3 and 7 hours, and absorption continues up to 15 hours. Bioavailability ranges between 22 and 50%. Amiodarone is distributed widely throughout the tissues of the body, including skin, subcutaneous fat, and muscle. The greatest concentration of amiodarone and its major metabolite (see below) is in the liver, followed in order by fat, lung, lymph tissue, myocardium, and skeletal muscle. The apparent volume of distribution is large, ranging between 20 and 160 liters/kg.

Elimination

Neither amiodarone nor major metabolites appear in the urine within 24 hours of a single dose. The distribution into several tissue compartments plays a key role in preventing or terminating dysrhythmias during the early phases of drug administration. During long-term therapy the half-life of amiodarone ranges between 13 and 100 days, and the drug is eliminated primarily by metabolism. The major metabolite, *N*-desethylamiodarone, may be antiarrhythmic, but such activity has not been reported. If oral dosing is started without a loading dose, up to 28 days may be required for antiarrhythmic effect. A loading dose may be antiarrhythmic by 10 days; intravenous administration does not reduce the lag time. The antiarrhythmic activity persists after the termination of drug therapy for up to 30–45 days.

ADVERSE EFFECTS

Amiodarone has few adverse hemodynamic effects; however, in the presence of SA or AV nodal dysfunction or impaired myocardial contractility, the drug may cause bradycardia or AV block or even depress contractility. Side effects, mostly mild, occur in more than 50% of patients, but the drug must be discontinued because of these effects in fewer than 10% of patients. Untoward reactions requiring discontinuance of the drug include thyroid dysfunction, visual disturbances, pulmonary infiltrates, ataxia, cardiac conduction disturbances, and drug interactions. The incidence rate of adverse reaction is related to serum amiodarone concentrations and to total dose received over time. Adverse reactions occur with serum values higher than 2.5 mg/liter; however, pulmonary complications can appear at any concentration. Amiodarone also has an arrhythmogenic potential. Exacerbation of existing arrhythmias occurs in approximately 3–5% of patients.

Pulmonary fibrosis and infiltrates are the most serious complication of amiodarone therapy. Three to five percent (in some series, up to 10%) of patients taking the drug have developed this complication, and it has been lethal. The mechanism of the pulmonary toxicity is unknown, but it resembles a drug-induced lysosomal storage disease, phospholipidosis. Pulmonary complications may resolve if the drug is continued. Corticosteroids have been shown to be consistently effective in accelerating the resolution of pulmonary infiltrations in improving hypoxia.

Nearly all patients receiving long-term amiodarone therapy experience corneal lipofuscin deposits. In general, these do not impair vision; however, some patients experience photophobia, colored halos around light, and a reduction in visual acuity.

Some patients also exhibit a bluish gray discoloration of the skin in the sun-exposed areas. A fraction of these patients experience photosensitivity reactions such as erythema and swelling, photodermatitis, melanodermatitis, and rashes. Some of these skin manifestations can be reduced by the appropriate use of sunscreen, usually with a sun protection factor (SPF) of 15.

Gastrointestinal symptoms including anorexia, nausea, vomiting, abdominal pain, and constipation have been reported. Central nervous system side effects, which are rare, include headache, insomnia, nightmares, hallucinations, ataxia, and peripheral neuropathy. Some cases of alopecia related to amiodarone use have been reported. Amiodarone may induce hypothyroidism. The chemical structure of amiodarone resembles that of, and may be, an antagonist of the thyroid hormone. Hypothyroidism may require replacement therapy. Increases in thyroxine T_4 are seen with long-term therapy, but clinical hyperthyroidism is not as commonly seen as is hypothyroidism.

PATIENT MONITORING

Patients receiving amiodarone should be carefully monitored to prevent the development of serious side effects. The ECG should be monitored at least every 3 months during office visits. Liver and thyroid function tests should be done at least at 6-month intervals. There is variability in practice among cardiologists and electrophysiologists regarding the use of chest x rays and pulmonary function tests in the early diagnosis of pulmonary complications. Many clinicians rely on history and physical examinations solely, while others obtain these tests at 6- to 12-month intervals. Other clinicians obtain these tests on a yearly basis.

PREPARATIONS AND DOSAGES

Oral: *Adult* — numerous dosage regimens are given in the literature; two representing the spectrum are given here. *Regimen 1:* 600 mg is given daily in three divided doses for 1 week, followed by 200–400 mg daily. Thereafter, the lowest effective dose should be given to minimize side effects. A maintenance dose of 200 mg on alternate days may be effective in some patients. Larger doses are recommended for ventricular arrhythmias: for example, 800–1200 mg daily initially, followed by 600–800 mg daily after 1 or 2 weeks. (See *AMA Drug Evaluations* 6, 1986.) *Regimen 2:* 2000 mg on day 1, given in divided doses, followed by 1400 mg/day for 3 days, followed by 1000 mg/day for 1 week, followed by 800 mg/day for 2 weeks, and finally 600 mg/day for at least the next 4 weeks. Maintenance doses of 200–400 mg/day may suffice in treating supraventricular arrhythmias; 400–600 mg/day may be required to control life-threatening ventricular arrhythmias.

IV: *Adult* — up to 5 mg/kg given over a 5-minute period; the dose should not be repeated within 15 minutes. Some clinicians prefer to infuse the dose over a 15-minute period to minimize the hypotension associated with one 5-minute infusion.

Bretylium Tosylate

PHARMACOLOGY

Bretylium is most commonly used by the intravenous route, and its pharmacologic effects can be best understood in terms of the chronology of hemodynamic and antiarrhythmic effects after an acute intravenous injection. Initially, bretylium is taken up into peripheral adrenergic nerve terminals and causes the release of the endogenous neurotransmitter norepinephrine. As a consequence, heart rate, cardiac output, peripheral resistance, and blood pressure may be elevated. Ventricular ectopic activity may also increase during this phase. Within 20–30 minutes after the injection, the initial hypertensive phase dissipates and is followed by a prolonged period of hypotension. Bretylium becomes concentrated in adrenergic nerve terminals, producing an adrenergic neuron blockade, a "chemical denervation." This latter antiadrenergic effect of bretylium may contribute to the antiarrhythmic action of the drug. However, its major antiarrhythmic effect is its direct electrophysiologic action on cardiac membrane. Characteristic of the class III agents, bretylium causes a marked prolongation of the AP duration and ERP. In canine hearts with infarcted areas, the drug decreases the disparity in AP duration between the normal and infarcted regions. These properties may be responsible for the ability of bretylium to lower the electrical threshold for successful defibrillation and to induce "chemical" defibrillation by itself.

THERAPEUTIC USE

Both the release of norepinephrine and the subsequent neuron blockade by bretylium result because this agent is taken up by nerve terminals by the catecholamine uptake process and concentrated. Pretreatment of the patient with drugs that block neuronal catecholamine uptake, such as protriptyline (tricyclic antidepressant), will prevent both the early hypertensive as well as the subsequent hypotensive phase while having no effect on the cardiac membrane actions of bretylium. Protection of the heart from the initial catecholamine released may also be provided by pretreatment with a beta blocker.

Bretylium is used for the treatment of ventricular tachycardia and other life-threatening arrhythmias refractory to other drug therapy or cardioversion. Bretylium may be used as a first-line drug in the treatment of ventricular fibrillation. It may terminate the fibrillation on its own — chemical defibrillation — or it may improve the efficacy of electrical cardioversion.

PHARMACOKINETICS

Bretylium is administered either IV or IM. Distribution after IV injection is almost immediate; however, the onset of antiarrhythmic action depends on accumulation of bretylium in myocardial tissue as well as the arrhythmia being treated. In ventricular fibrillation, onset of action is 5–10 minutes; in ventricular tachycardia, 20–120 minutes. Bretylium accumulates to high levels in sympathetic ganglia and postganglionic adrenergic neurons. Its volume of distribution is approximately 6 liters/kg.

Elimination

Bretylium is eliminated entirely by renal excretion of unchanged drug. The half-life is 8–12 hours but may increase to 16–32 hours in patients with impaired renal function.

ADVERSE EFFECTS

Bretylium causes increased ectopic activity and elevated blood pressure in the initial 20–30 minutes after IV injection. Subsequently, it causes hypotension, which is rarely symptomatic but may be accompanied by dizziness, lightheadedness, or fainting. Nausea and vomiting may occur, particularly when the drug is given by rapid intravenous injection. Bretylium should be used with caution in patients with aortic stenosis. The fall in peripheral resistance cannot be compensated for by an increase in cardiac output in these patients, and they may experience a marked hypotension.

PATIENT MONITORING

Hypersensitivity to infused catecholamines, such as dopamine and dobutamine, is seen presumably as a result of the impaired uptake of these catecholamines into nerve terminals. The patient should be carefully monitored as the dose of these agents may need to be reduced. Both ECG and blood pressure should be monitored throughout therapy.

PREPARATIONS AND DOSAGES

Injection: 50 mg/ml.
IV: *Adult* — for immediate control of life-threatening ventricular fibrillation, administer 5 mg/kg of undiluted bretylium by rapid injection. Dosage may be increased to 10 mg/kg and repeated as needed. For control of VT and other arrhythmias, 1 ampule (10 ml) is diluted with at least 50 ml of dextrose injection or sodium chloride injection. A dose of 5–10 mg/kg may be infused slowly over 8 or more minutes. This dose may be repeated in 1–2 hours. Maintenance — IV infusion of diluted solution may be given at a rate of 5–10 mg/kg body weight over a 10- to 30-minute period every 6–8 hours. Alternatively, bretylium may be administered by continuous IV infusion of the diluted solution at a rate of 1–2 mg/minute.
IM: *Adult* — initially, 5–10 mg/kg body weight administered undiluted. Dose may be repeated every 1–2 hours as needed. Maintenance — 5–10 mg/kg body weight administered undiluted every 6–8 hours.

Properties of Individual Class IV Antiarrhythmic Drugs

The class IV antiarrhythmic agents, the Ca^{2+} channel blockers, act by inhibiting the entry of Ca^{2+} into both cardiac and vascular smooth muscle cells via voltage-dependent Ca^{2+} channels. There are three Ca^{2+} antagonists currently available in the United States, all of which act by the same mechanism. However, there are important differences in effectiveness at different sites. For example, nifedipine blocks Ca^{2+} channels in vascular smooth muscle at concentrations approximately one-tenth those necessary to block Ca^{2+} channels in cardiac muscle. Thus, the most predominant effect of this agent in therapeutic concentrations is vasodilation. On the other hand, verapamil blocks Ca^{2+} channels in heart and vascular smooth muscle at the same concentration. Thus, this agent affects both heart and blood vessel function at therapeutic concentrations. Diltiazem is intermediate between verapamil and nifedipine, tending to resemble verapamil more closely. Since diltiazem and verapamil are qualitatively similar in their pharmacologic effects on the heart and are the two currently available Ca^{2+} channel blockers used to treat arrhythmias, the pharmacology and therapeutic use of these agents will be reviewed together.

DILTIAZEM HYDROCHLORIDE AND VERAPAMIL HYDROCHLORIDE

Pharmacology

The Ca^{2+} channel blocking agents block voltage-dependent Ca^{2+} channels of cardiac muscle, pacemaker, and conducting tissue. Thus, they reduce intracellular Ca^{2+} concentration and may decrease cardiac contractility. Such a blockade of the Ca^{2+} channel in myocardial cells becomes important in cases of preexisting depressed cardiac function. The Ca^{2+} channel blockers may reduce heart rate by decreasing the rate of entry during the 0 phase of the Ca^{2+}-dependent AP in the SA node, an effect that is modest in healthy subjects. The most dramatic, clinically important effect of Ca^{2+} channel blockers is on the AV node, where the rate of rise of the 0 phase of the AP is slowed, resulting in decreased AV nodal conduction and increased duration of the ERP. Thus, conduction through the AV node is slowed to the point of partial AV block by Ca^{2+} channel blockers. Total AV block may be seen as a component of the toxicity of these agents. The major effect of Ca^{2+} channel blockers on the ECG is a prolongation of the PR interval.

Therapeutic Use

The Ca^{2+} channel blockers have their greatest use in treatment of supraventricular tachyarrhythmias. PSVT is most commonly caused by AV nodal reentrant tachycardia involving a dual AV nodal pathway or an accessory AV bypass tract such as those seen in WPW syndrome, or it may result from sinus nodal reentrant tachycardia. The Ca^{2+} channel blockers are effective in interrupting these reentrant pathways by slowing conduction in the SA or AV node. Occasionally, these agents may increase conduction velocity along the accessory pathway and in patients with WPW syndrome and atrial tachycardia, flutter, or fibrillation, the ventricular rate may be increased to dangerous levels. Electrophysiologic testing must be performed to determine if the patient is susceptible to this adverse effect.

In the treatment of atrial flutter and fibrillation, the Ca^{2+} channel blockers cause reversion to normal sinus rhythm in a small fraction of the patients. In the remainder, these agents produce sufficient AV block to slow the ventricular response and thus provide protection for the ventricles.

Diltiazem Hydrochloride

PHARMACOKINETICS

Absorption and Distribution

Diltiazem is rapidly and nearly completely absorbed after oral administration. However, it undergoes extensive first-pass metabolism with a bioavailability of 40% initially. After continuous therapy, the bioavailability increases to 90%, indicating saturation of metabolism or negative feedback inhibition by metabolic products. The time to reach peak plasma concentration is quite variable, ranging between 30 minutes and 3 hours. Diltiazem is 70–80% plasma protein bound and exhibits a volume of distribution of 5.3 liters/kg.

Elimination

Diltiazem undergoes extensive metabolism with only a small fraction, 2–4%, being excreted in the urine unchanged. The half-life of diltiazem is 3–5 hours initially, and increases to 4–6 hours with continued therapy. The half-life is also increased in hepatic dysfunction.

ADVERSE EFFECTS

The major adverse effects of diltiazem relate to its cardiac effects and are generally observed only in patients with preexisting disease of pacemaker, conducting, or contractile tissue. These effects include second- or third-degree AV block, possibly leading to bradycardia; hypotension caused by severe reduction in cardiac contractility; and peripheral vasodilation and severe arrhythmias in patients with WPW syndrome. Rarely, SA node arrest is seen.

Other side effects — dizziness or lightheadedness; headache; nausea; swelling of the ankles, feet, or lower legs; and skin rash — occur rarely. This drug is fairly well tolerated, rarely requiring discontinuation because of side effects.

PREPARATIONS AND DOSAGES

Tablets: 30, 60, and 90 mg.
Oral: *Adults* — initially 30 mg 3 or 4 times daily. The dose may be increased gradually at 1- or 2-day intervals to a maximum of 240 mg daily (U.S.P.-DI) or 360 mg daily (AMA drug evaluations).

Verapamil Hydrochloride

PHARMACOKINETICS

Absorption and Distribution

Verapamil is rapidly, nearly completely absorbed from the gastrointestinal tract after oral administration. However, it undergoes marked first-pass metabolism. Consequently, oral availability may be only 10–35%. Peak plasma concentration is achieved in 1½–2½ hours. Verapamil is 90% plasma protein bound and exhibits a volume of distribution of 4 liters/kg.

Elimination

Only a small fraction of verapamil, 3–4%, is excreted in the urine unchanged. Verapamil undergoes N-dealkylation. The major metabolite is norverapamil, which has about 20% of the cardioactivity of verapamil. During long-term therapy, plasma levels of norverapamil exceed those of the parent compound, and the metabolite may contribute to the therapeutic effect. Verapamil has an initial half-life of 4–6 hours. However, it increases to 7–13 hours with chronic therapy and may be markedly prolonged in patients with liver disease.

ADVERSE EFFECTS

The major adverse effects of verapamil relate to its cardiac effects and are generally observed only in patients with preexisting disease of pacemaker, conducting, or contractile tissue. These effects include second- or third- degree AV block, possibly leading to bradycardia; hypotension caused by severe reduction in cardiac contractility; and peripheral vasodilation and severe arrhythmias in patients with WPW syndrome. Congestive heart failure can be worsened in patients with underlying left ventricular dysfunction.

Additional side effects occur frequently: unusual tiredness dizziness, or lightheadedness; headache; nausea; constipation; and swelling of the ankles, feet, or lower legs.

PREPARATIONS AND DOSAGES

Tablets: 80 and 120 mg.
Injection: 2.5 mg/ml.
Extended-release tablets: 120 mg.
IV: *Adults* — initially, 5–10 mg/kg body weight administered over a 2-minute period (Administer this dose over a 3-minute period in geriatric patients to minimize undesired effects.) Repeat in 5–10 minutes, if necessary. For maintenance, an infusion of 0.005 mg/kg/min may be used. *Pediatric* — infants up to 1 year of age, initially 0.1–0.2 mg/kg; children 1–15 years of age, initially 0.1–0.3 mg/kg body weight, not to exceed a total of 5 mg. For repeated dose, wait 30 minutes after initial dose and do not exceed 10 mg as a single dose.
Oral: Initially, dose is 80 mg every 6–8 hours, with titration every 24–48 hours for a maximum dose of 120 mg every 6 hours. With extended-release tablets, initial dose is 120 mg/day up to 480 mg/day.

Appendix
Antiarrhythmic Drug Interactions

Interacting drug	Drug interaction	Recommendation
Acecainide Hydrochloride (NAPA)		
Cimetidine	May reduce renal clearance of acecainide.	Monitor patient for adverse reactions and reduce acecainide dose if necessary.
Amiodarone Hydrochloride		
Beta blockers	Amiodarone may cause bradycardia, possibly by noncompetitive beta blockade. This action is additive with that of beta blockers. Combination may cause AV block or sinus arrest.	Avoid this combination, or monitor patient carefully throughout period of establishing stable dose of amiodarone for sinus arrhythmia, bradycardia, or progressive AV block.
Quinidine	Amiodarone increases serum levels of quinidine and may lead to quinidine toxicity including ventricular arrhythmias.	Monitor patient for signs of cardiotoxicity throughout time of stabilization of amiodarone dose and reduce quinidine dose as needed.
Digoxin	Amiodarone increases digoxin blood levels, possibly leading to symptoms of digitalis toxicity.	Monitor patient for signs of digitalis toxicity and reduce digoxin dosage as needed.
Beta Blockers		
Chlorpromazine (and possibly other phenothiazines)	Combination may lead to significant increase of bioavailability of propranolol. Mechanism is unknown, but may be result of decreased first-pass hepatic metabolism of propranolol.	Patients should be monitored for development of delirium, seizures, hypotension, or other adverse effects. It may be necessary to lower the dosage of either propranolol or chlorpromazine.

Interacting drug	Drug interaction	Recommendation
Ca^{2+} channel blocking agents	In patients with impaired AV or SA nodal function the drugs may produce hypotension, bradycardia, or AV block. A pharmacologic addition of Ca^{2+} channel blocking effects on AV and SA nodes plus beta blocking effect removes sympathetic tone.	Combination of Ca^{2+} channel blocking agents and beta blockers is therapeutically beneficial and does not result in adverse effects in patients without underlying disease. Patients should be carefully selected for combination therapy, and heart rate and blood pressure should be monitored in first few days of therapy.
Clonidine (interacts with propranolol and timolol, but not labetalol or, theoretically, cardioselective beta blockers, such as atenolol and metoprolol)	Clonidine and propranolol may be combined to treat hypertension. Adverse drug reaction occurs with rapid discontinuation of clonidine, resulting in sympathetic activity: tremor, insomnia, nausea, apprehension, flushing, headache, and rapid blood pressure elevation caused by rebound increase in sympathetic activity. Blood pressure elevation because of increased α-receptor-mediated vasoconstriction while β_2-adrenergic receptors are blocked.	When clonidine is to be combined with beta blocker, one should use cardioselective beta blockers or labetalol, which blocks both β- and α-receptors. Alternatively, when propranolol is used, propranolol therapy should be discontinued well in advance of discontinuing clonidine therapy.

Interacting drug	Drug interaction	Recommendation
Cimetidine (interacts with propranolol, metoprolol, labetalol, and other hepatically metabolized beta blockers)	Combination of cimetidine and propranolol results in substantial elevation of hepatic blood flow and may result in a reduction in the extraction metabolism of propranolol, leading to elevated propranolol blood levels.	Monitor patient for excessive beta blocking activity and reduce dose of either beta blocker or cimetidine as needed. Beta blockers that do not undergo extensive hepatic metabolism such as atenolol or pindolol may be preferred to propranolol in combination with cimetidine.
Epinephrine (ephedrine) (interacts with all nonselective beta blocking agents except labetolol) (phenylephrine)	Epinephrine administration in presence of propranolol may result in marked blood pressure elevation and reflex reduction in heart rate. Most likely mechanism involves activation of vascular α-receptors. Vasoconstriction and blood pressure elevation are marked because vasodilative β-receptors are blocked.	Combination of sympathomimetic agents with α-agonist activity plus propranolol or other nonselective beta blockers should be avoided. Possibility of hypertensive crisis is much less with cardioselective beta blockers.
Furosemide	Furosemide plus propranolol results in elevation of propranolol blood levels with increase in β-adrenergic blockade. Mechanism is unknown.	Combination of propranolol plus furosemide may be used; however, patients should be monitored for excess β-adrenergic blockade. Reduced dose of either agent may be necessary.

Interacting drug	Drug interaction	Recommendation
Insulin (interacts with nonselective beta blocking agents)	In hypoglycemic episode caused by insulin, propranolol will slow recovery from hypoglycemic event and mask symptoms such as heart rate and blood pressure increase. Propranolol may exacerbate hypertensive response some hypoglycemics experience. Mechanism may involve propranolol-induced block of insulin release from pancreatic cells.	If beta blocking drug is required in diabetic patient, cardioselective blocking agent is preferred. These have little effect on rate of recovery from hypoglycemic episode but may still mask cardiovascular symptoms of hypoglycemia.
Indomethacin (interacts with propranolol and, theoretically, all other beta blocking agents)	Indomethacin attenuates blood-pressure-lowering effect of propranolol. May do this by its ability to elevate blood pressure. Alternatively, indomethacin's ability to inhibit prostaglandin synthesis may reduce synthesis of vasodilator prostaglandin.	Patient's blood pressure must be monitored during combined therapy. Loss of blood pressure control will require either increase in propranolol dose or discontinuation of indomethacin.
Methyldopa (interacts with propranolol and other nonselective beta blocking agents)	Propranolol plus methyldopa may cause hypertensive crisis. Methyldopa converts to methylnorepinephrine in adrenergic nerve terminals, contributing to greater neurotransmitter release during sympathetic activity. β-Receptor blockade with unopposed α-receptor activity results in vasoconstriction.	This drug combination does not provide any particular therapeutic advantage and should be avoided.

Interacting drug	Drug interaction	Recommendation
Prazosin (interacts with propranolol and, theoretically, all other beta blocking agents)	Prazosin exhibits first-dose hypotensive reaction in a small percentage of patients. Propranolol may enhance hypotensive reaction. Beta blockers probably contribute to this response through reduced cardiac output.	Prazosin treatment should be initiated with dose of 0.5 mg or less and blood pressure monitored during first few hours of therapy. It is preferable to give first dose at bedtime.
Theophylline (and aminophylline) (interacts with propranolol and other nonselective beta blocking agents)	Theophylline is used to improve airway function in lungs. Beta blockers attenuate this action by blocking β-receptors in lungs and increasing bronchial resistance.	Therapeutic response to theophylline should be monitored and dose of theophylline increased as needed. Cardioselective beta blockers are less likely to interact in this way.
Thyroid (interacts with propranolol and metoprolol tartrate)	Hyperthyroid patients exhibit decreased bioavailability of propranolol and metoprolol. Thus, thyroid supplementation may have similar effect. This interaction is not seen with beta blockers that do not undergo major first-pass metabolism (atenolol, nadolol, and pindolol).	When thyroid and beta blocker therapy are used in combination, patient should be monitored for loss of therapeutic effect, and dose of beta blocking agent increased as needed. Alternatively, beta blockers that do not undergo major first-pass metabolism may be used.

Interacting drug	Drug interaction	Recommendation
Tobacco (interacts with propranolol and metoprolol)	Smoking increases propranolol clearance, possibly by induction of hepatic microsomal enzymes.	Patients receiving propranolol therapy who are smokers may require larger doses than nonsmokers. Adverse drug reaction occurs if patient stops smoking while taking propranolol. Metabolism of propranolol decreases and serum levels increase, necessitating reduction in propranolol dose.
Tubocurarine (and, theoretically, all other neuromuscular blocking agents) (interacts with propranolol and, theoretically, all other beta blocking agents)	Propranolol prolongs neuromuscular blockade produced by tubocurarine.	Patients receiving propranolol may exhibit unexpected prolongation of neuromuscular blockade leading to respiratory depression and apnea. Effects of neurotransmitter-blocking drugs may be reversed by administration of neostigmine (1–3 mg) with atropine (0.6–1.2 mg).
Bretylium Tosylate		
Digitalis	Bretylium causes norepinephrine release from adrenergic nerve terminals when it is first injected, and this may aggravate digitalis toxicity.	Avoid combination of bretylium and digitalis.

Interacting drug	Drug interaction	Recommendation
Ca^{2+} Channel Blockers		
Beta blockers (interact with diltiazem hydrochloride and verapamil hydrochloride)	Beta blockers prolong AV conduction by removing sympathetic tone to AV node. Ca^{2+} channel blockers also prolong AV conduction, and drug combination may produce substantial AV block.	When beta blockers and Ca^{2+} channel blockers are combined, ECG should be monitored regularly during early phase of therapy and intermittently thereafter. Alternatively, the Ca^{2+} channel blocker nifedipine may be substituted. Nifedipine has a much more marked effect on vasculature than heart at therapeutic doses and is less likely to affect AV nodal function.
Calcium gluconate	Ca^{2+} supplementation reduces or eliminates therapeutic effect of verapamil hydrochloride and other Ca^{2+} channel blockers, apparently because of direct competition between Ca^{2+} and verapamil hydrochloride at level of Ca^{2+} channel.	Patient should be monitored for possible reduction of therapeutic response to verapamil hydrochloride and dose of verapamil hydrochloride adjusted as necessary.
Digitalis glycosides	Digitalis glycosides prolong AV nodal induction and may induce AV block when combined with Ca^{2+} channel blocking agents. Excessive AV block or SA nodal depression may occur.	Monitor patient's ECG and reduce digitalis dose as necessary.

Interacting drug	Drug interaction	Recommendation
Disopyramide phosphate	Both disopyramide and Ca^{2+} channel blocking agents may exert a negative inotropic effect, particularly with underlying cardiac dysfunction. Combination may cause dramatic worsening of cardiac function or cardiac decompensation.	Avoid this combination.
Quinidine	See Quinidine below.	
Digoxin		
Verapamil hydrochloride, quinidine, amiodarone hydrochloride, nifedipine, flecainide acetate, propafenone	Clear and clinically important increases in serum digoxin concentration have been observed when digoxin was combined with quinidine or verapamil hydrochloride. There is evidence that amiodarone hydrochloride, nifedipine, flecainide acetate, and propafenone also increase serum digoxin levels, though clinical importance has not been established. These drugs decrease renal or nonrenal clearance (or both) of digoxin.	When digoxin and quinidine are combined, digoxin dose should be reduced up to 50%. While it may not be necessary to reduce digoxin dose with verapamil hydrochloride and other interacting antiarrhythmic agents, patient must be monitored for signs of digitalis toxicity, and serum digoxin levels should be assessed.
Disopyramide Phosphate		
Beta blockers	Beta blockers prolong AV conduction and decrease cardiac contractility. Both actions are shared by disopyramide and represent particular risk for patients with any degree of cardiac impairment. Total AV block or congestive heart failure or both may result.	Avoid this combination.

Interacting drug	Drug interaction	Recommendation
Ca^{2+} channel blocking agents	See Ca^{2+} Channel Blockers above.	
Lidocaine, procainamide, quinidine, tocainide	In patients with compromised cardiac function, disopyramide combined with any of these agents may exacerbate depressed cardiac function or AV block or both.	Monitor ECG and other measures of cardiac function during initial stages of combined therapy and intermittently thereafter.
Timolide	Combination may potentiate cardiac arrhythmias.	Avoid this combination.
Lidocaine		
Cimetidine	Combination results in reduction in lidocaine clearance and prolongation of lidocaine half-life. Lidocaine toxicity may result. Mechanism is unknown; however, metabolism of lidocaine may be reduced by either cimetidine-induced inhibition of microsomal enzymes or reduction in hepatic blood flow.	Patient should be monitored for increasing plasma concentrations of lidocaine and toxicity, and lidocaine dose should be reduced as necessary. Alternatively, ranitidine may be substituted for cimetidine.
Propranolol hydrochloride	Propranolol decreases metabolism and lidocaine clearance, leading to increase in lidocaine serum levels. This may lead to lidocaine toxicity. Mechanism is unknown; however, propranolol reduces lidocaine metabolism either through its beta blocking effect, by decreasing cardiac output and hepatic blood flow, or by inhibiting hepatic drug metabolism.	Infused dose of lidocaine given to patient receiving beta blocker therapy may need to be reduced. Serum concentrations of lidocaine should be monitored and dose reduced as needed.

Interacting drug	Drug interaction	Recommendation
Succinylcholine chloride	Lidocaine may prolong and increase neuromuscular blocking action of succinylcholine, thus prolonging apnea. Mechanism of interaction is unknown; however, respiratory depression caused by lidocaine acting in central nervous system may be important component.	Patients receiving both lidocaine and succinylcholine must be continually monitored to determine need for artificial ventilation.
Quinidine		
Phenobarbital, phenytoin, rifampin	All three drugs reduce half-life and plasma concentration of quinidine. Capacity of each of these drugs to induce hepatic microsomal enzymes, and therefore increase metabolism of quinidine, is probably underlying mechanism.	Quinidine plasma levels and antiarrhythmic effect should be monitored during combined therapy of quinidine plus any of these interacting drugs. Quinidine dose may be increased as needed. Potential risk of combined therapy lies in enhanced quinidine plasma concentration and resulting toxicity on withdrawal of interacting drug.
Verapamil hydrochloride	Quinidine plus verapamil may cause hypotension in patients with hypertrophic cardiomyopathy. As both drugs can decrease cardiac contractility, their pharmacologic actions are additive, resulting in worsening cardiac function and decrease in cardiac output. Capacity of quinidine to block α-adrenergic receptors may also contribute.	Avoid this combination.

Interacting drug	Drug interaction	Recommendation
Warfarin sodium (and other anticoagulant drugs that act by inhibiting vitamin K–dependent clotting factors)	Quinidine has mild anticoagulant action of its own, which may be based on its ability to inhibit production of vitamin K–dependent clotting factors. Thus pharmacologic actions of quinidine and warfarin sodium are additive, causing exaggerated prolongation of prothrombin time.	Avoid this combination. Use other antiarrhythmic agents that do not interact with warfarin sodium.

References

1. Ahlquist, R. P. A study of the adrenotropic receptors. *Am. J. Physiol.* 153:586, 1948.
2. Anderson, S., et al. The Esmolol vs Placebo Multicenter Study Group. *Am. Heart J.* 111:42, 1986.
3. Cranefield, D. F., and Aronson, R. S. Initiation of sustained rhythmic activity by single propagated action potentials in canine cardiac Purkinje fibers exposed to sodium-free solution or to ouabain. *Circ. Res.* 34:477, 1974.
4. Durrer, D., et al. Preexcitation revisited. *Am. J. Cardiol.* 25:690, 1970.
5. Jervall, A., and Lange-Nielsen, F. Congenital deaf mutism: Functional heart disease with prolongation of the QT interval and sudden death. *Am. Heart J.* 54:59, 1957.
6. Pelleg, A. Cardiac cellular electrophysiologic actions of adenosine and adenosine triphosphate. *Am. Heart J.* 110:688, 1985.
7. Romano, C., et al. Aritmie cardiache rare dell'eta pediatrica: II. Accessi sincopali per fibrillazone ventricolare parossistica. *Clin. Pediatr.* (Bolgona) 45:656, 1963.
8. Rossi, L. Conduction and nervous system of the heart in atrial arrhythmias: A clinicopathological study of 33 cases. *Acta Cardiol.* (Brux.) 21:34, 1966.
9. Schmitt, F. O., and Erlanger, J. Directional differences in the conduction of the impulse through heart muscle and their possible relation to extrasystolic and fibrillary contractions. *Am. J. Physiol.* 871:326, 1928–29.
10. Singh, B. N. Amiodarone: Historical development and pharmacologic profile. *Am. Heart J.* 106:788, 1983.
11. Ward, O. C. New familial cardiac syndrome in children. *J. Ir. Med. Assoc.* 54:103, 1964.
12. Wellens, H. J. J., et al. The management of preexcitation syndromes. *J.A.M.A.* 257:2325, 1987.
13. Zwerling, H. K. Does exogenous magnesium suppress myocardial irritability and tachyarrhythmias in the nondigitalized patient? *Am. Heart J.* 113:1046, 1987.

Selected Reading

ARTICLES

Dreifus, L. S. Cardiac arrhythmias in the elderly: Clinical aspects. *Cardiol. Clin.* 4:273, 1986.

Heger, J. J., et al. Clinical use and pharmacology of amiodarone. *Med. Clin. North Am.* 68:1339, 1984.

Kates, R. E. Metabolites of cardiac antiarrhythmic drugs: Their clinical role. *Ann. N.Y. Acad. Sci.* 75:89, 1984.

Williams, E. M. A classification of antiarrhythmic actions reassessed after a decade of new drugs. *J. Clin. Pharmacol.* 24:129, 1984.

BOOKS

American Medical Associaton. Drug Evaluations (6th ed.), 1986.

Dreifus, L.S. (ed.). *Cardiac Arrhythmias: Electrophysiologic Techniques and Management* (Vol. 16, No. 1). Philadelphia: Davis, 1985.

Levy, M. N., and Vassalle, M. (ed.). *Excitation and Neural Control of the Heart*. American Physiological Society, 1982.

3

Arterial Hypertension

Pathophysiology of Primary (Essential) Hypertension

A sustained elevation of arterial blood pressure (hypertension) is a common disease and is the most serious chronic disease in humans amenable to successful therapeutic management. In some populations, nearly 20% of all adults may have the disease; in the United States, by some estimates, at least 20 million people have hypertension. Epidemiologic studies generally concur that a reduced morbidity and mortality follows a lowering of elevated blood pressure to normotensive levels.

Episodic elevation of arterial blood pressure is part of the adaptation process of humans to their environment. Such elevations are brought about by interactions between the autonomic nervous and endocrine (neuroendocrine) systems that affect:

contractile properties of the heart
arterial and arteriolar contraction
volume of circulatory fluid

Aberrant neuroendocrine interactions affecting contractile properties of the heart, arterial and arteriolar contraction, and the volume of circulatory fluid may lead to a permanent elevation of arterial blood pressure.

The neuroendocrine processes that affect arterial blood pressure levels are:

I. Adrenergic neural impulse $\xrightarrow{\text{norepinephrine}}$ receptor
$\longrightarrow$ muscle cell (myocardial and/or arterial)

Higher levels of enzyme activities involved in the biosynthesis of tissue norepinephrine from hypertensive compared to normotensive men of similar age, along with elevated plasma norepinephrine and epinephrine levels in some hypertensives (which correlates in a positive manner with blood pressure increases), provide strong support for increased sympathetic activity in hypertension.

Baroreceptor reflexes may also play a role in the elevated sympathetic activity associated with hypertension. Blood pressure increases, detected by the baroreceptors of the aortic arch and carotid sinus, increase vagal activity and reduce sympathetic stimulation, while a decrease in baroreceptor sensitivity in hypertensive patients and in elderly patients reduces the response to blood pressure increases and results in a higher sympathetic outflow from the central nervous system.

II. Adrenergic neural impulse $\xrightarrow{\text{norepinephrine}}$ receptor $\xrightarrow{\text{renin}}{\text{substrate}}$ smooth muscle cell angiotensin II endocrine gland

In the type II neuroendocrine process, released norepinephrine interacts with receptors on specific cells of the juxtaglomerular apparatus located in the afferent renal arterial wall and causes the release of the proteolytic enzyme renin. Circulating renin acts on renin-substrate, α-2 globulin, and cleaves off a decapeptide, angiotensin I. Angiotensin I, in turn, is converted by angiotensin-converting enzyme to an octapeptide, angiotensin II (A-II). Angiotensin-converting enzyme is located on the plasma membranes of pulmonary vascular endothelial cells. While angiotensin I is essentially inert, A-II is a potent vasoconstrictor that can directly elevate blood pressure. In addition, A-II acts on peripheral adrenergic nerves to facilitate the release of norepinephrine and thereby amplifies the vasoconstrictor response of A-II. A-II may act in the central nervous system to enhance sympathetic outflow. All of these actions contribute to angiotensin's marked capacity to induce vasoconstriction.

A-II also stimulates aldosterone synthesis and release by the adrenal glomerulosa cells. Aldosterone acts on the distal tubule of the kidney, where it facilitates reabsorption of Na^+ in exchange for either K^+ or hydrogen (H^+) ion. The reabsorption of Na^+ is accompanied by an anion, usually chloride (Cl^-), which creates an osmotic drive for the reabsorption of water from the glomerular filtrate. Thus, a major consequence of the action of the renin-angiotensin–aldosterone axis is the expansion of plasma volume.

Plasma renin activity varies among patients with essential hypertension; approximately 20% will have low renin levels, while another 15% have high renin levels [7]. Recognition of plasma renin activity may be useful in drug selection for the treatment of hypertension. Other authors disagree about the utility of plasma renin activity measurements in the management of hypertension. The following categories of patients may benefit from plasma renin activity determinations [11]:

1. Patients who become refractory to medications because of the development of renovascular disease (resistant hypertension)
2. Young patients with target organ damage and severe hypertension
3. Patients in whom primary aldosteronism is suspected
4. Patients with severe hypertension.

The type III neuroendocrine process (Fig. 3-1) located in the phylogenetically "old" part of the brain, may play a key role in regulating the diurnal or circadian rhythms involved in fluid and electrolyte metabolism. The principal product, vasopressin or antidiuretic hormone (ADH), acts to prevent salt-free water loss in the renal tubule by stimulating water and sodium uptake by renal cells as well as by cells in general. Both type II and III neuroendocrine processes are involved in regulating the circulatory plasma volume.

Fig. 3-1. Neuroendocrine process involved in regulating plasma volume.

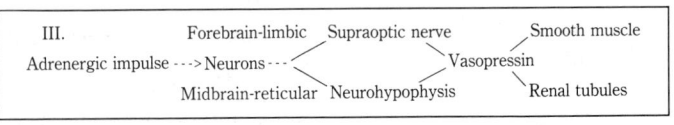

```
III.              Forebrain-limbic   Supraoptic nerve          Smooth muscle
Adrenergic impulse --->Neurons ---<                  Vasopressin
                  Midbrain-reticular  Neurohypophysis          Renal tubules
```

Nearly all studies agree that, in hypertension, plasma volume declines with increasing peripheral resistance, while interstitial fluid volume and blood pressure levels increase in parallel. Such increases in interstitial fluid volume may reflect parallel rises in arteriolar and venular smooth muscle tone and capillary filtration pressure, thereby causing outward movement of fluid from the plasma.

HEMODYNAMIC CONSEQUENCES OF ABERRANT TYPE I, II, AND III NEUROENDOCRINE PROCESSES IN HYPERTENSION

While there are variations in hemodynamic patterns between hypertensive patients, cardiac output and heart rate tend to be higher, in part caused by increased adrenergic autonomic activity and a larger central blood volume in mild or borderline hypertension. In this setting, the time for cardiac filling is prolonged and, eventually, stroke volume is reduced. In more severe hypertension, medial muscle and intimal layer thickening in arteries reduces the capacity of the vessel and sustains an elevated peripheral resistance. Hypertrophic changes in the heart then restore cardiac output to normal. With hypertension, the plasma volume tends to be increased initially in the central pulmonary area as a result of high venular tone. An increased central blood volume increases cardiac output in early hypertension by enhancing left ventricular preload.

DIVALENT CATIONS, CALCIUM AND MAGNESIUM, AND PRIMARY HYPERTENSION

In some manner, the levels of serum ionized calcium (Ca^{2+}) and magnesium (Mg^{2+}) are related to plasma renin activity in patients with hypertension. The range of plasma renin activity is negatively related to serum Mg^{2+} and positively related to serum Ca^{2+} and low blood pressure values [13]. It was subsequently learned that with low plasma renin hypertension, low serum Ca^{2+} levels, and dietary salt sensitivity (in black and elderly hypertensive patients), Ca^{2+} supplementation may lower the blood pressure, thereby suggesting linkages between serum Ca^{2+}, the renin-aldosterone system, and Na^+ metabolism.

CHANGES IN SPECIFIC ORGANS AND SYSTEMS WITH HYPERTENSION

Heart

Cardiac hypertrophy is a compensatory mechanism for hypertension, caused in part by raised preloads and afterloads and increased work. However, cardiac diastolic dysfunction, as reflected by a delayed rate of rapid left ventricle filling, occurs before changes in the ejection fraction, cardiac output, and peak left ventricular ejection rates appear. Neither blood pressure nor an increase in left ventricle mass explains the delayed rate of rapid left ventricle filling. A compelling body of evidence suggests participation of the heart in some manner with hypertension regulation and, in turn, that the heart itself is affected by hypertension. [16]. The heart modulates norepinephrine release by the autonomic nervous system by generating positive feedback hypertensive reflexes and influencing adrenergic suppressor reflexes from the cardiopulmonary area; levels of endogenous catecholamines may regulate the subsequent left ventricle mass in hypertension [18]. Additional evidence suggests an alpha adrenoceptor participation in maintaining cardiac hypertrophy; left ventricular hypertrophy in hypertensive patients treated with diuretics and beta blockers regressed with prazosin but not with hydralazine [8].

Progression of cardiac hypertrophy can be followed by echocardiography, even in cases with minimal blood pressure elevations. Hypertrophy begins in the septum and is followed by changes in posterior wall thickness. The hypertrophy is considered physiologic in that ventricular function is increased to overcome the increased afterload characteristic of hypertension. However, hypertrophy may slow the rate of ventricular relaxation (reduced diastolic function) (see Chap. 1), which, in turn, reduces stroke volume. However, this reduction is compensated in part as central blood volume is increased to raise ventricular preloading. In more severe hypertension, as the ventricle dilates, both the ejection fraction and stroke volume are reduced. Further dilatation ultimately results in congestive heart failure.

Left ventricular hypertrophy may also contribute to coronary artery disease. Progressive hypertension is almost invariably accompanied by atherosclerosis of the coronary arteries [4], reducing blood flow to the myocardium. The effects of atherosclerosis are compounded by the substantially greater oxygen requirement of the hypertrophied muscle mass, and angina and other forms of ischemic disease are likely to appear. Left ventricular hypertrophy (as revealed by electrocardiogram or echocardiogram) may increase the risk of sudden death. The mechanism underlying sudden death appears to be complex ventricular arrhythmias [10].

Arteries

Arteries change both structurally and functionally with the development of hypertension. Structurally, the wall thickens and the ratio of wall thickness to lumen diameter increases, while, functionally, peripheral resistance is higher in hypertensives than in normals, even after maximum vasodilation with autonomic blockade. Increased artery wall thickness of hypertension may be partially reversed by antihypertensive therapy, but, if untreated, hypertension induces fibrinoid necrosis and hyaline degeneration of the arterial medial layer. These structural changes extend from large- to small-sized arteries and render the arterial walls less compliant.

In addition to structural changes, vascular smooth muscle is often hyperactive to stimuli in the hypertensive patient. The mechanism of this hyperresponsiveness is likely to involve the increased "leakiness" of the vascular smooth muscle cell membrane, losses of intracellular K^+, and increases of intracellular Na^+. The increased intracellular Na^+, in turn, may lead to an ion exchange in which Na^+ moves out of the cell and Ca^{2+} moves in via the Na^+-Ca^{2+} exchange carrier.

Kidneys

In contrast to other organs, the kidneys experience a disproportionate decline in blood flow as hypertension progresses. The reduced blood flow is due to hypertrophy and increased responsiveness to vasoconstrictor substances of all blood vessels, including the renal vascular bed, as well as increased sympathetic neurogenic activity and circulating levels of angiotensin II. Atherosclerosis-mediated luminal reduction of large-sized renal arteries, as well as narrowing of afferent arterioles, contributes to a reduction in renal blood flow.

Reduction in blood flow, leading ultimately to renal dysfunction, is reflected by nocturia and albuminuria initially, but, with time, as glomeruli hyalinize and tubules atrophy, the glomerular filtration rate is reduced, and blood urea nitrogen and creatinine levels are elevated.

Pressure-natriuresis is a property of kidney function whereby elevations in blood pressure and, therefore, perfusion of the kidneys increases Na^+ and water excretion. The resultant fluid volume reduction serves to return elevated blood pressure levels to normal. However, in primary hypertension, natriuresis occurs at a relatively high arteriolar pressure [6]. With pressure-induced natriuresis, the reduced plasma volume lowers blood pressure, but not below the hypertension range. The resetting of the pressure-natriuresis relationship to a higher pressure range may involve increases in the extent of the renal efferent arteriole vasoconstriction and in the fraction of blood undergoing glomerular filtration. Thus, the relatively large quantities of water and salt leaving the blood increases the oncotic pressure of blood entering the peritubular capillary system and augments the reabsorption of salt and water back into the blood compartment.

Such evidence suggests a renal defect as a primary mechanism in the pathogenesis of hypertension. Epidemiologic evidence suggests that this defect is revealed in societies that consume large quantities of salt. In the United States, a typical 24-hour urine Na^+ excretion is approximately 200 mEq; while in third world peoples, such as the New Guinea Highlanders and Yanamamo Indians, 15 mEq or less is excreted over a 24-hour period, and hypertension is rare and does not correlate with age.

Arterial Hypertension Types

Hypertension in humans is not a single disease. At least four types of hypertension can be recognized at present, the most common being essential or primary hypertension. To further complicate matters, the clinical course of primary hypertension may be protracted (chronic) or rapid (malignant). Such clinical variations require a cautious therapeutic strategy on one hand, or an aggressive anticrisis approach on the other. Hypertension secondary to neurogenic renovascular, organic renal parenchymal, or endocrine (including an adrenal tumor) disorders or coarctation of the aorta may have a chronic or a malignant clinical course.

The major focus of this chapter is the treatment of essential or primary hypertension. First, normal arterial blood pressure and recognition of hypertensive subtypes by clinical means are addressed.

DIAGNOSIS AND CLASSIFICATION OF HYPERTENSION

Both systolic and diastolic arterial pressures (mm Hg) increase with age in males and females (117 ± 12 systolic and 73 ± 10 diastolic [mean $\pm$ standard deviation] at 16 years vs. 143 ± 22 and 85 ± 12 at 60–64 years). The major incremental rise in and frequency of blood pressure increases occurs after age 45. In general, the greatest range in arterial pressure is found in the older ages and among women. The lower limits for hypertension are given as 140 and 190 systolic and 90 and 110 diastolic at 16 and 60–64 years, respectively.

Once hypertension is identified, the subtypes related to the clinical course can be recognized by ophthalmoscopic findings. According to Wagner-Keith (more commonly referred to as K-W) [20], fundoscopic criteria provide a useful index of the fate of hypertensive patients. Table 3-1 lists K-W ophthalmoscopic criteria.

Group IV hypertension is properly named *malignant hypertension* due to the short life expectancy associated with this disease.

An additional element in the evaluation of patients with primary hypertension is an objective evaluation of the status of target organs of an elevated systemic arterial pressure. These include an electrocardiogram (ECG), chest x-ray and echocardiogram,

Table 3-1. K-W ophthalmoscopic criteria for hypertension groups

Group	Fundi	Prognosis (if untreated)
I	Narrowing of arterioles	Limited or no influence on life expectancy
II	Spasm and narrowing of arterioles; AV nicking with bulging of some veins; sclerosis of arteries; "copper wire" effect	Slight reduction of life expectancy
III	Changes of II + hemorrhaging and exudates; optic disc poorly defined	Definite reduction of life expectancy
IV	Changes of II and II + papilledema	1–2 years

urinalysis, blood creatinine or blood urea nitrogen (BUN), and possibly intravenous pyelography.

The questions of whether or not to treat mild to moderate (groups I and II) hypertension and at what level of blood pressure therapy should be initiated are answered largely by national epidemiologic study results. The Veterans Administration Cooperative Study [19] was the first to establish that antihypertensive therapy prevents deaths from strokes, congestive heart failure, and kidney disease. A clear reduction in morbidity and mortality was observed among middle-aged and elderly men with diastolic pressures between 90 and 114 mm Hg. The results of a second major study initiated in 1972 by the National Heart, Lung, and Blood Institute, which were released in 1979, provided the first direct evidence that treatment of high blood pressure is worthwhile in blacks, women, and younger people as well. The finding that patients with borderline hypertension (between 140/90 and 160/95) experienced a 20% lower mortality rate from all causes was particularly interesting.

GOALS OF THERAPY

The overall goal of therapy in the treatment of hypertension, therefore, is to reduce or prevent end-organ damage and other consequences of high blood pressure itself, and to eliminate elevated blood pressure as one of several factors operating to increase the overall risk of hypertensive cardiovascular disease. The specific goal is to lower the diastolic level of blood pressure to below 90 mm Hg. Given that essential hypertension is symptomless for most patients, an additional specific goal is to identify appropriate antihypertensive agents that not only lower blood pressure, but also cause few or no side effects, since therapy is generally lifelong and patient compliance is extremely important.

Two additional factors that are not yet goals of current drug therapy warrant consideration. The first concerns the effects of antihypertensive agents on plasma lipids. For example, the thiazide diuretics elevate low-density lipoprotein (LDL), cholesterol, and triglycerides, and beta blockers lower high-density lipoprotein (HDL) cholesterol. These drug-induced changes in lipid profile mimic those associated with increases in the overall risk factors of cardiovascular disease (see Chap. 5).

Does treatment with thiazide diuretics or beta blockers merely exchange one risk factor, high blood pressure, for another, high serum lipids? Presently, there is no answer to this important question; however, the thiazide diuretics and beta blockers have played a large role in the marked reduction in morbidity and mortality from essential hypertension that has occurred over the last two decades. Most authorities continue to recommend the use of these agents as significant components of the antihypertensive drug spectrum.

As discussed above, left ventricular hypertrophy invariably accompanies the development of hypertension and appears early in the disease. Left ventricular hypertrophy may be important as a risk factor, as it relates or contributes to ischemic heart disease.

Given that left ventricular hypertrophy is a risk factor for cardiovascular disease, should reduction of ventricular muscle mass be an additional goal of antihypertensive drug therapy? Several drugs, such as prazosin, clonidine, and methyldopa, the angiotensin-converting enzyme inhibitors, and possibly beta blocking agents may reduce left ventricular hypertrophy; however, the effect is seen only in approximately 50% of patients. Presently, no epidemiologic data are available to indicate life expectancy benefits from the reduction of left ventricular hypertrophy in essential hypertension.

Treatment of Primary (Essential) Hypertension

In selecting a therapeutic regimen for a given hypertensive patient, consideration should be given to the potential of drug-induced modification in the quality of life. Recently three relatively equivalent antihypertensive drugs — captopril, methyldopa, and propranolol — were compared for their effects on the quality of life in patients with mild to moderate hypertension. Captopril use was accompanied by improvement in the greatest number of quality of life measurements [2].

NUTRITIONAL THERAPY

Some less severe forms of hypertension (group I K-W) may be controlled by weight reduction, restriction of dietary salt, and perhaps supplemental calcium. Nearly 40% success with nutritional therapy alone was reported in a recent series [14].

CATEGORIES OF DRUGS

There are five major categories of antihypertensive drugs and scores of drugs are available within each category in most cases. This wide choice of drugs almost ensures that with careful selection, appropriate therapy can be identified for nearly all patients; that is, in each patient, the blood pressure will be lowered into normal range, side effects will be minimal or nonexistent, and compliance will be high. The categories of drugs are as follows:

Diuretics
    Thiazides
    Loop diuretics
    K^+-sparing diuretics
Sympathetic depressant drugs
    Centrally acting (i.e., methyldopa, clonidine)
    Peripherally acting (i.e., reserpine, guanethidine)
    Beta blockers (i.e., propranolol, metoprolol)
    Alpha blockers (i.e., prazosin)
Vasodilators (i.e., hydralazine, minoxidil)
Angiotensin converting enzyme (ACE) inhibitors (i.e., captopril, enalapril)

Calcium channel antagonists (i.e., verapamil, diltiazem, nifedipine)

GENERAL GUIDELINES FOR MONO-DRUG THERAPY (MONOTHERAPY)

Monotherapy, or treatment with one antihypertensive agent, is highly desirable because it is less confusing, has the highest likelihood of compliance, and reduces or eliminates the incidence of adverse drug interactions. A number of drugs may be effective as monotherapy, such as:

Thiazides
Beta blockers
Clonidine and guanabenz
ACE inhibitors
Calcium (Ca^{2+}) channel antagonists

GENERAL GUIDELINES FOR COMBINATION DRUG THERAPY

Certain drugs are not generally successful when used as monotherapy, for example, reserpine, guanethidine, and methyldopa. These sympathetic depressant drugs lower blood pressure initially but induce a "pseudo tolerance" over time, that is, an increase in plasma volume, which tends to elevate the blood pressure back to pretreatment levels. Consequently, these drugs are almost always used in combination with a diuretic.

Vasodilators, such as hydralazine, also induce an increase in plasma volume. In addition, these agents lower blood pressure by reducing peripheral resistance and, thereby, induce a reflex increase in cardiac output and heart rate. The vasodilators are almost always used in combination with a diuretic to lower plasma volume and a beta blocker to prevent the reflex cardiac effects.

THE "STEPPED CARE" APPROACH

Two or three decades ago, in the early days of antihypertensive therapy, the thiazides; the sympathetic depressant drugs, reserpine, methyldopa, and guanethidine; and the vasodilator hydralazine were the main therapeutic agents available. Accordingly, the "stepped care" approach utilized the drugs in the following schedule:

Step 1 — thiazide diuretics
Step 2 — sympathetic depressant drugs
Step 3 — vasodilator (hydralazine)
Step 4 — guanethidine

Step 1 was found sufficient in many cases of mild hypertension (diastolic—90–104 mm Hg). The addition of a second drug in step 2 was generally required for moderate hypertension (105–119 mm Hg). However, in some cases, a third drug was required (step 3). Severe hypertension (> 120 mm Hg) generally required a step 3 level treatment and possibly the addition of an adrenergic neuron blocking drug. Steps 2, 3, and 4 were combined for the management of malignant hypertension. As originally conceived, the stepped care approach involved initiating therapy at each step and increasing the dose of the drug until a maximal blood pressure lowering effect was obtained or side effects prevented further increases in dose. A drug from the next step was then added, and the dose was, again, increased to maximum effect; additional steps were added until the blood pressure was brought under control.

The stepped care approach continues to be used but has been dramatically modified. First, **only low doses are used at each step,** since, in many cases, the dose-pressor response to an antihypertensive agent is flat. Thus, little advantage is gained by increasing the dose. Second, **diuretics may not be the drug of choice as a first step.** Beta blockers or drugs from other categories may be used, followed by diuretics as the second step. The places of each drug in the current version of the stepped care approach is discussed in the section on the properties of individual antihypertensive agents.

Factors influencing the choice of diuretics over beta blockers are:

Less expensive
Fewer side effects
Greater efficacy in the elderly ($>$ 65 years of age)
Greater efficacy in blacks
Fewer drug interactions

Factors affecting the choice of beta blockers over diuretics are:

Particular efficacy in the young with systolic hypertension
Greater efficacy in patients with recent myocardial infarction or migraine headaches

An appropriate plan in considering antihypertensive drug therapy is to first outline a list of drugs, taking into account the age, sex, and ethnicity of the patient, and the severity of the Primary Hypertension as judged by the level of blood pressure and fundoscopic findings using the accepted K-W criteria.

GROUPS I AND II (K-W) PRIMARY HYPERTENSION

Patients with group 1 or 2 primary hypertension have mild hypertension — 90–99 mm Hg diastolic pressure — and low or normal plasma renin levels and are best treated by the following regimen:

Genuine effort to normalize blood pressure with non-drug treatment for a 3- to 6-month period (dietary regimen of Na^+ restriction and weight regulation)
If control is not achieved with a non-drug regimen, **then administer** β-adrenoceptor antagonists (beta blockers) for young whites; patients with a recent myocardial infarction or a hyperkinetic cardiovascular system (tachyarrhythmias); individuals with angina pectoris, who are volume contracted, and/or who have history of hypokalemia, migraine, or gout
ACE-inhibitor drugs, which are potent and effective antihypertensive agents and are used with increasing frequency as a

monotherapy for young whites. Blacks respond less well than whites to ACE-inhibitor, because blacks have a higher prevalence of low-renin hypertension than whites

Thiazide diuretics for the black, fluid-expanded patient with a history of hypoglycemia, asthma, congestive heart failure, and/or cardiac conduction disturbance

Prazosin, α methyldopa, hydralazine, or clonidine as add-on drugs

MANAGEMENT OF THE ELDERLY HYPERTENSIVE PATIENT

Successful therapy reduces cardiovascular morbidity and mortality, particularly in males with elevated diastolic pressure levels. Evidence in support of treatment for elevated diastolic pressure comes from the results of a number of multicenter and international studies. The goals of therapy for diastolic hypertension in elderly patients are similar to those for young patients.

Therapy requires careful considerations of risk versus benefit as well as the simplicity of regimens because of the psychosocial problems of many elderly patients. Uniformity exists for the recommendation that blood pressures in excess of 160/100 (on at least two occasions) and unresponsive to nonantihypertensive regimens require treatment. However, age influences the pharmacokinetic processes affecting antihypertensive drugs, gastrointestinal absorption, the "first-pass" phenomenon of liver metabolism, the density or affinity of adrenoceptors, and the renal elimination of drugs, and thereby limits the usefulness of drugs such as beta blockers in the management of the elderly hypertensive patient.

Effective antihypertensive regimens for elderly patients, as judged by two recently reported prospective, placebo-controlled, and well-designed studies include:

Hydrochlorothiazide plus triamterene initially and methyldopa addition, if required (840 patients) [1]

Low-dose hydrochlorothiazide (12.5 mg) plus metoprolol (100 mg) (562 patients) [21]

Ca^{2+} channel blockers may be particularly effective as antihypertensive drugs in elderly patients, many of whom have low renin levels. However, the long-term effects of Ca^{2+} channel blockers on the morbidity and mortality of hypertension in the elderly as monotherapy are presently unknown.

REMISSION OF GROUPS I AND II PRIMARY HYPERTENSION

Hypertension, once diagnosed as mild in nature, does not necessarily require a lifetime commitment to drugs. From anecdotal accounts, drug-induced reduction in arterial blood pressure may down-regulate baroreceptor responses and normalize pressures for indefinite periods. While virtually all hypertensive patients eventually relapse, a small group experiences normotensive levels for 4, 8, and 12 years [3].

GROUP III PRIMARY HYPERTENSION

Patients with group III primary hypertension exhibit group III K-W fundoscopic changes and diastolic blood pressures ranging from 110–112 mm Hg. In this setting, an antihypertensive drug regimen should be instituted concomitantly with the dietary program. Selection of the initial drug will be influenced by age, sex, ethnicity, and symptoms and signs. ACE inhibitors, beta blockers, and Ca^{2+} channel blockers with relatively large initial doses should be considered as monotherapy.

GROUP IV PRIMARY MALIGNANT HYPERTENSION

Patients with group IV primary malignant hypertension exhibit group IV fundoscopic changes and diastolic pressures exceeding 130 mm Hg. Eighty percent of patients with untreated malignant hypertension die within one year; 90% can be expected to die within two years. Practically all forms of hypertension (primary or secondary) may be complicated by a malignant phase. The risk for a malignant phase is greater in younger than in elderly subjects, with the greatest incidence occurring in 50–54-year-old males and 45–54-year-old females. Absolute levels of blood pressure elevation are less diagnostic of malignant hypertension than the presence of papilledema. Malignant hypertension is an emergency situation that requires hospitalization for complete diagnostic workup to rule out secondary forms of hypertension and to reduce the blood pressure within hours.

Emergencies of Hypertension (Blood Pressure Reduction in Hours)

The emergencies [16] of malignant forms of primary as well as secondary hypertension require blood pressure reduction within hours [5]. The emergency situations are as follows:

Severe accelerated (malignant) hypertension
Encephalopathy
Hypertension complicated by:
   Acute left ventricular failure
   Intracranial hemorrhage
   Aortic dissection
   Postoperative bleeding
Progressing renal failure
Eclampsia with convulsions or fetal distress
Extensive burns
Hypertensive crisis of pheochromocytoma or during monamine
   oxidase inhibitor therapy.

HYPERTENSIVE ENCEPHALOPATHY

The course of hypertension is occasionally punctuated by encephalopathies. The encephalopathy is ushered in by the subacute onset of alteration in consciousness progressing from drowsiness to stupor and disorientation, and finally to coma. These developments are accompanied by severe headache, nausea, vomiting, visual blurring, and transient neurologic disturbances. Characteristically, the blood pressure is spectacularly elevated (> 259/150 mm Hg).

The drugs recommended for hospital management of hypertensive emergencies are:

Sodium nitroprusside (Nipride) and **furosemide** (20 mg IV) and **propranolol** (1–2 mg IV bolus q6h to offset reflex tachycardia). Infuse nitroprusside at 0.5 µg/kg/min and titrate upward until arterial pressure is in the normal range. Do not exceed 10 µg/kg/min. (see Chap. 1 for pharmacology and use of sodium nitroprusside). This regimen is inappropriate in eclampsia or renal failure because of cyanide toxicity.

Diazoxide (small dose of 30–100 mg as IV bolus) is usually not used in patients older than 65 years of age, patients with known cerebral or coronary arterial insufficiency, or toxemic patients with a viable fetus. If other antihypertensive drugs are in use, diazoxide must be administered with caution because of its incremental and often sudden hypotensive effect. Diazoxide may exacerbate angina pectoris or a dissecting aneurysm by rapidly raising cardiac work and output.

Trimethaphan camsylate is used for a dissecting aortic aneurysm or subarachnoid hemorrhage, as it reduces blood pressure promptly by lowering peripheral resistance (1–5 mg/min). The drug has formidable side effects and is rarely used.

Hydralazine (bolus dose of 5–25 mg) is used in treating patients with severe toxemia of pregnancy.

To affect a smooth transition from the emergency to a convalescent condition, combination therapy is usually employed. These include ACE plus a diuretic and, in some cases, a beta blocker.

Urgencies of Hypertension

Hypertensive patients in whom blood pressure reduction should be accomplished within 24 hours [16] include those with:

Severe or accelerated hypertension without evidence of end-organ dysfunction
Perioperative hypertension

The drugs recommended for urgencies include:

Clonidine
Nifedipine
ACE
Labetalol (contraindicated with asthma or congestive heart failure)
Loop diuretics (small doses [20–40 mg furosemide, IV] as a secondary drug)
Reserpine (1–5 mg IM; methyldopa (250 mg IV over 30–60 minutes). Both drugs cause somnolence and have a delayed response.

Resistant Hypertension

Severe hypertension (diastolic pressure > 120 mm Hg) is more likely to become resistant hypertension than mild (groups I and II) hypertension. It is defined as a failure to control blood pressure with a combination of a diuretic, a beta blocker, and a vasodilator [15]. The common causes of resistant hypertension are:

Poor drug compliance
Ineffective drug dose level
Excessive salt intake
Pressor mechanisms related to primary disease (i.e., pheochromocytoma), compensatory reaction to the antihypertensive drugs (i.e., secondary aldosteronism to diuretic use, fluid retention of beta blockers and vasodilators, and high plasma renin levels)
Complications of hypertension (i.e., renal artery stenosing disease, advance nephrosclerosis, myocardial ischemia)
Drug interactions (i.e., chiefly nonsteroidal anti-inflammatory drugs, tricyclic antidepressants, amphetamines, chlorpromazine, and possibly aspirin)

Antihypertensive Drugs as Monotherapy or Combined Therapy

In the remainder of this chapter, each antihypertensive agent is evaluated in terms of its usefulness in monotherapy and as a part of combined or "stepped care approach." A summary of a modern version of the stepped care approach is given and specific drugs are identified that may have particular utility in the hypertensive patient with an additional disease manifestation such as congestive heart failure or coronary artery disease.

DIURETICS

The classes of diuretics used in the treatment of hypertension are the thiazides, thiazide-related diuretics, and the "loop" diuretics (Fig. 3-2). These agents cause diuresis by inhibiting active transport processes involved in the reabsorption of ions from the lumen of the renal tubule. Thus, they increase the renal excretion of Na^+, K^+, H^+, Mg^{2+}, bicarbonate ($^-HCO_3$), Cl^-, and other ions. The presence of higher concentrations of ions in the tubular lumen creates the osmotic gradient responsible for the increased volume of water that also remains in the tubular lumen and is ultimately excreted as urine.

THIAZIDES

Thiazides are the most commonly used antihypertensive agents. They are often effective alone in the treatment of mild to moderate hypertension. However, thiazides exert a synergistic blood pressure lowering effect when combined with virtually any of the other available antihypertensive agents. Some agents, particularly certain sympathetic depressant drugs and the vaso-

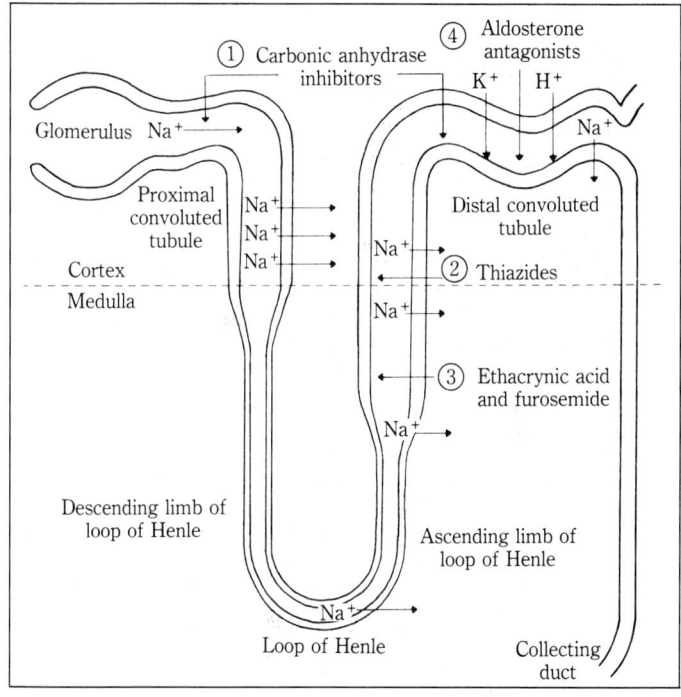

Fig. 3-2. Drugs acting along the proximal convoluted tubule (carbonic anhydrase inhibitor), the ascending limb of Henle's loop (furosemide and ethacrynic acid), the distal convoluted tubule (thiazides, carbonic anhydrase inhibitors), and the more distal convoluted tubule (aldosterone antagonists) to effect a diuresis of sodium (Na^+) and a retention of potassium (K^+) as well as magnesium (Mg^{2+}, not shown). (Modified from M. Sokolow and M. B. McIlroy. *Clinical Cardiology* [2nd ed.]. Los Altos, CA: Lange, 1979.)

dilators, tend to cause plasma volume expansion and therefore must be combined with a thiazide diuretic to retain their blood pressure lowering effect. A hallmark of the modern use of thiazides as well as other antihypertensive agents is low-dose therapy. Since the dose-response curve for the antihypertensive effect of thiazides is flat, increasing the dose produces minimal blood pressure lowering, while raising the likelihood of adverse effects, such as hypokalemia, which has a relatively steep dose-response curve.

Mechanism and Site of Action

The thiazide diuretics inhibit Na^+ and Cl^- reabsorption in the early distal tubule or cortical diluting segment of the renal tubule, thereby causing more ions and water to appear in the urine. As a result, plasma and extracellular fluid volume are reduced, thereby decreasing venous return and cardiac output. Acutely, this accounts for the reduction in blood pressure. With chronic use, plasma volume increases slightly but remains below pretreatment levels, peripheral resistance decreases, and, thereby, thiazides exert an antihypertensive effect with long-term use. The mechanism of reduced peripheral resistance is unknown. However, vascular reactivity to pressor stimuli is reduced during diuretic therapy. There is evidence that diuretics reduce intracellular Na^+, and, since vascular smooth muscle membrane possesses a carrier that cotransports Na^+ and Ca^{2+} in opposite directions, a lower intracellular Na^+ level enhances Na^+ entry and Ca^{2+} extrusion. Intracellular Ca^{2+} levels are the signal that mediates smooth muscle contraction. On the long term, thiazide diuretics reduce both plasma and extracellular fluid volume and peripheral resistance. Cardiac output is also slightly reduced, but the heart rate is usually unchanged. Thiazide diuretics exert their greatest effect in blacks, women, the elderly, and the obese. Their antihypertensive effect is noted after 3 weeks.

Adverse Effects

Hypokalemia

Long-term therapy with thiazide diuretics reduces plasma K^+ concentrations in virtually all patients. However, only a small percentage achieve a plasma level below 3.5 mEq/liter, the level generally considered clinically significant.

Potassium (K^+) is the most exchangeable cation in the body. It exists primarily as an intracellular ion at concentrations of 140–150 mEq/liter. The kidneys are the principal regulators of K^+ homeostasis. Renal regulation of K^+ was outlined by Thier [17] as follows:

I. Increased K^+ excretion
   A. High intracellular K^+
      1. High K^+ intake
      2. Alkalemia
      3. Aldosterone
   B. Favorable chemical or electrical gradient
      1. Increased urine flow to distal tubule
      2. Increased nonreabsorbable anion accompanying Na^+
      3. Decreased distal Cl^- delivery
   C. Diuretics — proximal, loop, and cortical diluting segment diuretics
II. Decreased K^+ excretion
   A. Decreased intracellular K^+
      1. Dietary intake
      2. Acute acidemia
   B. Unfavorable chemical or electrical gradient
      1. Decreased distal urine flow
      2. Decreased distal Na^+ delivery or reabsorption
   C. Hormone effect — β_2-catecholamines
   D. Impaired cell integrity
   E. Diuretics
      1. Inhibitors of distal Na^+ channels — amiloride and triamterene
      2. Inhibitors of aldosterone

Thiazide diuretics cause hypokalemia by blocking reabsorption in the early distal tubule, thereby causing a large Na^+ load to appear at the distal tubule. Na^+ is reabsorbed in the late distal tubule by exchange with K^+ and/or H^+ ions. Thus, the larger Na^+ load in the late distal tubule causes more Na^+ to be reabsorbed and more K^+ to be secreted into the filtrate and eliminated in the urine. This mechanism also contributes to a self-limiting effect of thiazide diuretics on their own antihypertensive effect. Thiazides cause Na^+ depletion, a major stimulus to the renin-angiotensin system. This, in turn, stimulates the release of aldosterone from the adrenal cortex, which enhances the reabsorption of Na^+ in the late distal tubule. This action of aldosterone operates in the direction of expanding plasma volume, thereby opposing the antihypertensive effect of the thiazides. In addition, it further contributes to K^+ loss via the Na^+/K^+ exchange in the late distal tubule. The effect of Na^+ load on the late distal tubule underscores the value of dietary Na^+ restriction. Reduced Na^+ intake during thiazide diuretic therapy presents a lower Na^+ load at the distal tubule, which enhances the antihypertensive effect of the thiazide and reduces the hypokalemia.

When is hypokalemia clinically significant? In most hypertensive patients, hypokalemia has no significant effects and does not require treatment. However, even minimal hypokalemia represents a risk to patients receiving either digitalis or corticosteroids. Hypokalemia sensitizes the heart to the effects of digitalis and is the most common cause of digitalis toxicity. More marked hypokalemia, less than 3.5 mEq/liter, has been associated with ventricular ectopic beats. An increased incidence rate of mortality is associated with thiazide diuretics because of hypokalemia-induced ventricular dysrhythmias.

Patients receiving a diuretic plus digitalis or who exhibit plasma K^+ levels below 3.5 mEq/liter should have their hypokalemia corrected. This may be accomplished by increased dietary K^+ intake (bananas, orange juice, proteins, and so forth) or by K^+ supplementation with either liquid or microencapsulated KCl. Alternatively, thiazide plus a K^+-sparing diuretic (see below) may be used. The K^+-sparing diuretics act in the late distal tubule to interfere with Na^+/K^+ exchange.

Hypomagnesemia

Hypomagnesemia may be the result of either malabsorption states, alcoholism, or dialysis. However, as with hypokalemia, the most frequent cause is diuretic therapy. The incidence of hypomagnesemia is not known, and it has only become recognized in recent years that Mg^{2+}, as well as K^+, may become depleted during diuretic therapy. Moreover, K^+ supplementation alone may not correct hypokalemia in the Mg^{2+}-deficient patient. Coadministration of K^+ plus Mg^{2+} may be required to increase cellular K^+ content. This effect of Mg^{2+} is not mediated by an action on the Na^+-K^+-ATPase enzyme. Rather, Mg^{2+} prevents a cellular K^+ loss, possibly by decreasing K^+ conductance via a specific membrane K^+ channel.

Two options appear to be available for the treatment of hypomagnesemia/hypokalemia associated with diuretic therapy. One is the concomitant supplementation of both ions. Magnesium aspartate is a potentially useful orally effective preparation and is under investigation in the United States. Oral magnesium salts are available, such as milk of magnesia; a teaspoonful or so per day may be tolerated without gastrointestinal distress. The other option is to add a "K^+-sparing" diuretic (particularly the Mg^{2+}-sparing amiloride) to the therapy.

Hyperuricemia

Hyperuricemia may develop in 25–35% of all untreated essential hypertensives and is recognized by serum uric acid levels greater than 7.0 mg/dl in males and postmenopausal females, and greater than 6.0 mg/dl in premenopausal females.

Thiazide diuretics approximately double the number of patients experiencing hyperuricemia. Two factors underlie the thiazide-induced elevated serum uric acid levels: (1) a reduced plasma volume and (2) competitive inhibition by the diuretic of tubular secretion of uric acid.

When and how should thiazide-induced hyperuricemia be treated? In most patients, thiazide-induced hyperuricemia is asymptomatic. However, a small percentage may develop acute gouty attacks or renal uric acid stones. Patients should be monitored intermittently for uric acid levels, and therapy should be considered for patients with values greater than 10 mg/dl. However, some authorities recommend waiting for symptoms to arise from hyperuricemia, such as the development of a kidney stone, before instituting therapy. Colchicine is used to treat acute gouty attacks. Probenecid is the drug of choice for lowering plasma uric acid levels. Allopurinol should be used cautiously in patients receiving thiazide diuretics who have known or possible renal function impairment. Severe hypersensitivity reactions to allopurinol may occur, possibly resulting from an increase in serum oxipurinol, the active metabolite of allopurinol.

Hyperglycemia

Thiazide therapy may cause a slight elevation of fasting blood glucose in most patients. However, a worsening of glucose tolerance is usually not observed, except in those patients who have an elevation of pretreatment glucose levels and/or a preexisting tendency toward glucose intolerance.

The mechanism of thiazide-induced hyperglycemia is not known. However, it has been suggested to be related to an interference with the release of insulin from the pancreas. Some studies, but not all, have shown that hypokalemia may also play a role in hyperglycemia, since a return of plasma K^+ levels to normal is often accompanied by an improved glucose tolerance.

When and how should hyperglycemia be treated? Generally, no treatment of hyperglycemia is required. In patients with preexisting glucose intolerance, blood glucose levels should be monitored and hypoglycemic medication adjusted accordingly.

Hyperlipidemia

Thiazide therapy has been shown to cause an increase in total serum cholesterol, LDL-cholesterol, and triglycerides and may cause a slight decrease in HDL-cholesterol. Lipids participate as a risk factor for cardiovascular disease, and these thiazide-induced changes are in the direction of greater risk. Thus, the benefits of lowering blood pressure as a risk factor may be offset by the thiazide-induced changes in plasma lipids. While no epidemiologic information is available that demonstrates such increased risk, several recommendations can be made. The physician should monitor lipid levels periodically and use low doses of diuretics. Other classes of antihypertensive agents are available that do not adversely affect lipid levels (see below).

Additional Adverse Effects from Thiazides

Most other adverse effects are relatively rare and include the following: Hyponatremia is signalled by nausea and vomiting as initial symptoms, followed rapidly by central nervous system dysfunction related to encephalopathy and diffuse cerebral edema. Sensitivity reactions, such as skin rash or hives, may occur in patients intolerant of sulfonamide-type medications. Hematologic effects include thrombocytopenia and, possibly, hemolytic anemia and cytosis. Hepatic dysfunction may be detected by a yellowing of the eyes or skin. Cholecystitis and pancreatitis may result in stomach pain with nausea and vomiting.

Pharmacokinetics

Thiazide diuretics are absorbed relatively rapidly and completely after oral administration. Many of the thiazides exhibit high plasma protein binding. The majority of thiazide and thiazide-like diuretics are excreted unchanged, almost totally via the kidneys. Metolazone undergoes some enterohepatic recycling, with small amounts of the drug excreted in the bile. Other factors relating to pharmacokinetics will be presented with the individual drugs (see below).

Individual Thiazide Diuretic Drugs

Chlorothiazide: Diuril, SK-Chlorothiazide

DOSAGE FORMS AND STRENGTHS AVAILABLE

Chlorothiazide oral suspension: 50 mg/ml.
Chlorothiazide tablets: 250 and 500 mg.

DOSAGES

Adult: initially, 250 mg daily; may be increased to 500 mg.
Children: 10–20 mg/kg daily in 2 divided doses.
Onset of action: 2 hours.
Time to peak effect: 4 hours.
Duration of action: 6–12 hours.

Hydrochlorothiazide: Esidrix, Hydrodiuril, Oretic, Generic

DOSAGE FORMS AND STRENGTHS AVAILABLE

Oral solution: 10 and 100 mg per milliliter.
Tablets: 25, 50, and 100 mg.

DOSAGES

Adult: initially, 25 mg daily; may be increased to 50 mg daily.
Children: 1–2 mg/kg daily in 2 divided doses.
Onset of action: 2 hours.
Time to peak effect: 4 hours.
Duration of action: 6–12 hours.

Bendroflumethiazide: Naturetin

DOSAGE FORMS AND STRENGTHS AVAILABLE

Tablets: 2.5, 5, and 10 mg.

DOSAGES

Adult: initially, 2.5 mg daily; may be increased up to 5 mg daily.
Children: initially, 0.1 mg/kg daily in 1 or 2 doses; for maintenance, 0.05 to 0.3 mg/kg daily in 1 or 2 doses.
Onset of action: 1–2 hours.
Time to peak effect: 6–12 hours.
Duration of action: more than 18 hours.

Benzthiazide: Aquatag, Exna, Proaqua, Generic

DOSAGE FORMS AND STRENGTHS AVAILABLE

Tablets: 25 and 50 mg.

DOSAGES

Adult: initially, 25 mg daily; may be increased to 50 mg daily.
Children: 1–4 mg/kg daily in 3 doses.
Onset of action: 2 hours.
Time to peak effect: 4–6 hours.
Duration of action: 12 18 hours.

Cyclothiazide: Anhydron

DOSAGE FORMS AND STRENGTHS AVAILABLE

Tablets: 2 mg.

DOSAGES

Adult: initially, 1 mg daily; may be increased to 2 mg daily.
Children: 0.02–0.04 mg/kg once daily.
Onset of action: less than 6 hours.
Time to peak effect: 7–12 hours.
Duration of action: 18–24 hours.

Hydroflumethiazide: Diurcardin, Saluron, Generic

DOSAGE FORMS AND STRENGTHS AVAILABLE

Tablets: 50 mg.

DOSAGES

Adult: initially, 25 mg daily; may be increased to 50 mg daily.
Children: 1 mg/kg daily.
Onset of action: 1–2 hours.
Time to peak effect: 3–4 hours.
Duration of action: 18–24 hours.

Methyclothiazide: Aquatensen, Enduron, Generic

DOSAGE FORMS AND STRENGTHS AVAILABLE

Tablets: 2.5 and 5 mg.

DOSAGES

Adult: initially, 2.5 mg daily; may be increased to 5 mg daily.
Children: 0.05–0.2 mg/kg daily.
Onset of action: 2 hours.
Time to peak effect: 6 hours.
Duration of action: more than 24 hours.

Polythiazide: Renese

DOSAGE FORMS AND STRENGTHS AVAILABLE

Tablets: 1, 2, and 4 mg.

DOSAGES

Adult: initially, 2 mg daily; may be increased to 4 mg daily.
Children: 0.02–0.08 mg/kg daily.
Onset of action: 2 hours.
Time to peak effect: 6 hours.
Duration of action: 24–48 hours.

Trichlormethiazide: Metahydrin, Naqua, Generic

DOSAGE FORMS AND STRENGTHS AVAILABLE

Tablets: 2 and 4 mg.

DOSAGES

Adult: initially, 2 mg daily; may be increased to 4 mg once daily.
Children: 0.07 mg/kg once daily or in divided doses.
Onset of action: 2 hours.
Time to peak effect: 6 hours.
Duration of action: up to 24 hours.

Individual Thiazidelike Diuretic Drugs

Chlorthalidone: Hygroton, Generic

DOSAGE FORMS AND STRENGTHS AVAILABLE

Tablets: 25, 50, and 100 mg.

DOSAGES

Adult: initially, 25 mg daily; may be increased to 50 mg daily.
Children: 1 mg/kg daily.
Onset of action: 2 hours.
Time to peak effect: 2 hours.
Duration of action: 24–72 hours.

Indapamide: Lozol

Indapamide differs from other thiazide diuretics in a number of ways. First, it is metabolized by the liver and therefore should be used cautiously in patients with liver disease. Second, while indapamide is a diuretic, it may exert an antihypertensive effect at concentrations below the diuretic effect, apparently due to a reduction in peripheral resistance. Experience to date suggests that indapamide might be different from the other thiazide diuretics in that it appears not to alter either glucose tolerance or lipoprotein profiles. If these findings are confirmed over long-term use, these important differences may represent a distinct advantage of indapamide over other thiazide diuretics.

DOSAGE FORMS AND STRENGTHS AVAILABLE

Tablets: 2.5 mg.

DOSAGES
Adult: initially, 2.5 mg daily; may be increased to 5 mg daily.

Metolazone: Diulo, Zaroxyolyn

Metolazone differs from other thiazide diuretics in possessing an intrinsically greater diuretic capacity. Not only does this agent act at the cortical diluting segment, but it appears to inhibit sodium reabsorption in the proximal tubule as well. Thus, metolazone retains diuretic activity even when the glomerular filtration rate decreases to below 25 ml/minute.

DOSAGE FORMS AND STRENGTHS AVAILABLE
Tablets: 2.5, 5, and 10 mg.

DOSAGES
Adult: initially, 2.5 mg daily; may be increased to 5 mg daily.
Onset of action: 1 hour.
Time to peak effect: 2 hours.
Duration of action: 12–24 hours.

Quinethazone: Hydromox

DOSAGE FORMS AND STRENGTHS AVAILABLE
Tablets: 50 mg.

DOSAGES
Adult: initially, 50 mg daily; may be increased to 100 mg daily.
Onset of action: 2 hours.
Time to peak effect: 6 hours.
Duration of action: 18–24 hours.

Loop Diuretics

The loop diuretics are not the first drugs of choice in the treatment of hypertension. In part, this is due to the relatively short duration of action of these agents, approximately 6–8 hours. This works against being able to maintain the sustained slight reduction in plasma volume required for the antihypertensive effect. However, the loop diuretics are indicated in the treatment of hypertension with impaired renal function and are usually used in combination with other antihypertensives. The loop diuretics have a greater intrinsic capacity to induce diuresis and therefore are effective even when the glomerular filtration rate is less than 25 ml/minute.

MECHANISM AND SITE OF ACTION

The loop diuretics block the reabsorption of Cl^- and therefore Na^+ ions in the thick ascending limb of the loop of Henle. Fully 30% of the glomerular filtrate reaches the thick ascending limb and therefore is acted on by the loop diuretics. This explains the much greater intrinsic diuretic capacity of these agents compared to the thiazides, which have only 10% of the filtrate to act on at their sites of action, the cortical diluting segment and the early distal tubule. It should be noted that the greater blockade of Na^+ and Cl^- reabsorption by the loop diuretics presents a greater Na^+ load at the distal tubule for exchange with K^+, and, therefore, the loop diuretics possess a greater potential for producing hypokalemia.

Furosemide: Lasix, SK-Furosemide

Furosemide is one of the three currently available loop diuretics. It is selected over ethacrynic acid because of less severe ototoxicity. Furosemide does not appear to be qualitatively different from bumetanide, a more recently introduced diuretic.

PHARMACOKINETICS

Furosemide is absorbed well and quickly in the gastrointestinal tract. Approximately 60–70% of an oral dose is absorbed, but this may be reduced in patients with severe renal disease or with edematous bowel caused by severe congestive heart failure. Intravenous (IV) administration is recommended in these patients. The onset of action of furosemide is 30–60 minutes after oral administration and 5 minutes after IV administration. Time to peak effect is 1–2 hours after oral administration and ⅓ to 1 hour after IV administration. The duration of action is 6–8 hours after oral administration and 2 hours after IV administration. Furosemide is excreted primarily unchanged, 88% by the renal route and 12% by the biliary route. In severe renal insufficiency, biliary excretion increases dramatically.

ADVERSE EFFECTS

The most common side effects are volume depletion, hyperuricemia, and hypokalemia. In addition, hypotension, hyperglycemia, and hypochloremic alkalosis may also occur. Transient deafness has been reported with furosemide. The level of ototoxicity, however, is less with furosemide than with ethacrynic acid (see below).

DOSAGE FORMS AND STRENGTHS AVAILABLE

Oral solution: 10 mg/ml.
Tablets: 20, 40, and 80 mg.
Injection: 10 mg/ml.

DOSAGES

Adult: initially, 40 mg twice daily. If an adequate response is not obtained, dosage may be increased gradually up to 480 mg daily in two doses.
Children: 1–2 mg/kg.

Ethacrynic Acid: Edecrin

PHARMACOKINETICS

Ethacrynic acid is readily absorbed from the gastrointestinal tract and is extensively plasma-protein bound. About two-thirds of a dose of ethacrynic acid is excreted by the kidneys, and the remainder is metabolized by the liver. Ethacrynic acid appears in the urine as an unchanged drug and as conjugates of cysteine and N-acetylcysteine. The onset of action of ethacrynic acid is 30 minutes after oral administration, and 5 minutes after IV administration. The respective times to peak effect are 2 hours and 15–30 minutes, while the respective durations of action are 6–8 hours and 2 hours.

ADVERSE EFFECTS

Ethacrynic acid exhibits many of the same side effects as those listed for furosemide (see above). This agent has the greatest potential of all the loop diuretics for ototoxicity; therefore, furosemide therapy is often chosen over ethacrynic acid.

DOSAGE FORMS AND STRENGTHS AVAILABLE

Tablets: 25 and 50 mg.
Ethacrynate sodium for injection: the equivalent of ethacrynic acid — 50 mg.

DOSAGES

Adult: initially, 25 mg twice daily; may be increased to 200 mg daily in 2 divided doses.

Bumetanide: Bumex

Bumetanide is a relatively recently released loop diuretic. It is approximately 40 times more potent than furosemide. However, in equivalent doses, its pharmacologic and therapeutic properties closely resemble those of furosemide.

PHARMACOKINETICS

Bumetanide is rapidly and almost completely absorbed from the gastrointestinal tract and is extensively plasma-protein bound. Bumetanide is excreted primarily via the kidney and is 45% unchanged. The onset of action is 30–60 minutes after oral administration and within minutes after IV administration. The respective times to peak effect are 1–2 hours and 15–30 minutes. The respective durations of action are 4 hours (this may increase with higher doses) and 3.5–4.0 hours.

ADVERSE EFFECTS

The side effects of bumetanide are nearly identical to those listed for furosemide (see above).

DOSAGE FORMS AND STRENGTHS AVAILABLE

Tablets: 500 µg (0.5 mg) and 1 mg.
Injection: 250 µg (0.25 mg) per milliliter.

DOSAGES

Adult: initially, 0.5 mg daily; may be increased to 10 mg daily in 2 divided doses.

MODIFYING FACTORS FOR DIURETIC-INDUCED HYPOKALEMIA

Diuretic itself
Duration of diuretic therapy
K^+ concentration prior to diuretic therapy
Status of renin-angiotensin-aldosterone system
Status of renal function
Complicating medical conditions (congestive heart failure, hypertension, cirrhosis, and quantity of fluid to be mobilized)

Potassium-Sparing Diuretics

The K^+-sparing diuretics, spironolactone, amiloride, and triamterene, block Na^+/K^+ exchange in the distal convoluted tubule where only 1–2% of the filtered Na^+ load appears at this site. Therefore, these agents possess a low intrinsic capacity to cause diuresis. Nonetheless, they do cause a mild diuresis and, at least in the case of spironolactone and amiloride, exert a mild, sustained antihypertensive effect. The unique property of these agents is their capacity to cause K^+ retention. This capacity underlies their most common use, which is in combination with thiazide diuretics to prevent thiazide-induced hypokalemia. The most significant adverse reaction to these agents is hyperkalemia, which occurs in approximately 10% of patients receiving amiloride alone and in up to 26% of patients receiving spironolactone, even when it is combined with thiazide diuretics.

MECHANISM OF ACTION OF THE POTASSIUM-SPARING DIURETICS

Spironolactone

Spironolactone is a 17-spirolactone steroid and is a direct competitive antagonist of aldosterone and other mineralocorticoids.

The receptor for aldosterone is a soluble, cytoplasmic protein, which, when occupied by aldosterone, changes to an active conformation, initiating a chain of biochemical events leading to the synthesis of transport proteins responsible for mediating the exchange of Na^+ and K^+ in the distal convoluted tubule. When spironolactone occupies the aldosterone receptor, it fails to change conformation, thus blocking the subsequent biochemical events.

Amiloride and Triamterene

Amiloride and triamterene are not aldosterone antagonists but act directly in the distal tubule to block Na^+-K^+ ion exchange across the membrane.

MECHANISM OF POTASSIUM CONSERVATION

Hypokalemia occurs with the use of both thiazide and loop diuretics, which cause a much larger Na^+ load to appear at the distal convoluted tubule. This increases the Na^+ concentration gradient for reabsorption in exchange for K^+. However, the K^+-sparing diuretics block Na^+-K^+ exchange in the distal tubule, leading to Na^+ loss and K^+ conservation.

ADVERSE EFFECTS

Hyperkalemia

Hyperkalemia, serum K^+ levels over 5.5 mEq/liter, is one of the most significant adverse reactions to the potassium-sparing diuretics. It may occur even when these agents are used in combination with thiazides, which tend to cause hypokalemia. Potassium supplementation is specifically contraindicated in patients who are also receiving potassium-sparing diuretics. In addition, impaired renal function is also a contraindication to the use of potassium-sparing diuretics, as this disease entity sharply increases the risk of hyperkalemia. Symptoms of hyperkalemia include one or more of the following: confusion; irregular heart beat; numbness or tingling of hands, feet, or lips; shortness of breath or difficulty in breathing; nervousness; unusual tiredness or weakness; and weakness or heaviness of legs. Periodic determination of serum electrolytes, especially potassium, should be carried out during therapy with potassium-sparing diuretics.

ADDITIONAL ADVERSE EFFECTS

Amiloride and triamterene cause relatively few other side effects. These include nausea, vomiting, leg cramps, dizziness, diarrhea, and headache. Spironolactone causes gynecomastia and amenorrhea. However, these effects are dose-related and occur rarely when the recommended low doses are used.

Spironolactone: Aldactone, Generic

The most common use of spironolactone in the treatment of hypertension is as a K^+-sparing diuretic in combination with a thiazide. However, spironolactone does exert an antihypertensive effect when used by itself and has been considered an alternative for those patients who are unable to take thiazide diuretics.

DOSAGE FORMS AND STRENGTHS AVAILABLE

Tablets: 25, 50, and 100 mg.

DOSAGES

Adult: initially, 50 mg daily; may be increased to 100 mg daily in a single dose or 2 divided doses. Dosage should be adjusted according to blood pressure response and serum K^+ level.
Children: 1–2 mg/kg daily in 2 doses.
Time to peak effect: 2–3 days (after multiple doses).
Duration of action: 2–3 days (after multiple doses).

Amiloride: Mirador

DOSAGE FORMS AND STRENGTHS AVAILABLE

Tablets: 5 mg.

DOSAGES

Adults: initially, 5 mg daily, not to exceed 10 mg daily. Adjust dose according to blood pressure response and serum K^+ level.
Onset of action: within 2 hours.
Time to peak effect: 6–10 hours.
Duration of action: 24 hours.

Triamterene: Dyrenium

DOSAGE FORMS AND STRENGTHS AVAILABLE

Capsules: 50 and 100 mg.

DOSAGES

Adult: initially, 50 mg daily; may be increased to 100 mg daily in a single dose or 2 divided doses. Should be given after meals. Adjust dose according to blood pressure response and serum K^+ level.
Onset of action: 2–4 hours.
Time to peak effect: 1 to several days (multiple doses).
Duration of action: 7–9 hours (single dose).

Fixed Combinations of Potassium-Sparing and Thiazide Diuretics

Fixed dose combinations have the advantage of simplifying administration of the medication and may enhance patient compliance. However, fixed dose combinations cannot be recommended unless the strengths of each component are optimal.

Spironolactone and Hydrochlorothiazide Tablets

Aldactazide: 25 mg and 25 mg, or 50 mg and 50 mg.

Amiloride and Hydrochlorothiazide Tablets

Moduretic: 5 mg and 50 mg.

Triamterene and Hydrochlorothiazide Capsules

Dyazide: 50 mg and 25 mg.
Maxzide: 75 mg and 50 mg.

Diuretic Drug Interactions

THIAZIDE DIURETICS PLUS ADRENOCORTICOSTEROIDS/CORTICOTROPIN/AMPHOTERICIN B

The thiazides induce hypokalemia. Adrenocorticosteroids and corticotropin act in the kidney to enhance K^+ excretion by an aldosteronelike action. Amphotericin B also causes K^+ depletion. When these agents are combined with the thiazides, their pharmacologic effects on K^+ blood levels are additive, causing a much more severe K^+ depletion. When the thiazides are combined with any of these agents, plasma concentrations of K^+ must be monitored, and K^+ supplementation must be given as needed.

THIAZIDE DIURETICS PLUS LITHIUM

The thiazide diuretics reduce the renal clearance of lithium, possibly causing lithium plasma concentrations to increase and lithium-induced cardiotoxicity and neurotoxicity to occur. Lithium is also nephrotoxic. In general, these agents should not be used concurrently. The K^+-sparing diuretics, spironolactone, triamterene, and amiloride, do not affect serum lithium concentrations and may be used instead of the thiazides.

THIAZIDE DIURETICS PLUS INDOMETHACIN

Indomethacin tends to reduce the blood pressure lowering effects of the thiazide diuretics. This may involve an indomethacin-induced inhibition of vasodilator prostaglandin synthesis. When these agents are combined, the patient's blood pressure should be monitored and the dose of the thiazide increased as needed.

THIAZIDE DIURETICS PLUS DIGITALIS

One of the most important drug interactions is that between the thiazide diuretics and the digitalis glycosides. The thiazides induce K^+ depletion, which, in turn, enhances the digitalis action, possibly leading to digitalis toxicity. This interaction is based on a competition between K^+ and digitalis. Plasma concentrations should be monitored intermittently, and the patient should be assessed for either changes in therapeutic response or possible signs of digitalis toxicity. K^+ supplementation or the use of a K^+-sparing diuretic may prevent this adverse drug interaction.

THIAZIDE DIURETICS PLUS METHENAMINE

The thiazide diuretics may alkalinize the urine, preventing the conversion of methenamine to formaldehyde, the active antibacterial agent. Thiazides and methenamine should not be combined.

LOOP DIURETICS PLUS ADRENOCORTICOSTEROIDS/CORTICOTROPIN/AMPHOTERICIN B

The loop diuretics induce hypokalemia. Adrenocorticosteroids and corticotropin act in the kidney to enhance K^+ excretion by an aldosteronelike action. Amphotericin B also causes K^+ depletion. When these agents are combined with the loop diuretics, their pharmacologic effects on K^+ blood levels are additive, causing a much more severe K^+ depletion. When these agents are combined, plasma concentrations of K^+ must be monitored and K^+ supplementation must be given as needed.

LOOP DIURETICS PLUS LITHIUM

The loop diuretics reduce the renal clearance of lithium, causing lithium plasma concentrations to increase and lithium-induced cardiotoxicity and neurotoxicity to occur. Lithium is also nephrotoxic. In general, these agents should not be used concurrently. The K^+-sparing diuretics, spironolactone, triamterene, and amiloride, do not affect serum lithium concentrations and may be used instead of the loop diuretics.

ETHACRYNIC ACID PLUS WARFARIN AND OTHER COUMARIN ANTICOAGULANTS

Ethacrynic acid is highly plasma-protein bound and displaces warfarin from plasma proteins, increasing free anticoagulant blood concentrations and the risk of hemorrhage. In patients stabilized on warfarin, the prothrombin activity should be monitored when either adding or withdrawing a loop diuretic from the regimen. The dose of warfarin should be adjusted accordingly.

ETHACRYNIC ACID PLUS CISPLATIN

Both ethacrynic acid and cisplatin are ototoxic, and, when combined, this toxicity is additive. When it is necessary to use these agents in combination, the eighth cranial nerve function must be monitored and lower doses of ethacrynic acid used to reduce the potential for an interaction. Bumetanide and furosemide are less ototoxic and may represent a better choice when it is necessary to combine a loop diuretic and cisplatin.

SPIRONOLACTONE/AMILORIDE/TRIAMTERENE PLUS K$^+$-CONTAINING BLOOD (FROM A BLOOD BANK), MILK, MEDICATIONS, SALT SUPPLEMENTS, AND CAPTOPRIL

By definition, the K$^+$-sparing diuretics conserve K$^+$ and may cause hyperkalemia. Thus, other sources of K$^+$ must be avoided to prevent severe hyperkalemia. According to the United States Pharmacopeia Drug Information (USP DI), blood from a blood bank may contain up to 30 mEq of K$^+$ per liter or up to 65 mEq per liter of whole blood when stored for more than 10 days. Low-salt milk may contain up to 60 mEq of K$^+$ per liter. Captopril, which reduces plasma aldosterone levels, also conserves K$^+$ and could lead to a marked hyperkalemia when combined with a K$^+$-sparing diuretic.

SPIRONOLACTONE PLUS DIGOXIN

The combination of spironolactone plus digoxin increases digoxin plasma concentrations due to a reduced renal clearance of digoxin. Both K$^+$ and digoxin plasma concentrations should be monitored intermittently, and the patient should be assessed for either changes in therapeutic response or possible signs of digoxin toxicity.

TRIAMTERENE PLUS INDOMETHACIN

The combination of triamterene and indomethacin may lead to reversible acute renal failure. Triamterene appears to stimulate the synthesis of prostaglandin E$_2$, while indomethacin inhibits this synthesis. These actions probably account for this adverse drug interaction. When it is necessary to combine these agents, renal functions must be monitored. Deterioration of renal function would require the discontinuation of one or both agents.

Sympathetic Depressant Drugs — Beta Adrenoceptor Blockers, Beta Blockers

The beta blockers have revolutionized the treatment of a broad range of cardiovascular diseases. In addition to hypertension, these agents are effective in the treatment of angina and cardiac arrhythmias (see Chaps. 2 and 4). Beta blockers also offer substantial protection against the reoccurrence of a myocardial infarction (see Chap. 4).

The beta blockers have substantially advanced the therapy of hypertension. When used according to the original stepped care approach, the beta blockers emerged as the drugs of choice for step 2. More recently, they have become recognized as efficacious

Table 3-2. Pharmacologic properties of the beta blockers

Beta blocker	Cardio-selectivity	Intrinsic sympathethomimetic activity	Membrane stabilizing properties	Lipophilic[a] properties
Acebutolol	+	+	+	+
Atenolol	+	−	−	−
Labetalol[b]	−	−	+	−
Metoprolol	+	−	−	+
Nadolol	−	−	−	−
Oxprenolol	−	+	+	+
Pindolol	−	+	+	+
Propranolol	−	−	+	+
Timolol	−	−	−	−

[a] Enter central nervous system more readily than nonlipophilic beta blockers.
[b] Unique, possesses α-adrenergic blocking activity in the same concentration range as its β-blocking action; beta:alpha = 7:1–3:1.
Key: + = property present; − = property absent.

monotherapy and as a possible step 1 drug in the updated versions of the stepped care approach.

In addition to beta blockade, individual blockers exhibit a variety of pharmacologic properties including cardioselectivity (preferential blockade of cardiac β_1-receptors), intrinsic sympathomimetic activity, lipid versus water solubility, and membrane stabilization. Table 3-2 lists beta blockers, indicating whether each exhibits one or more of these properties.

There are only two properties that all beta blockers share in common, namely, (1) blockade, or at least occupation, of cardiac β-receptors and (2) nearly equal antihypertensive efficacy. Given this, the primary basis for selecting one beta blocker over another is to reduce or avoid side effects and therefore to increase patient compliance.

MECHANISM OF ANTIHYPERTENSIVE ACTION OF BETA BLOCKERS

The mechanism of the antihypertensive effect of beta blockers is unknown. However, while the beta blocker propranolol decreases heart rate and cardiac output almost immediately, the reduction in blood pressure begins after 2–4 days and reaches optimal lowering in about 2 or 3 weeks. This suggests that the mechanism of its antihypertensive effect involves an adaptive change in response to beta blockade in the heart. Prichard and Gillam [12] proposed that because propranolol reduces the cardiac components of pressor responses, **baroreceptors reset** over the first 3 weeks to regulate blood pressure at a lower level. Lewis [9] suggested that it was not a reduction in cardiac components of pressor response but a damping or reduction in the fluctuation of cardiac activity. Beta blockade sharply reduces or eliminates responses to nerve stimulation or circulating catecholamines. The reduced fluctuation in cardiac activity results in a **damping of autonomic afferent input** to the central nervous system (CNS) blood pressure control centers, which results in a physiologic adaptation underlying a decline in sympathetic tone.

HEMODYNAMIC EFFECTS OF BETA BLOCKERS WITHOUT INTRINSIC SYMPATHOMIMETIC ACTIVITY

As the prototype beta blocker, propranolol causes approximately a 20% reduction in cardiac output in most patients shortly after initiation of therapy, and this reduction is maintained until the drug is withdrawn. Peripheral resistance increases acutely, and within the first few hours to days there is little or no change in blood pressure (there are exceptions to this in the case of certain high-renin hypertensive subjects). Beginning around the third day of propranolol therapy, peripheral resistance begins to decline slowly, with a maximal reduction in approximately 2–3 weeks. The reduction in blood pressure parallels changes in peripheral resistance.

HEMODYNAMIC EFFECTS OF BETA BLOCKERS WITH INTRINSIC SYMPATHOMIMETIC ACTIVITY

Pindolol possesses intrinsic sympathomimetic activity (ISA) or partial agonist activity. Thus, at rest, when the heart is receiving minimal sympathetic stimulation, the introduction of pindolol does not change the heart rate or cardiac output. However, the heart rate and cardiac output increase only modestly during exercise, indicating that pindolol is occupying cardiac β-receptors, preventing the increased sympathetic activity from stimulating the heart. Since cardiac output does not change initially on pindolol therapy, peripheral resistance is also unchanged, and blood pressure is generally unaffected. However, over the course of several hours to 3 days, peripheral resistance and, therefore, blood pressure begins to fall. Maximum blood pressure lowering requires 1–3 weeks.

ROLE OF SPECIFIC ORGAN SYSTEMS IN THE ANTIHYPERTENSIVE EFFECT OF BETA BLOCKERS

Since the mechanism of the blood pressure lowering effect of beta blockers is unknown, numerous proposals have been put forward. Following is a summary of evidence against a direct role of a number of organ systems in beta blocker-induced blood pressure lowering.

Heart

Cardiac output falls with propranolol and other agents lacking ISA. However, the decrease in cardiac output occurs immediately, while the decrease in blood pressure begins between several hours and 3 days after the initiation of therapy. Furthermore, with beta blockers possessing ISA, the decrease in cardiac output is either reduced or absent. Nonetheless, these drugs are equally effective as antihypertensive agents. Because beta blockers with

ISA tend not to reduce the inotropic response of the heart at rest, these agents have much less effect on exercise capacity than those lacking ISA.

Plasma Renin Activity

Renin secretion from the kidneys results, in part, from neurogenic stimulation of β_1-receptors. Propranolol blocks these receptors and thus inhibits renin release. This action may play a role in the treatment of malignant or high-renin hypertension. However, in most cases of primary hypertension:

1. A single oral dose of propranolol reduces plasma renin activity within 4 hours, whereas arterial pressure is unchanged.
2. A single oral dose of pindolol does not affect plasma renin activity but reduces blood pressure.
3. During prolonged treatment, there is no correlation between the decrease in blood pressure and the decrease in plasma renin activity by beta blockade.

Central Nervous System

From animal experimentation, there is evidence that beta blockers, injected into the CNS, lower blood pressure. Furthermore, there is electroencephalographic and other evidence in humans that propranolol enters the CNS. However, highly lipophobic agents such as sotolol cross the blood-brain barrier poorly and, therefore, achieve very low concentrations in the brain. Nevertheless, these agents are equally effective as propranolol as antihypertensive agents.

PHARMACOLOGIC PROPERTIES OF BETA BLOCKERS

Since avoidance of adverse reactions is one of the major bases for selection between beta blockers, the different pharmacologic properties of individual beta blockers are reviewed in terms of their adverse effects. Among the most common of these are fatigue, bronchospasm, Raynaud's-like cold extremities, and central side effects, including vivid dreams and hallucinations. Life-threatening adverse reactions include bradycardia, heart block, hypotension, and congestive heart failure. Beta blockers also delay the recovery from hypoglycemia in diabetics, as well as in normal subjects, and diminish the normal cardiovascular response to hypoglycemia. In addition, beta blockers elevate serum triglycerides and lower HDL-cholesterol.

Cardioselectivity

It is now well established that β-adrenergic receptors exist in two subtypes, β_1 in the heart and kidney (juxtaglomerular apparatus) and β_2 in the lung (bronchiolar smooth muscle), blood vessels, pancreatic β-cells (mediating insulin release), and lipid and other cells mediating lipolysis. In predisposed individuals, the nonselective β_2 blockers may induce bronchospasm, cold extremities, and an inappropriate response to hypoglycemia. In addition, most subjects experience an adverse effect on lipid profile. While several beta blockers are cardioselective and exert a preferential effect on cardiac β_1-receptors, some degree of β_2-receptor blockade can be expected within the normal antihypertensive dosage range. Nevertheless, the incidence and severity of bronchospasm in asthmatics and cold extremities, inappropriate response to hypoglycemia, and lipid profile derangement in other patients is reduced. It should be noted that in those individuals receiving a cardioselective beta blocker who experience bronchospasm, reversal of the spasm is relatively easily achieved using β_2-selective agonists.

Intrinsic Sympathomimetic Activity

Certain beta blockers, including acebutolol, oxprenolol, and pindolol, possess ISA; that is, they are partial agonists of beta receptors. Their intrinsic capacity to stimulate the receptor is much less than that of epinephrine or isoproterenol. However, since these agents do not alter resting heart rate or cardiac output, this implies that they stimulate the beta receptors of the heart to an extent that approximates resting sympathetic tone. However, when sympathetic stimulation to the heart is increased by exercise, for example, heart rate does not increase to the extent expected, indicating an occupancy of beta receptors by the beta blocker.

Benefits of Beta Blockers with Intrinsic Sympathomimetic Activity on the Heart

Beta blockers lacking ISA remove all sympathetic drive to the heart. Thus, sinoatrial (SA) nodal rate and, therefore, heart rate is reduced, as is the conduction rate through the atrioventricular (AV) node and other cardiac tissues. Finally, the strength of contraction or inotropic response is reduced. Thus, in pathologic conditions involving bradycardia, conduction defects or congestive heart failure, the sympathetic drive is decisive in maintaining function, and beta blockers, in general, are contraindicated, as they remove the sympathetic drive. In spite of this relative contraindication, whenever beta blocker therapy is to be used, beta blockers possessing ISA are the drugs of choice. Their inherent agonist activity replaces the sympathetic tone, minimizing the reduction in "sympathetic drive."

Benefits of Beta Blockers with Intrinsic Sympathomimetic Activity in Patients with Cold Extremities

Cold extremities are caused by a reduced blood flow to the body parts. When beta blocker therapy is given to a patient susceptible to cold extremities, the symptoms become much more marked. By removing β-receptor mediated vasodilation through a beta blockade, the unopposed α-receptors mediate vasoconstriction. The use of beta blockers with ISA reduces this problem. The partial agonist activity at vascular β-receptors restores β-receptor mediated vasodilation and operates in the direction of improving blood flow.

Effects on Lipid Profile

In general, beta blockers raise serum triglycerides and lower HDL-cholesterol. This effect is seen less often with cardioselective agents and may be absent with beta blockers possessing either ISA or concomitant alpha blocking activity (labetalol).

Membrane Stabilization

At high doses, certain beta blockers, including acebutolol, pindolol, and propranolol, stabilize cell membranes. In this respect, beta blockers resemble the actions of antiarrhythmic compounds, such as quinidine on Na^{2+} channel function (see Chap. 2). Presently, membrane stabilization is considered to have little clinical consequence in the use of beta blockers in the treatment of hypertension or other cardiovascular disorders. One unique consequence of membrane stabilization is that when beta blockers are applied to the eye in the high concentrations necessary to treat glaucoma, they produce conjunctival anesthesia. Three beta blockers, betaxolol, levobunolol, and timolol, lack membrane stabilizing activity and can be used in the treatment of glaucoma because they fail to produce conjunctival anesthesia.

Water and Lipid Solubility

The solubility of beta blockers in lipid versus water influences both metabolism and entry into the CNS. Lipid-soluble blockers, such as propranolol and metoprolol, undergo extensive first-pass metabolism in the liver, thereby drecreasing their bioavailability. Such beta blockers can also cross the blood-brain barrier more easily to achieve higher concentrations in the CNS and, in susceptible individuals, may account for the CNS side effects. Water-soluble beta blockers, that is, atenolol, nadolol, and timolol, do not undergo first-pass metabolism and, therefore, have a longer plasma half-life. In addition, these agents enter the CNS to only a limited extent and tend to produce less neurologic side effects.

Combined Beta and Alpha Adrenergic Activity

Labetalol is the first of a unique class of compounds exhibiting both α- and β-adrenergic blocking activity. The agent is approximately 3–7 times more potent against the β-receptor than the α-receptor. Labetalol exhibits a different hemodynamic profile in that both cardiac output and peripheral resistance are reduced acutely and over long-term therapy. Thus, blood pressure is also lowered very shortly after the initiation of labetalol therapy. Labetalol also has less tendency to exacerbate cold extremities because it blocks alpha adrenoceptor-mediated vasoconstriction.

SPECIFIC USES OF BETA BLOCKERS AS ANTIHYPERTENSIVES

Patients with coexisting angina pectoris

Patients with cardiac arrhythmias, particularly super- and ventricular tachyarrhythmias

Patients on tricyclic antidepressants and antipsychotic agents, although caution is advised since propranolol (and other lipophilic beta blockers) may produce depression

Patients with marked hyperuricemia (i.e., diuretic-induced gout-prone individuals)

Patients with hyperkinetic hypertension — beta blockers are particularly effective in individuals with a higher cardiac output, tachycardia, and palpitations.

ADVERSE EFFECTS OF BETA BLOCKER THERAPY

The most common side effects include fatigue, bronchospasm, cold extremities, and vivid dreams. The most life-threatening side effects are bradycardia, heart block, hypotension, and congestive heart failure. Additional side effects include sleep disturbances, mental depression, dizziness, paresthesia, hallucinations, muscle cramps, blurring of vision, gastrointestinal disorders (diarrhea), and dry mouth.

These side effects are characteristic of beta blockers as a class of drugs. However, side effects occur with different degrees of severity and incidence among beta blockers with the different pharmacologic properties reviewed above. A summary of side effects of beta blockers and of the basis for selecting beta blockers to minimize these side effects follows.

Bronchospasm

Cardioselective beta blockers preferentially block cardiac β_1-receptors rather than β_2-receptors in the lung. Thus, there is less potential to cause bronchospasm with these agents. Furthermore, patients who develop asthma while taking a cardioselective beta blocker will respond readily with bronchodilation to standard doses of β_2-stimulant drugs, whereas patients taking a nonselective beta blocker will not.

Cold Extremities

Nonselective beta blockers can cause cold extremities or Raynaud's phenomenon-like symptoms. Cardioselective beta blockers are less likely to exhibit this side effect, as vascular β-receptors are the β_2-subtype. Labetalol, which possesses α-antagonist activity, also tends to lack this side effect.

Central Nervous System

Vivid dreams, blurring of vision, mental depression, and other central side effects occur to a greater extent with lipophilic beta blockers that cross the blood-brain barrier. In patients exhibiting central side effects, lipophobic beta blockers, which do not cross the blood-brain barrier readily, should be used.

Congestive Heart Failure, Bradycardia, Conduction Defects

Function in the impaired heart is often maintained by increased sympathetic activity. Thus, in general, beta blockers are relatively contraindicated in these cases, since sympathetic drive will be removed, exacerbating the cardiac dysfunction. However, in those cases where beta blocker therapy is judged appropriate, beta blockers with ISA should be used, since their partial agonist activity provides some stimulus to the heart, thereby replacing the sympathetic drive and minimizing further deterioration of cardiac function.

PHARMACOKINETICS OF BETA BLOCKERS

Beta Blockers That Undergo Liver Metabolism

Acebutolol, labetalol, metoprolol, oxprenolol, and propranolol undergo extensive first-pass metabolism, which reduces the bioavailability of these compounds. While pindolol does not undergo first-pass metabolism, liver metabolism is its major route of inactivation, as is the case with the other beta blockers. As a consequence, the half-lives of these compounds are short and necessitate at least two doses of drug per day. In addition, the half-lives of these beta blockers are increased in patients with liver disease, possibly requiring an adjustment of dose.

Nonmetabolized Beta Blockers

Atenolol and nadolol undergo little or no hepatic metabolism; consequently, their longer half-lives permit daily dosage for effective hypertension treatment. The half-lives of these beta blockers are increased with renal impairment and may require a down-adjustment of the dose.

Individual Beta Blockers

Beta blockers may be used as monotherapy in the treatment of hypertension or in combination with a diuretic. Certain fixed dose combinations of a beta blocker plus a diuretic are available and are listed at the end of this section.

Acebutolol: Sectral

PHARMACOKINETICS

While acebutolol undergoes first-pass metabolism, the acetylated metabolite, diacetolol, has pharmacologic activity and is present at steady state in concentrations 2.7 times that of acebutolol. Thus, while bioavailability is reduced, the beta blocking effect is not. The half-life is 2.7 hours.

DOSAGE FORMS AND STRENGTHS AVAILABLE

Capsules: 200 and 400 mg.

DOSAGES

Adult: initially, 400 mg as a single dose or in 2 divided doses. Maintenance, 200–800 mg daily (some patients may require up to 1.2 gm daily in two divided doses). It is recommended that the dose of acebutolol be reduced in patients with renal impairment; if creatinine clearance is less than 50 ml/min, 50% of the normal dose is used and if less than 25 ml/min, 25% of the normal dose is used.

Atenolol: Tenormin

PHARMACOKINETICS

Atenolol undergoes only minimal hepatic metabolism and is excreted unchanged in the urine. Its half-life is 6.3 hours and is increased in renal impairment.

DOSAGE FORMS AND STRENGTHS AVAILABLE
Tablets: 50 and 100 mg.

DOSAGES
Adult: initially, 25 mg once daily; may be increased to 50 or 100 mg daily. With severe renal impairment, the following maximum doses are recommended: When creatinine clearance is between 15 and 35 ml/min, 50 mg/day and when less than 15 ml/min, 50 mg every second day (USP DI).

Labetalol: Normodyne, Trandate

Labetalol is a competitive antagonist at both α- and β-adrenergic (3:1 to 7:1 β:α) receptors and acts somewhat like a combination of propranolol and prazosin. Thus, it reduces heart rate, cardiac output, and peripheral resistance, particularly with chronic use and rapid position changes. Labetalol differs from the classic beta blockers in that it appears to beneficially affect the plasma lipid profile. In addition, while classic beta blockers are more effective antihypertensive agents in white patients than in black patients, labetalol is equally effective in both [9].

PHARMACOKINETICS

Labetalol, with a half-life of 5.2 hours, undergoes extensive first-pass metabolism and is eliminated primarily by liver metabolism. Plasma-protein binding is 50%.

DOSAGE FORMS AND STRENGTHS AVAILABLE
Tablets: 100, 200, and 300 mg.
Injection: 5 mg/ml.

DOSAGES
Adult: initially, 100 mg twice daily; maintenance, 400–800 mg for mild to moderate hypertension. In severe hypertension, up to 1.2 gm daily in 2 or 3 divided doses may be required.

Metoprolol: Lopressor

Metoprolol acts preferentially on β_1-receptors.

PHARMACOKINETICS

Metoprolol undergoes extensive first-pass metabolism and has a half-life of 3.2 hours.

DOSAGE FORMS AND STRENGTHS AVAILABLE

Tablets: 50 and 100 mg.
Injection: 1 mg/ml.

DOSAGES

Adult: initially, 50 mg daily; maintenance, 100–300 mg daily in 1 or 2 doses. Some patients may require the total daily dose to be given in 3 separate doses to maintain satisfactory blood pressure control.

Nadolol: Corgard

Because of its long half-life, nadolol may serve as a one-a-day beta blocker.

PHARMACOKINETICS

Nadolol is eliminated primarily unchanged, by renal excretion, and has a half-life of 16 hours.

DOSAGE FORMS AND STRENGTHS AVAILABLE

Tablets: 40, 80, 120, 160 mg.

DOSAGES

Adult: initially, 20 mg once daily. Maintenance, 40–80 mg. Total daily dosage may be increased to 240 mg if needed. In patients with renal impairment, the dosage interval should be increased as creatinine clearance decreases according to the following:

Creatinine Clearance (ml/min)	Dosage Interval (hours)
> 50	24
31–50	24–36
10–30	24–48
> 10	40–60

Oxprenolol: Trasicor, Slow-Trasicor

Oxprenolol exhibits moderate ISA.

PHARMACOKINETICS

Oxyprenolol undergoes extensive first-pass metabolism.

DOSAGE FORMS AND STRENGTHS AVAILABLE

Tablets: 20, 40, and 80 mg.
Extended-release tablets: 80 and 160 mg.

DOSAGES

Adult: initially, 20 mg 3 times daily; may be increased to an upper limit of 480 mg/day. Twice daily dosing may be sufficient once the optimal daily dose is established. For maintenance, extended-release tablets may be taken once daily in the morning.

Pindolol: Visken

Pindolol is a nonselective beta blocker with ISA properties.

PHARMACOKINETICS

Pindolol is eliminated unchanged and is removed approximately equally by liver metabolism and by kidney excretion. It undergoes little or no first-pass metabolism and has a 3.6-hour half-life and plasma-protein binding of 51%.

DOSAGE FORMS AND STRENGTHS AVAILABLE

Tablets: 5 and 10 mg.

DOSAGES

Adult: initially, 10 mg twice daily or 5 mg 3 times daily. Dosage may be increased to an upper limit of 60 mg daily to obtain satisfactory blood pressure control. When optimal daily dose is established, once daily dosing may be used.

Propranolol: Inderal, Inderal LA, Detensol, Generic

Propranolol, the first clinically useful beta blocker, is nonselective and does not exhibit ISA.

PHARMACOKINETICS

Propranolol undergoes extensive first-pass metabolism and has a half-life of 3.9 hours. Plasma-protein binding is greater than 90%.

DOSAGE FORMS AND STRENGTHS AVAILABLE

Tablets: 10, 20, 40, 60, 80, 90, and 120 mg.
Extended-release capsules: 80, 120, and 160 mg.
Injection: 1 mg/ml.

DOSAGES

Adult: initially, 40 mg twice daily (may be increased to a total dose of up to 640 mg daily). Extended-release capsules may be administered once a day for maintenance of previously established dosage requirements.
Children: 1 mg/kg four times daily.

Timolol: Blocadren

PHARMACOKINETICS

Timolol undergoes extensive first-pass metabolism and has a 4-hour half-life. Oral timolol is the same drug as Timoptic, which is used in treatment of glaucoma by conjunctival instillation. Consequently, timolol is readily absorbed through conjunctival membranes and may raise plasma levels sufficiently to induce bradycardia and bronchospasm. Oral timolol may lower intraocular pressure. It is water soluble and less likely to affect the CNS than the lipophilic beta blockers.

DOSAGE FORMS AND STRENGTHS AVAILABLE

Tablets: 5, 10, and 20 mg

DOSAGES

Adults: initially, 10 mg twice daily; maintenance, 20–40 mg/day up to a maximum 60 mg/day in 2 divided doses.

Fixed Dose Combinations of Beta Blockers and Diuretics

Several fixed dose combinations of a beta blocker and a diuretic are available. These preparations simplify the use of these medications and may increase patient compliance where they can be used. However, such combinations should only be used when they contain the optimal amounts of each ingredient. The following is a list of the dosage forms and strengths available of such combinations.

Atenolol and Chlorthalidone
Tablets: Tenoretic

Atenolol (mg)	Chlorthalidone (mg)
50	25 (Tenoretic 50)
100	25 (Tenoretic 100)

Metoprolol Tartrate and Hydrochlorothiazide Tablets: Lopressor HCT

Metoprolol (mg)	Hydrochlorothiazide (mg)
50	25
100	25
100	50

Nadolol and Bendroflumethiazide Tablets: Corzide

Nadolol (mg)	Bendroflumethiazide (mg)
40	5
80	5

Pindolol Hydrochloride and Hydrochlorothiazide Tablets: Viskenzide

Pindolol (mg)	Hydrochlorothiazide (mg)
10	25
10	50

Propranolol Hydrochloride and Hydrochlorothiazide Tablets: Inderide

Propranolol (mg)	Hydrochlorothiazide (mg)
40	25
80	25

Timolol Maleate and Hydrochlorothiazide Tablets: Timolide

Timolol, 10 mg; hydrochlorothiazide, 25 mg.

Beta Blockers — Drug Interactions

PROPRANOLOL/LABETALOL/NADOLOL/PINDOLOL/TIMOLOL PLUS AMINOPHYLLINE/THEOPHYLLINE

Nonselective beta blockers antagonize the actions of theophylline in the lung and may increase bronchial resistance. Propranolol and other hepatically metabolized beta blockers may also reduce theophylline clearance and, thereby, increase theophylline blood levels. When these beta blockers and theophylline are combined, theophylline blood levels and the therapeutic response must be monitored, and the dose of theophylline should be adjusted as needed.

PROPRANOLOL AND OTHER BETA BLOCKERS PLUS VERAPAMIL/DILTIAZEM

The combination of a beta blocker and either of the two Ca^{2+} channel blockers may cause hypotension, bradycardia, and/or atrioventricular block. Both classes of agents decrease heart rate and AV conduction by different pharmacologic mechanisms, and their effects are additive.

The combination of these agents is common in the treatment of angina pectoris but should be avoided in patients with preexisting SA or AV nodal dysfunction. Cardiac function must be monitored frequently in the early stages of combination therapy and intermittently thereafter.

PROPRANOLOL AND OTHER BETA BLOCKERS PLUS CHLORPROMAZINE

When propranolol and other beta blockers and chlorpromazine are combined, the oral bioavailability of propranolol increases, apparently because of a reduction in first-pass metabolism of propranolol by chlorpromazine. Other phenothiazines may also exhibit a similar enhancing effect, and other beta blockers, such as labetalol and metoprolol, may also undergo an enhanced bioavailability when combined with chlorpromazine. Patients receiving the combination should be monitored for adverse effects, such as delirium, seizures, or hypotension, and the dose of propranolol and/or chlorpromazine should be reduced as needed.

PROPRANOLOL AND OTHER BETA BLOCKERS PLUS CLONIDINE

When clonidine is rapidly discontinued in a patient receiving both clonidine and propranolol, severe symptoms of sympathetic hyperactivity and blood pressure elevations occur within 24–72 hours. However, slowly decreasing the clonidine dosage over 7 days and concurrently reducing the propranolol dosage over several days may prevent this adverse interaction.

The discontinuation of clonidine is thought to result in a rebound increase in sympathetic activity. While the β_2-receptor-mediated vasodilation is blocked in patients receiving a nonselective beta blocker, the α-receptor-mediated vasoconstriction is unopposed. It is recommended that labetalol, which possesses alpha blocking activity, or one of the cardioselective beta blocking agents may be used instead of a nonselective agent, or that propranolol therapy may be discontinued well in advance of stopping clonidine therapy.

PROPRANOLOL/METOPROLOL/LABETALOL PLUS CIMETIDINE

The combination of hepatically metabolized beta blockers plus cimetidine results in as much as a twofold increase in plasma concentrations of the beta blocker. Cimetidine appears to reduce both first-pass and subsequent metabolism of the beta blocker by its ability to reduce hepatic blood flow and/or directly inhibit the metabolism of the beta blockers by the liver. Blood levels and the therapeutic response to the beta blocker should be monitored and the dose adjusted as needed. Alternatively, the use of a beta blocker such as atenolol, which does not undergo substantial hepatic metabolism, may be used.

PROPRANOLOL AND OTHER NONSELECTIVE BETA BLOCKERS PLUS EPINEPHRINE

The intravenous administration of epinephrine in a patient receiving propranolol will lead to a marked elevation of blood pressure plus a reflex reduction in heart rate. In the presence of the beta blocker, vasodilator β-receptors are blocked leaving vasoconstrictor α-receptors unopposed. Peripheral resistance and, therefore, blood pressure increases, causing a reflex increase in vagal stimulation to the heart. The use of epinephrine and other α-agonists should be avoided in patients receiving a nonselective beta blocker.

PROPRANOLOL AND OTHER NONSELECTIVE BETA BLOCKERS PLUS FUROSEMIDE

The combination of furosemide plus propranolol causes an elevation of blood levels of propranolol by unknown mechanisms. Blood levels and the therapeutic response to propranolol should be monitored, and the propranolol dose should be adjusted as needed.

PROPRANOLOL AND OTHER NONSELECTIVE BETA BLOCKERS PLUS INDOMETHACIN

Indomethacin reduces the antihypertensive effectiveness of propranolol. This may involve the indomethacin-induced inhibition of a vasodilator prostaglandin. The blood pressure should be monitored and either the propranolol dose increased or the indomethacin discontinued.

PROPRANOLOL AND OTHER NONSELECTIVE BETA BLOCKERS PLUS INSULIN

Hypoglycemia occasionally accompanies the use of insulin in diabetic patients. Propranolol slows the rate of return of glucose to normal blood levels and also prevents palpitations and other signs that indicate the diabetic is experiencing a hypoglycemia attack. Thus, the combination of insulin plus propranolol or other nonselective beta blockers represents an important risk for the diabetic patient. The modification of the hypoglycemic response by beta blockers involves primarily the $β_2$-receptor. Thus, when a beta blocking agent is indicated, a cardioselective agent should be used. The danger of unrecognized hypoglycemia in the insulin-dependent diabetic who is taking propranolol (and also cardioselective beta blockers) can be reduced if the patient is aware of the associated diaphoretic response.

LABETALOL PLUS HALOTHANE

In patients receiving labetalol, administration of halothane may cause myocardial depression; a decrease in arterial pressure, cardiac output, heart rate, and peripheral resistance; and an increase in central venous pressure. This interaction is due to a synergism between labetalol's α- and β-receptor blockade and halothane's myocardial depressant activity. This interaction between labetalol and halothane may be useful in cases in which reduced blood pressure without tachycardia is desirable. In those cases in which it is not desirable, the concentration of halothane may need to be reduced or another anesthetic may need to be substituted.

METOPROLOL PLUS PENTOBARBITAL/RIFAMPIN

The plasma concentration and bioavailability of orally administered metoprolol are reduced by coadministration of pentobarbital. This appears to involve a pentobarbital-induced induction of liver microsomal enzymes. Other beta blockers, such as propranolol and labetalol, which also undergo substantial first-pass and systemic metabolism, are likely to be similarly affected. Other barbiturates and rifampin, which are capable of inducing liver enzymes, may also interact in a similar manner. When these drugs are used in combination, the dose of metoprolol may have to be increased. Alternatively, drugs such as atenolol, nadolol, and pindolol that undergo little hepatic metabolism may be unaffected by coadministration with pentobarbital.

PROPRANOLOL PLUS THYROID

The bioavailability of propranolol is decreased in hyperthyroid patients. This results from enhanced first-pass metabolism and suggests that metoprolol and labetalol, which also undergo first-pass metabolism, would be similarly affected. Thus, in patients being treated for a thyroid abnormality, the dose of beta blocker may need to be increased. Alternatively, beta blockers that do not undergo first-pass metabolism may be used.

Sympathetic Nervous System Depressant Drugs

Drugs that lower blood pressure by depressing sympathetic activity act at numerous sites including the CNS, autonomic ganglia, adrenergic nerve terminals, and postsynaptic α- and β-adrenergic receptors. Beta blockers are included in this drug class. The remaining drugs in this class are reviewed in chronological order, since this corresponds with the growth in our understanding of antihypertensive drug action as well as the changing trends in the use of these agents. Reserpine and guanethidine were among the earliest antihypertensive agents available. Alpha-methyldopa soon followed, and the use of these three agents as antihypertension drugs established the following general characteristics of the sympathetic nervous system depressant drugs:

1. Effective in the treatment of mild to severe hypertension
2. Tend to cause plasma volume expansion, which attenuates their antihypertensive effect: "pseudo tolerance"
3. Used as "step 2" agents in the stepped care approach because:
   a. The step 1 diuretic prevents sympathetic depressant drug-induced plasma volume expansion
   b. Blood pressure lowering effects of the diuretics and the sympathetic depressant drugs are additive (exception: guanethidine is a step 4 agent)
4. Prevents the reflex sympathetic stimulation and cardiac hyperactivity caused by the step 3 agents, the vasodilators
5. Reduces plasma renin activity by lowering the sympathetic drive that mediates renin release from the kidneys
6. Can cause postural hypotension — for example, guanethidine causes venodilation, preventing the venoconstrictor response that maintains venous return to the heart and cardiac output when the patient changes from a supine to standing position
7. Can influence sexual dysfunction

While the above-listed adverse characteristics (numbers 2, 6, and 7) hold true for such sympathetic depressant drugs as reserpine, guanethidine, and α-methyldopa, they are much less representative or are absent in the case of the more recently introduced centrally acting α-agonists and the peripherally acting α_1-selective antagonist, prazosin. These agents exhibit little or no plasma volume expansion and leave both baroreceptor reflexes and venoconstrictor responses intact, greatly reducing the incidence and severity of postural hypotensive responses. However, it should be pointed out that the antihypertensive effects of these agents are also enhanced by combination with a thiazide diuretic.

Properties of Individual Sympathetic Nervous System Depressant Drugs

Reserpine: Sandril, Serpasil, SK-Reserpine, Generic

THERAPEUTIC USE

Reserpine is derived from *Rauwolfia serpentina* and has been used extensively as an antihypertensive agent since the 1950s. While some of the newer agents have certain advantages, reserpine still has a place in current therapy.

Reserpine is effective in mild to moderate hypertension. It has the potential to lower blood pressure very markedly and can be effective in more severe hypertension. However, the doses required to achieve this also elicit severe effects. The overriding consideration should be to use the lowest therapeutically effective doses in order to avoid all side effects.

Reserpine causes plasma volume expansion. Thus, it is almost always used in combination with a diuretic, which will potentiate its antihypertensive effect.

Reserpine has advantages that make its use recommended under particular circumstances, namely, when either cost or patient compliance is a concern. When combined with a diuretic, a low dose of reserpine can control blood pressure in most cases, with a low incidence of side effects, no greater than that observed with a diuretic plus a beta blocker. Reserpine is also effective when administered once daily, and it is inexpensive. All of these factors combine to improve patient compliance and overall therapeutic response. Numerous fixed dosage combinations of reserpine plus a diuretic are available. Selection of such a combination, provided that it contains the optimal dose of each drug, will further simplify drug therapy.

MECHANISM OF ACTION

Reserpine causes neurotransmitter depletion in peripheral adrenergic nerves, in the adrenal medulla, and in catecholaminergic and other monoaminergic nerves in the central nervous system. In the periphery, the depletion results in an impairment of adrenergic neurotransmission, and this is thought to be responsible for the antihypertensive effect. Reserpine-induced depletion of neurotransmitter in the CNS may also decrease sympathetic outflow. The overall effect is to reduce sympathetic activity in the cardiovascular system, with an attendant reduction in blood pressure.

ADVERSE EFFECTS

Reserpine can induce numerous side effects of modest to marked severity, and these effects are dose dependent. Using low but therapeutically effective doses, the incidence of side effects is comparable to that of α-methyldopa or beta blockers.

Some side effects of reserpine resulting from the depletion of CNS neurotransmitters include a decrease in mental alertness, headache, sedation, depression, and, rarely, extrapyramidal symptoms. Depression is of particular concern, since in sensitive individuals, the effect can be severe. Reserpine is contraindicated in patients with a history of depressive episodes.

Depression of the sympathetic nervous system by reserpine can cause nasal stuffiness, postural hypotension, and impotence. However, the incidence and severity of these symptoms is generally low. Sympathetic depression can also cause a phenomenon called *parasympathetic predominance*. This manifests primarily as gastrointestinal hyperactivity and can be the underlying cause of abdominal cramps, diarrhea, and gastro-hypersecretion. Reserpine should be used cautiously in patients with gall stones, peptic ulcer, or ulcerative colitis.

PHARMACOKINETICS

Reserpine is rapidly and easily absorbed after oral administration. It is taken up into lipid structures and uniformly distributed throughout the brain. The half-life initially is 4½ hours. However, the antihypertensive effect of reserpine is independent of blood levels. Reserpine becomes bound to the neurotransmitter storage granules in sympathetic adrenergic nerves, the adrenal medulla, and monamine systems in the brain. In normal antihypertensive doses, the drug slows neurotransmitter synthesis by an action at one step in this process, and depletion occurs as a consequence of normal sympathetic nerve activity plus slowed repletion by synthesis. The onset of antihypertensive action is seen after several days and reaches peak effect between 3 and 6 weeks. Return to normal sympathetic function also takes several weeks after termination to reserpine therapy. Elimination of reserpine is primarily by liver metabolism.

DOSAGE FORMS AND STRENGTHS AVAILABLE

Tablets: 0.1, 0.25, 0.5, and 1 mg.
Timed-release capsules (Releserp-5): 0.5 mg.

DOSAGES

Adults and children: initially and for maintenance, 0.05–0.1 mg once daily. Daily dose should not exceed 0.25 mg.

Other rauwolfia alkaloids are also available. The reader is referred to either American Medical Association drug evaluations or USP DI.

The following fixed combinations of reserpine and diuretic are also available:

Diupres-250–500

Reserpine (mg)	Chlorothiazide (mg)
0.125	250
0.125	500

Diutensin-R

Reserpine, 0.1 mg; methyclothiazide, 2.5 mg.

Hydromox-R

Reserpine, 0.125 mg; quinethazone, 50 mg.

Hydropres-25–50

Reserpine (mg)	Hydrochlorothiazide (mg)
0.125	25
0.125	50

Metatensin

Reserpine (mg)	Trichlormethiazide (mg)
0.1	2
0.1	4

Naquival

Reserpine, 0.1 mg; trichlormethiazide, 4 mg.

Regroton

Reserpine, 0.125 mg; chlorthalidone, 25 mg.

Demi-Regroton

Reserpine, 0.25 mg; chlorthalidone, 50 mg.

Renese-R

Reserpine, 0.25 mg; polythiazide, 2 mg.

Salutensin

Reserpin, 0.125 mg; hydroflumethiazide, 25 mg.

Salutensin-Demi

Reserpine, 0.125 mg; hydroflumethiazide, 50 mg.

Serpasil-Esidrix No. 1, No. 2

Reserpine (mg)	Hydrochlorothiazide (mg)
No. 1 0.1	25
No. 2 0.1	50

Guanethidine: Ismelin

THERAPEUTIC USES

Among the sympathetic depressant drugs, guanethidine has the greatest capacity to lower blood pressure. This agent is almost always used in combination with other drugs to control severe hypertension. The greater efficacy of guanethidine is also responsible, in part, for its greater tendency to expand plasma volume and induce postural hypotension.

Guanethidine is used for the treatment of moderate to severe hypertension. It is considered a step 4 drug. As one example of this approach, guanethidine could be combined with a diuretic, a beta blocker, and a vasodilator. At the very least, guanethidine should be combined with a diuretic to counteract its marked ability to expand plasma volume.

MECHANISM OF ACTION

Guanethidine is taken up into peripheral adrenergic nerve terminals, where it is concentrated and exerts a local anestheticlike nerve block. Thus, it impairs adrenergic neurotransmission and depresses sympathetic activity in the cardiovascular system. This, in turn, underlies the drug's blood pressure-lowering effect. In addition, guanethidine is taken up into intraneuronal storage granules and displaces norepinephrine from these sites. This leads to neurotransmitter depletion, which also contributes to the antihypertensive action of the drug. Guanethidine has little or no effect on adrenal medullary function and does not cross the blood-brain barrier.

HEMODYNAMIC EFFECTS

Guanethidine decreases both cardiac output and peripheral resistance. Peripheral resistance is decreased because of reduced sympathetic tone on the arterial side. Cardiac output is decreased because of reduced sympathetic tone in the heart and veins; this increases venous capacitance and reduces venous return to the heart, thereby reducing cardiac output. Guanethidine also reduces heart rate.

ADVERSE EFFECTS

The adverse effects of guanethidine are due primarily to adrenergic neuron blockade. This results in postural hypotensive effects such as dizziness or lightheadedness. These side effects are common, and the patient must be advised not to stand up rapidly from a sitting or lying position. Other side effects include nasal stuffiness, tiredness or weakness, and difficulty in ejaculation. The impairment of sympathetic activity also allows parasympathetic predominance, which leads to diarrhea or an increase in bowel movements and, rarely, nausea and vomiting. The high degree of sympathetic depression caused by guanethidine can induce the development of supersensitivity in the cardiovascular system. Thus, high circulating levels of catecholamines can cause a hypertensive crisis. For this reason, guanethidine is contraindicated in pheochromocytoma.

PHARMACOKINETICS

Guanethidine undergoes highly variable absorption among patients, ranging between 3% and 30% of an oral dose. Approximately half of the drug is excreted unchanged, while the other half is metabolized. Guanethidine has a half-life of approximately 5 days.

The antihypertensive effect of guanethidine is independent of fluctuations in plasma levels, since its antihypertensive effect depends on the uptake and storage of guanethidine in peripheral adrenergic nerve terminals. The onset of its effect occurs within a few hours, and full therapeutic effects are observed after 1–3 weeks. A similar 1- to 3-week period is required for recovery from the effects of guanethidine after withdrawal of therapy.

TITRATION OF DOSE

The dose of guanethidine must be carefully titrated in each patient for several reasons. First, its absorption after oral administration ranges between 3% and 30%. Second, the full therapeutic effect is not obtained until 1–3 weeks after the initiation of therapy. Third, the therapeutic endpoint is complex. Due to the postural hypotensive effect of guanethidine, blood pressure lowering is greater in the standing position and during exercise than it is in the supine position. The goal is to obtain adequate blood pressure lowering in the supine position without excessive postural hypotensive effects in the standing position. During titration of the drug, the dose should be increased no more often than every 5–7 days.

DOSAGE FORMS AND STRENGTHS AVAILABLE

Tablets: 10 and 25 mg.

Adult: ambulatory patients: initially 10 or 12.5 mg once daily. The daily dosage may be increased by 10 or 12.5 mg at 5–7 intervals. An upper limit is 300 mg/day. However, it is rarely necessary to go above 100 mg daily, since guanethidine is combined with other antihypertensive agents.
Adult: hospitalized patients: initially 25–50 mg once daily; may be increased by 25–50 mg at daily intervals or every other day as needed for control of blood pressure.
Children: 0.2 mg/kg of body weight daily; may be increased by 0.2 mg/kg at 7- to 10-day intervals as needed.

Guanadrel: Hylorel

THERAPEUTIC USE

Guanadrel is chemically related to guanethidine and lowers blood pressure by the same mechanism. Its duration of action is shorter, and this may result in a lower incidence or severity of morning postural hypotension than is experienced with guanethidine.

Guanadrel has the capacity to lower blood pressure dramatically and can be used in a manner similar to that used for guanethidine. Nevertheless, it has been evaluated primarily in comparison with α-methyldopa and other drugs of similar potency. It is considered a step 2 drug and should be used in combination with a diuretic to treat moderate to severe hypertension.

MECHANISM OF ACTION

Guanadrel is concentrated in peripheral adrenergic nerve terminals, where it exerts a local anesthetic-like nerve block. It also displaces endogenous norepinephrine from intraneuronal granular storage sites, resulting in neurotransmitter depletion. Overall, sympathetic neurotransmission is impaired, and this underlies the pressure-lowering effect of the drug. Guanadrel has little or no effect on adrenal medulla and does not cross the blood-brain barrier.

HEMODYNAMIC EFFECTS

Guanadrel decreases both cardiac output and peripheral resistance. Peripheral resistance is decreased because of reduced sympathetic tone on the arterial side. Cardiac output is decreased because of reduced sympathetic tone in the heart and veins. This increases venous capacitance and reduces venous return to the heart, thereby reducing cardiac output. Guanadrel also reduces heart rate.

ADVERSE EFFECTS

The adverse effects of guanadrel are due primarily to adrenergic blockade. Like guanethidine, guanadrel can cause postural hypotension, dizziness, lightheadedness, impotence, difficulty in ejaculation, and diarrhea. Morning postural hypotension and diarrhea may be less than is seen with guanethidine, and this is due to the shorter duration of action of guanadrel.

PHARMACOKINETICS

Guanadrel is rapidly absorbed from the gastrointestinal tract. Onset of antihypertensive action occurs at approximately 2 hours and reaches a peak effect between 4 and 6 hours. Duration of effect ranges between 4 and 14 hours after a single dose. Approximately 40% of guanadrel is excreted unchanged, and the remainder undergoes hepatic metabolism.

DOSAGE FORMS AND STRENGTHS AVAILABLE

Tablets: 10 and 25 mg.

DOSAGES

Adults: initially, 10 mg daily; may be increased daily, weekly, or monthly until blood pressure control is obtained. Maintenance, usually 25–75 mg daily. The total dose may be given in 2 divided doses.

Alpha-Methyldopa: Aldomet

THERAPEUTIC USE

Alpha-methyldopa has been used extensively and successfully for the last 20 years in the treatment of mild to moderate hypertension. It has less capacity to lower blood pressure than guanethidine, but it also causes much less postural hypotension, impotence, and gastrointestinal symptoms associated with parasympathetic predominance.

Alpha-methyldopa is indicated for the treatment of mild to moderate hypertension. Since this agent can induce salt and water retention during long-term use, it is almost always used in combination with a diuretic, which enhances its blood-pressure lowering effect.

MECHANISM OF ACTION

Alpha-methyldopa distributes throughout the body, including the brain, since it readily crosses the blood-brain barrier. It is taken up into all catecholaminergic nerve terminals and converted to α-methylnorepinephrine. Its site of antihypertensive action is the medulla of the brain stem, where its synthesis product, α-methylnorepinephrine, acts to decrease sympathetic outflow to the heart and vasculature. This results in decreased cardiac output and peripheral resistance and, thus, in lowered blood pressure.

ADVERSE EFFECTS

The most common adverse effects include dizziness, drowsiness, dry mouth, and headache. Mental depression can occur occasionally. Most patients receiving long-term alpha-methyldopa as sole therapy will experience fluid retention, weight gain, and edema. Ten to 20% of patients exhibit a positive Coombs' test. However, only a small fraction of these experience hemolytic anemia. Nevertheless, alpha-methyldopa should not be used in patients with a history of autoimmune hemolytic anemia. Thrombocytopenia, leukopenia, and hepatic dysfunction have also been reported to occur rarely.

The incidence of severe adverse effects with alpha-methyldopa is low. Nevertheless, to avoid these, it is recommended that blood cell counts and hepatic function determinations be performed before initiating therapy and again intermittently during therapy. The occurrence of side effects with alpha-methyldopa is dose related and may be substantially reduced or eliminated by using the smallest therapeutically effective dose, in the range of 125–150 mg twice daily.

PHARMACOKINETICS

Alpha-methyldopa's rate of absorption from the gastrointestinal tract approximates 50%, and it has a plasma half-life of 1.8 hours.

Alpha-methyldopa appears 20–55% unchanged in the urine. The remainder undergoes hepatic metabolism. Its antihypertensive effect is unrelated to the plasma half-life, since the drug acts by crossing the blood-brain barrier, being taken up into central adrenergic neurons and converted to α-methylnorepinephrine. While an antihypertensive effect can be seen within a few hours, peak blood pressure lowering effect is obtained after 2–3 days.

DOSAGE FORMS AND STRENGTHS AVAILABLE

Oral suspension: 50 mg/ml.
Tablets: 125, 250, 500 mg.
Methyldopate hydrochloride injection: 50 mg/ml.

DOSAGES

Adult: initially, 250 mg at bedtime; may be increased to 250 mg twice daily after 1 week. Dosage may then be increased as needed to a maximum daily dose of 2 gm.

Children: initially, 10 mg/kg daily in 2–4 divided doses. Dose should be adjusted at 2 day- or longer intervals for proper blood pressure control. The maximum daily dose is 65 mg/kg.

Clonidine: Catapres

THERAPEUTIC USE

Clonidine is the first of a different class of antihypertensive agents, the centrally acting α_2-agonists. A particular advantage of these drugs is that they have little or no effect on postural reflexes, allowing effective blood pressure lowering without postural or exercise hypotension.

The therapeutic use of clonidine has changed due to the clinical experience gained over the decade since its introduction. In contrast to alpha-methyldopa, clonidine has been found effective as monotherapy in mild to moderate hypertension. It is especially useful in the elderly, who benefit from the lack of effect on postural reflexes. Clonidine appears to have an increased efficacy in certain other subgroups of hypertensive patients, such as adolescents and borderline hypertensives. In addition, since clonidine lowers blood pressure without altering either renal blood flow or glucose tolerance, this agent has particular usefulness in hypertensives with renal failure or diabetes.

RISK OF REBOUND HYPERTENSION

The risk of rebound hypertension on abrupt withdrawal of clonidine appears to be greater with doses above 1.2 mg/day. Certain precautions can be taken to avoid this adverse effect. Missed doses should be taken as soon as possible, and the patient should be instructed to check with the physician if 2 or more doses are missed. The patient should always have enough medication for weekends or vacations.

The side effects of clonidine are dose dependent and are substantially reduced or eliminated by low-dose therapy. When such doses do not sufficiently lower blood pressure, it is recommended to add a low dose of a second agent, rather than increase the clonidine dose. An increased antihypertensive effect is obtained while avoiding the side effects of either agent. For example, the combination of clonidine plus a diuretic has an additive effect on blood pressure. Clonidine has also been found to be an effective alternative to beta blockers in a triple-drug combination with a diuretic and a vasodilator.

MECHANISM OF ACTION

The site of antihypertensive action of clonidine is the medulla of the brain stem in the region of the nucleus tractus solitarius and the vasomotor control center. Clonidine activates α_2-receptors in this region, leading to a decreased sympathetic outflow to the cardiovascular system. In the standing position, cardiac output is reduced due to both decreased heart rate and diminished venous return to the heart. In the supine position, total peripheral resistance is reduced. These hemodynamic changes underlie the reduction of blood pressure caused by clonidine.

ADVERSE EFFECTS

The most common side effects are drowsiness, dry mouth, and dizziness. Fluid retention, leading to swelling in the lower extremities, occurs occasionally in long-term therapy, and mental depression occurs rarely. Rebound hypertension may occur upon abruptly stopping clonidine therapy, especially if very high doses have been used (greater than 1.2 mg/day); within 12–48 hours, the blood pressure may return to or rise above pretreatment levels. Some patients experience symptoms characteristic of increased sympathetic activity: insomnia, restlessness, tremor, anxiety, sweating, and palpitations.

PHARMACOKINETICS

Clonidine is well absorbed from the gastrointestinal tract. It has a half-life of approximately 12 hours but ranges widely from 6–23 hours and increases to a range of 25–37 hours with renal function impairment. Clonidine undergoes hepatic metabolism, and 65% of the drug is excreted via the kidneys as unchanged drug and metabolites. Twenty percent is excreted by the biliary tract. The onset of antihypertensive effect of clonidine is at 30–60 minutes and reaches a peak between 2 and 4 hours. The antihypertensive effects last up to 8 hours.

DOSAGE FORMS AND STRENGTHS AVAILABLE

Tablets: 0.1, 0.2 and 0.3 mg.

Transdermal clonidine (Catapres-TTS-1, -2, -3): Transdermal delivery systems are applied to the skin and designed to deliver clonidine 0.1, 0.2, and 0.3 mg/day, respectively. (These preparations may have the advantage of delivering a constant blood level of clonidine that does not fluctuate either into the toxic range or into the range that is below therapeutic efficacy. The preparations are designed to be applied for a 7-day interval. There is some report of skin irritation accompanying this mode of administration.)

DOSAGES

Adult: initially, 0.1 mg once daily at bedtime for several weeks, followed by 0.1 mg twice daily. Dosage may be increased gradually by 0.1 or 0.2 mg. Maintenance, 0.2–0.8 mg in 2–4 divided daily doses.

Treatment of severe hypertension in the urgent but not emergency situation — loading dose: PO, 0.2 mg, followed by 0.1 mg every hour until diastolic pressure is controlled or a total of 0.7 mg has been given. The patient is then controlled on a normal maintenance dose.

Guanabenz: Wytensin

THERAPEUTIC USE

Guanabenz is a newer member of the central α_2-agonist class of hypertensive agents. It is a derivative of aminoguanadine and also possesses some peripheral adrenergic neuron-blocking action similar to that of guanethidine. The long-term use of guanabenz has not been associated with any deleterious effects on either serum cholesterol or triglyceride levels.

Guanabenz is effective in treating mild to moderate hypertension. It appears to lack the potential to induce salt and water retention. In fact, many patients experience a mild natriuresis and weight loss during long-term therapy. Thus, guanabenz is clearly effective as monotherapy. However, its blood pressure lowering effect is enhanced by the addition of a diuretic, and many patients who fail to respond to guanabenz alone exhibit satisfactory blood pressure control with the combination of guanabenz plus a diuretic.

MECHANISM OF ACTION

Guanabenz activates α_2-receptors in the medulla of the brain stem, resulting in a decreased sympathetic outflow in the cardiovascular system. Initially, blood pressure is lowered by a reduction in cardiac output; a reduction in total peripheral resistance lowers blood pressure during long-term therapy.

ADVERSE EFFECTS

The most frequently reported side effects of guanabenz are sedation, dry mouth, weakness, and dizziness. Sexual dysfunction occurs rarely. Rebound hypertension on abrupt withdrawal has been reported to occur but is rare and appears to occur with doses above 32 mg per day. The associated symptoms include insomnia, restlessness, tremor, anxiety, sweating, and palpitations.

PHARMACOKINETICS

Guanabenz is approximately 75% absorbed from the gastrointestinal tract, but it undergoes extensive first-pass metabolism. Elimination is also primarily by hepatic metabolism. Guanabenz is approximately 90% plasma-protein bound and has a half-life of about 6 hours. Onset of its antihypertensive effect occurs within 60 minutes, reaches peak effect in 2–4 hours, and lasts for approximately 12 hours.

DOSAGE FORMS AND STRENGTHS AVAILABLE

Tablets: 4 and 8 mg.

DOSAGES

Adult: initially, 4 mg twice daily. The dose may be increased gradually up to 32 mg twice daily.

Guanfacine (Investigational Drug)

THERAPEUTIC USE

Guanfacine closely resembles clonidine in many of its therapeutic and pharmacologic properties. However, guanfacine enters and leaves the brain more slowly than clonidine and has a somewhat longer half-life. For this reason, it may have the advantage of being effective on once a day dosing.

MECHANISM OF ACTION

The site of antihypertensive action of guanfacine is the medulla of the brainstem in the region of the nucleus tractus solitarius and the vasomotor control center. Guanfacine activates α_2-receptors in this region, leading to a decreased sympathetic outflow to the cardiovascular system. In the standing position, cardiac output is reduced due to both decreased heart rate and diminished venous return to the heart. In the supine position, total peripheral resistance is reduced. These hemodynamic changes underlie the reduction of blood pressure caused by guanfacine.

ADVERSE EFFECTS

The adverse effects of guanfacine resemble those of clonidine: Dry mouth, sedation, and dizziness are the most common side effects. Fluid retention requiring concomitant use of a diuretic may occur. Rebound hypertension may also occur on sudden withdrawal of the medication.

PHARMACOKINETICS

Guanfacine is rapidly and almost completely absorbed from the gastrointestinal tract. It has a half-life of 16–20 hours and is eliminated by renal excretion of unchanged drug and by hepatic metabolism.

DOSAGE FORMS AND STRENGTHS AVAILABLE

Capsules: 0.5, 1, 2, and 3 mg.

DOSAGES

Adult: initially, 0.5 mg twice daily; may be increased gradually as needed; maintenance, usually 1–3 mg may be given as a single dose or in 2 divided doses.

Prazosin: Minipress

THERAPEUTIC USE

The early experience with α-antagonists as antihypertensive agents was disappointing. Phentolamine, used to treat essential hypertension, caused marked postural hypotension, increased heart rate, increased plasma renin activity, and increased salt and water retention. In light of this finding, it was surprising that prazosin, also an α-antagonist, is not only an effective antihypertensive agent but essentially lacks these side effects. One factor that may account for the difference between phentolamine and prazosin is that the former is nonselective, whereas the latter selectively blocks the postsynaptic α_1-receptor.

Prazosin is effective as monotherapy in the treatment of mild to moderate hypertension and may be particularly useful in those patients who cannot tolerate either diuretics or beta blockers. On the other hand, combining prazosin with a diuretic or a beta blocker provides greater blood pressure control than that with prazosin alone. The combination of all three drugs provides even greater blood pressure control and is effective in the treatment of moderate to severe hypertension. Thus, prazosin can be used as a step 1, step 2, or step 3 drug. Prazosin appears to be a unique hypertensive drug for reversing left ventricular hypertrophy.

The first-dose postural hypotensive reaction to prazosin occurs in only a small fraction of patients. In addition, this phenomenon may be avoided by initiating the prazosin therapy with a subtherapeutic dose of 1 mg taken at bedtime for the first few doses. Subsequently, the normal 2 or 3 times daily dosing may be undertaken.

Long-term therapy with prazosin is associated with lowered LDL levels and elevated HDL levels. Thiazide diuretics and beta blockers tend to increase LDL, but this action is attenuated when these agents are combined with prazosin.

MECHANISM OF ACTION

Prazosin is a selective α_1-antagonist. The α_1-receptor is located on the smooth muscle cells of both arteries and veins and mediates vasoconstriction. Prazosin blocks this receptor, causing both vasodilation and venodilation. Total peripheral resistance decreases, and this underlies the blood pressure-lowering effect of the drug. Prazosin has little or no effect on heart rate, cardiac output, or plasma renin activity. Since α_1-receptors are located on both arterial and venous sites, prazosin decreases both afterload and preload on the heart and is useful in the treatment of congestive heart disease.

α_2-presynaptic adrenoceptors are located on adrenergic nerve terminals and mediate a negative feedback inhibition of neurotransmitter release. Blocking these receptors, as with phentolamine, markedly enhances neurotransmitter release. However, prazosin has little or no effect on these presynaptic receptors. This, in part, may account for the fact that prazosin generally does not increase either heart rate or cardiac output. α_2-postsynaptic receptors have been identified on both the arterial and venous side of the vasculature. These receptors mediate vasoconstriction. However, prazosin has much less blocking effect on these receptors than on the α_1-adrenoceptor. Thus, the venoconstrictor response to standing from a supine position remains intact, probably mediated by postsynaptic α_2-mediated venoconstriction to enhance sympathetic activity.

ADVERSE EFFECTS

In general, the adverse effects of prazosin are relatively mild and rarely necessitate discontinuation of the drug. The most common side effects are related to postural reflexes; these include dizziness or lightheadedness, particularly on standing up rapidly from a sitting or lying position. Patients with sodium depletion or those already receiving beta blocker therapy are predisposed to these symptoms. Other less common side effects include drowsiness, headache, lack of energy, and edema of the lower extremities. A small fraction of patients experience a first-dose postural hypotensive reaction, characterized by excessive postural hypotension, very rapid heart rate, and syncope. This may be avoided by appropriate initial titration of the dose.

PHARMACOKINETICS

Prazosin is well absorbed from the gastrointestinal tract and undergoes first-pass metabolism. The plasma half-life of prazosin is 2–3 hours. However, the antihypertensive effect lasts much longer, up to 10 hours. The initial blood pressure lowering effect of prazosin occurs within 2–4 hours of the first dose. However, up to 3–4 weeks may be required for optimal effect. Prazosin is eliminated primarily in bile and feces. The drug undergoes enterohepatic circulation, and approximately 90% is metabolized in the liver. Five to 11% is eliminated as unchanged drug. Prazosin is approximately 95% plasma-protein bound.

DOSAGE FORMS AND STRENGTHS AVAILABLE

Capsules: 0.5 (not available in the United States), 1, 2, and 5 mg.

DOSAGES

Adult: to minimize the danger of syncopal reaction, the first dose should not exceed 1 mg and should be given at bedtime. The patient should be instructed to remain in bed for several hours. Thereafter, 1 mg may be given 2 times daily and increased to 3 times daily later, as needed.

Prazosin should be added cautiously to the regimen of patients receiving a beta blocker or other sympathetic depressants. When other antihypertensive drugs are added to the regimen, the dose of prazosin should be reduced to 1 or 2 mg and the optimal amount determined again on the basis of patient response.

The normal maintenance dose is 6–15 mg daily in 2 or 3 divided doses. The upper-normal maintenance dose is 20 mg daily, given in 2 or 3 divided doses. However, some patients respond to up to 40 mg daily.

Children: 7–12 years of age — PO, initially 0.5 mg 2 or 3 times daily, adjusted according to response.

Fixed Dose Combinations of Sympathetic Depressant Drugs and Diuretics

Several sympathetic depressant drugs are available in fixed dose combinations with diuretics. Those with reserpine are listed above, and additional combinations with clonidine, alpha-methyldopa, guanethidine, and prazosin are listed below. It is important to remember that these combinations should only be used if the dosages of both components are optimal. If so, these combinations simplify taking medicine and may improve patient compliance.

Clonidine Hydrochloride and Chlorthalidone Tablets: Combipres

Clonidine (mg)	Chlorthalidone (mg)
0.1	15
0.2	15
0.3	15

Methyldopa and Chlorothiazide Tablets: Aldoclor

Methyldopa (mg)	Chlorothiazide (mg)
250	150 (Aldoclor-150)
250	250 (Aldoclor-250)

Methyldopa and Hydrochlorothiazide Tablets: Aldoril

Methyldopa (mg)	Hydrochlorothiazide (mg)
250	15 (Aldoril-15)
250	25 (Aldoril-25)
500	30 (Aldoril D30)
500	50 (Aldoril D50)

Sympathetic Nervous Tissue Depressant-Drug Interactions

CLONIDINE PLUS PROPRANOLOL

See propranolol plus clonidine above.

GUANETHIDINE/GUANADREL PLUS CHLORPROMAZINE

Chlorpromazine may attenuate or reverse the antihypertensive effects of guanethidine. Guanethidine exerts its antihypertensive affect by being taken up into adrenergic nerve terminals, where it exerts a neuron blockade. Chlorpromazine blocks the neuronal uptake process and, thereby, the action of guanethidine. Other phenothiazines are less potent as norepinephrine uptake blockers. Nevertheless, they may also interact with guanethidine. Guanethidine and chlorpromazine should not be used in combination. Other antihypertensive agents that do not interact with chlorpromazine should be used.

GUANETHIDINE/GUANADREL PLUS DESIPRAMINE

Desipramine and other tricyclic antidepressants are inhibitors of the adrenergic neuronal uptake process for norepinephrine. Guanethidine acts by being taken up into the adrenergic neuron by the same uptake process. Thus, desipramine reverses the antihypertensive effect of guanethidine by blocking its uptake into adrenergic neurons. The combination of guanethidine plus desipramine or other tricyclic antidepressants should be avoided. Other antihypertensive agents that do not interact with the tricyclic antidepressants should be used.

GUANETHIDINE/GUANADREL PLUS DEXTROAMPHETAMINE

Guanethidine and guanadrel lower blood pressure by inducing adrenergic neuron blockade. These agents exert their actions by being taken up and concentrated into the adrenergic neuron. Dextroamphetamine exerts its action by being taken up into the adrenergic neuron and causing the displacement or release of endogenous neurotransmitter, norepinephrine. Dextroamphetamine reverses the antihypertensive effects of guanethidine and guanadrel by inhibiting their uptake into the adrenergic neuron and causing their displacement from intraneuronal storage sites. The combination of guanethidine or guanadrel plus dextroamphetamine should be avoided. Alternative antihypertensive agents may be used.

GUANETHIDINE/GUANADREL PLUS MINOXIDIL

The combined administration of guanethidine or guanadrel plus minoxidil may cause a profound orthostatic hypotension. The mechanism of this interaction is unknown. However, guanethidine causes orthostatic hypotension and minoxidil, which lacks this action itself, appears to enhance the orthostatic hypotensive effect of guanethidine. When starting minoxidil therapy, guanethidine administration should be stopped at least one week in advance or the drugs should be coadministered in a hospital setting.

GUANETHIDINE/GUANADREL PLUS INSULIN

Guanethidine improves glucose tolerance over long-term therapy, necessitating a reduction in insulin dose in diabetic patients. Diabetic patient response to insulin must be monitored and the dose adjusted as needed whenever guanethidine is added or removed from the drug regimen.

GUANETHIDINE/GUANADREL PLUS MAZINDOL

The combination of guanethidine/guanadrel and mazindol reverses the antihypertensive effect of either guanethidine or guanadrel. Mazindol possesses indirect sympathomimetic activity; that is, it is taken up into adrenergic nerve terminals and causes the displacement of endogenous neurotransmitter. Mazindol may either block the uptake of guanethidine/guanadrel into adrenergic nerve terminals and/or cause its displacement from the nerve terminal. Avoid this drug combination.

GUANETHIDINE/GUANADREL PLUS PHENELZINE AND OTHER MONOAMINE OXIDASE INHIBITORS

The addition of a monoamine oxidase inhibitor to guanethidine therapy markedly attenuates or reverses the antihypertensive effect of guanethidine. This combination should be avoided.

GUANETHIDINE/GUANADREL PLUS PHENYLEPHRINE AND OTHER DIRECT ACTING α-AGONISTS

α-agonists or direct acting sympathomimetic agents attenuate the antihypertensive actions of guanethidine and guanadrel. This may be due to a supersensitivity of vascular smooth muscle that results from long-term guanethidine therapy. The use of direct sympathomimetic agents should be avoided in patients receiving guanethidine.

METHYLDOPA PLUS NOREPINEPHRINE

In patients receiving methyldopa therapy, the pressure response to norepinephrine is increased and prolonged. Thus, when norepinephrine is to be used in such a patient, the dose should be initially reduced and titrated upward to achieve the appropriate therapeutic effect.

RESERPINE PLUS EPHEDRINE

Ephedrine is an indirect sympathomimetic. Thus, in a reserpine treated patient whose adrenergic nerve terminals have been at least partially depleted of catecholamines, ephedrine's action is attenuated or absent. It is recommended that a direct sympathomimetic agent, such as norepinephrine or phenylephrine, be used instead of ephedrine.

RESERPINE PLUS THIOPENTAL

Patients on reserpine who receive thiopental in preparation for surgery may experience hypotension and bradycardia. Should this interaction occur and require treatment, a direct sympathomimetic agent should be used to treat the hypotension.

RESERPINE PLUS LEVODOPA

Reserpine causes depletion of dopamine in the central nervous system and can cause Parkinson-like symptoms. In a Parkinson patient, reserpine will decrease the therapeutic effects of levodopa. The dosages of either or both drugs may need to be adjusted to maintain adequate therapeutic response.

RESERPINE PLUS MONOAMINE OXIDASE INHIBITORS

The combination of reserpine plus monoamine oxidase inhibitors (MAOI) may cause a moderate to sudden and severe hypertension and hyperpyrexia. This drug combination should be avoided.

PRAZOSIN PLUS INDOMETHACIN

Indomethacin attenuates the blood pressure lowering affect of prazosin, possibly through the inhibition of the synthesis of a vasodilator prostaglandin. When these agents are combined, the blood pressure must be monitored and the prazosin dose increased as needed.

PRAZOSIN PLUS PROPRANOLOL

Prazosin exhibits a first-dose postural hypotensive reaction in some patients. This reaction is enhanced in patients simultaneously receiving propranolol and prazosin. Prazosin therapy should be initiated with doses of 0.5 mg or less.

Vasodilators

Several drug classes exert their primary hemodynamic and antihypertensive effects by vasodilation. The present section addresses the direct vasodilators, hydralazine and minoxidil. The indirect vasodilators include the α_1-blocker prazosin, discussed in the previous section, and the converting enzyme inhibitors and calcium channel antagonists discussed in the next section.

MODE OF ACTION AND REFLEX RESPONSES TO VASODILATOR THERAPY

The primary site of action of these vasodilators used for the chronic treatment of hypertension is arteriolar smooth muscle. These agents can markedly reduce total peripheral resistance. On the other hand, they have little or no effect on capacitance vessels (venules and small veins). Vasodilation stimulates marked compensatory responses. The consequent reduction in blood pressure is detected by baroreceptors in the aortic arch and carotid sinus, leading to increased sympathetic activity throughout the cardiovascular system. The heart rate and strength of contraction is increased, leading to an increase in cardiac output. In addition, venoconstriction occurs, increasing venous return to the heart and contributing to the increased cardiac output. Increased sympathetic stimulation in the kidneys leads to elevated plasma renin activity (which contributes to fluid volume expansion; see below).

In addition to reflex cardiac stimulation, vasodilation induces intravascular volume expansion and, eventually, total fluid volume expansion. Reduction of the blood pressure by vasodilation reduces capillary hydrostatic pressure, causing the movement of fluid from the extracellular to the intravascular compartment, that is, plasma volume expansion occurs. In addition, vasodilation induces sodium and water retention by two mechanisms. First, lowering the blood pressure reduces the pressure-induced natriuresis, conserving both salt and water. Second, the reflex sympathetic stimulation caused by vasodilation stimulates renin release, leads to angiotensin and, subsequently, aldosterone formation, and ultimately, the conservation of Na^+ and water in the distal tubule of the kidney.

THERAPEUTIC USE OF THE VASODILATORS

Vasodilators used in the chronic treatment of hypertension are step 3 drugs. In general, vasodilators should not be used alone. Vasodilators should be used in combination with a diuretic to prevent fluid volume expansion and a beta blocker to prevent sympathetic stimulation of the heart and kidneys. Other agents, such as clonidine, which reduces sympathetic outflow from the central nervous system, may be used in place of the beta blocker.

When used in "triple therapy" (diuretic, beta blocker, and vasodilator), vasodilators are effective in the treatment of moderate to severe hypertension. The antihypertensive effects of the three classes of drugs are synergistic. Furthermore, combining these agents allows the use of low doses of each, yet it still provides good blood pressure control in the vast majority of patients.

Individual Vasodilator Agents

Hydralazine: Apresoline, Generic

MECHANISM OF ACTION

Hydralazine directly relaxes arteriolar smooth muscle, thereby reducing total peripheral resistance. Hydralazine does not act uniformly throughout the vasculature but causes a greater degree of vasodilation in the coronary, splanchnic, cerebral, and renal vasculatures.

ADVERSE EFFECTS

As reviewed above, hydralazine and other vasodilators cause plasma volume expansion, increased renin release, increased heart rate, and increased cardiac output. In addition, hydralazine can cause a number of adverse reactions related to the drug rather than the vasodilation. These include headache, palpitation, anorexia, nausea, dizziness, sweating, flushing, conjunctivitis, tremors, muscle cramps, and drug fever. In addition, a delayed form of toxic response to hydralazine is a drug-induced rheumatoid arthritislike syndrome, which can evolve into systemic lupus erythematosus syndrome. This syndrome is accompanied by a positive antinuclear antibody test, fever, myalgia, arthralgia, splenomegaly, edema, and lupus erythematosus cells in the peripheral blood.

Most, if not all, of the adverse reactions to hydralazine are dose related. In the early days of the use of hydralazine, total daily doses above 400 mg were commonly used and were accompanied by a fairly high incidence of side effects. Present experience indicates that use of total daily doses less than 200 mg is accompanied by a marked reduction in both the incidence and severity of side effects. Furthermore, since hydralazine is used in combination with a diuretic and a beta blocker or another sympathetic depressant drug, good blood pressure control can be obtained in the majority of patients within this upper limit of hydralazine dosage.

PHARMACOKINETICS

Up to 90% of hydralazine is absorbed after oral administration and undergoes extensive first-pass metabolism. It has a half-life of less than 1 hour. However, the half-life of the antihypertensive effect is much longer, probably due to accumulation of hydralazine in vascular smooth muscle. The duration of blood pressure lowering effect from a single dose ranges between 3 and 8 hours. Hydralazine is extensively metabolized by acetylation, hydroxylation, and conjugation with glucuronic acid. Most of the drug and its metabolites are excreted via the kidneys; however, 10% is lost through the feces. Systemic accumulation of hydralazine may occur in patients with renal dysfunction, requiring a reduction of the dosage. Hydralazine is extensively bound to plasma proteins.

DOSAGE FORMS AND STRENGTHS AVAILABLE

Tablets: 10, 25, 50, and 100 mg.
Oral solution: not commercially available; may be compounded using hydralazine hydrochloride injection to make a solution containing 10 mg/ml (see USP DI).
Injection: 20 mg/ml.

DOSAGES

Adult: initially, 10–25 mg 2 or 3 times daily. Dosage may be increased by 10–25 mg until the blood pressure is controlled. The maximum daily dose should not exceed 200 mg in 2 or more divided doses.
Children: initially, 0.75 mg/kg daily in 4 divided doses. The dosage may be increased over 3–4 weeks to a maximum of 7.5 mg/kg daily.

Minoxidil: Loniten

MECHANISM OF ACTION

Minoxidil acts directly on arterioles to reduce peripheral resistance. It has little or no effect on capacitance vessels (venules and small veins).

THERAPEUTIC USE

Minoxidil has a greater intrinsic capacity to vasodilate than hydralazine and, therefore, a greater capacity to cause reflex stimulation of the heart and plasma volume expansion. Minoxidil is reserved for the treatment of severe or accelerated hypertension after other oral drugs have been unsuccessful. It must be given in combination with a diuretic and a beta blocker.

ADVERSE EFFECTS

The major adverse effects of minoxidil are related to reflex stimulation of the heart and fluid retention. Minoxidil causes marked **sodium and water retention** leading to swelling of feet or lower legs and an unusually rapid weight gain of more than 5 pounds in adults or 2 pounds in children (USP DI). The increased plasma volume attenuates the antihypertensive effect of minoxidil and can lead to cardiac decompensation. The reflex stimulation of the heart increases both heart rate and cardiac output and can lead to an unusually fast or irregular heart beat and, occasionally, chest pains. Pericardial effusion occurs rarely. The reflex effects of minoxidil on heart and sodium and water retention are substantially reduced by combining this agent with a beta blocker and a diuretic.

Another major side effect of minoxidil is **hypertrichosis or excessive hair growth,** which occurs usually on the face, arms, and back. The extent of hair growth may be marked, tending to decrease patient compliance, particularly among women and children. Hypertrichosis is reversible upon stopping the drug.

PHARMACOKINETICS

Minoxidil is rapidly and nearly completely absorbed from the gastrointestinal tract. Only 12% of the drug is excreted in the urine unchanged, while the remainder undergoes liver metabolism, primarily conjugation with glucuronic acid. The half-life of minoxidil is approximately 3 hours. The time to onset of action is 30 minutes, the time to peak effect is 2–3 hours, and the duration of antihypertensive effect is 24–48 hours.

DOSAGE FORMS AND STRENGTHS AVAILABLE

Tablets: 2.5 and 10 mg.

DOSAGES

Adults and children over 12: initially, 5 mg once daily. Dosage may be increased gradually to 10, 20, and then 40 mg daily in single or divided doses, as needed. Maximum daily dose: 100 mg.

Children under 12: initially, 0.2 mg/kg daily as a single dose. Dosages may be increased as needed in increments of 0.1–0.2 mg/kg until control is achieved or a maximum dose of 50 mg/day is achieved.

Angiotensin-Converting Enzyme Inhibitors

The renin-angiotensin-aldosterone axis is described earlier in this chapter. In short, the angiotensin-converting enzyme (ACE) inhibitors block the enzyme responsible for converting angiotensin I to A-II. As a consequence, A-II and aldosterone plasma levels decline, while renin and angiotensin I levels increase. The use of the ACE inhibitors is also accompanied by small but significant increases in serum potassium and associated decreases in urinary potassium excretion, probably related to the decrease in plasma aldosterone.

MECHANISM OF ACTION

The blood pressure lowering effect of the angiotensin-converting enzyme inhibitors increases with the severity of the hypertension. This effect is probably related to increased plasma renin activity in severe hypertension. The ACE inhibitors are also more effective in white hypertensive patients, who tend to have higher plasma renin activities, and is less effective in black hypertensive patients, who characteristically have low plasma renin activity.

In large part, the ACE inhibitors reduce arterial pressure by reducing the generation of A-II. A-II elevates blood pressure by acting directly on vascular smooth muscle to cause constriction by enhancing sympathoadrenal activity and by stimulating the release of aldosterone from the adrenal cortex. Reduction of A-II reduces all of these activities.

While the inhibition of ACE is a major mechanism underlying the antihypertensive effect of the converting enzyme inhibitors, these agents are also effective in approximately 50% of low renin hypertensive patients, where converting enzyme inhibition is likely to have little effect. The antihypertensive mechanism(s) in these cases is unknown. However, ACE is also responsible for the inactivation of a powerful naturally occurring vasodilator, bradykinin. Thus, converting enzyme inhibition may prolong the plasma life of this peptide, thereby contributing to blood pressure lowering. In addition, it has been suggested that the converting enzyme inhibitors may increase the production of vasodilator prostaglandins.

HEMODYNAMICS

The converting enzyme inhibitors lower blood pressure primarily by vasodilating the peripheral vasculature, thereby reducing peripheral resistance. Cardiac output, heart rate, and plasma fluid volume are little changed. The converting enzyme inhibitors characteristically cause vasodilation in the kidney vasculature, accompanied by increased kidney blood flow. Blood flow in the cerebral and coronary vascular beds are generally well maintained. Finally, baroreceptor function and responses to postural changes and exercise are little affected by converting enzyme inhibition.

THERAPEUTIC USE

The angiotensin-converting enzyme inhibitors are especially effective in the treatment of renal, renovascular, accelerated, and malignant hypertension; these inhibitors are also effective in mild to moderate hypertension. These agents are effective as monotherapy in mild through severe hypertension. In patients with mild to moderate hypertension, the blood pressure lowering effect of converting enzyme inhibitors is enhanced by adding a diuretic to the regimen. Not only are the antihypertensive effects of the two classes of agents additive, but the diuretic stimulates renin secretion, further enhancing the antihypertensive effect of the converting enzyme inhibitor. In more severe levels of hypertension, the converting enzyme inhibitors have also been used as step 3 in combination with thiazide diuretic and a beta blocker in the stepped-care approach.

FEWER SIDE EFFECTS WITH THE CONVERTING ENZYME INHIBITORS

Individual converting enzyme inhibitors are discussed below, together with their respective adverse effects. However, when compared to the diuretics, beta blockers, sympathetic depressant agents, and vasodilators, the converting enzyme inhibitors do not cause the following adverse reactions: fatigue, sexual dysfunction, bronchospasm, depression, hypokalemia, hyperuricemia, and hyperglycemia.

Individual Angiotensin-Converting Enzyme Inhibitors

Captopril: Capoten

Captopril was the first orally effective converting enzyme inhibitor to be introduced. It was found to have dramatic antihypertensive effects in many, but not all, patients with severe hypertension. In the early stages of clinical investigation, captopril was used in a wide range of dosages, including those above the currently recommended maximum. As a consequence, captopril was observed to cause certain adverse reactions such as rash, taste disturbances, proteinuria, and leukopenia, which are dose dependent and are now seen with much less frequency, since lower doses (150 mg daily or less) are presently used.

ADVERSE EFFECTS

Initially, captopril may cause a precipitous fall in blood pressure in patients with severe hypertension who have been volume depleted by diuretic therapy. Patients with congestive heart failure may also experience a marked fall in blood pressure with the first doses of captopril. In these cases, low initial doses of captopril should be used initially.

Skin rash, occasionally accompanied by itching or fever, occurs during the first few weeks of captopril therapy and usually disappears with dosage reduction or withdrawal. Reversible loss or disturbance of taste also occurs with captopril therapy. Both rash and taste disturbance are dose dependent and have been attributed to the sulfhydryl group of the captopril molecule.

Neutropenia and agranulocytosis occur rarely but can lead to life-threatening infections signaled by fever and chills or sore throat. Leukocyte count determinations should be made prior to captopril therapy, every 2 weeks for the first 3 months of therapy and at periodic intervals thereafter.

Proteinuria has occurred in less than 2% of patients, usually within the first 8 months of captopril therapy. Urinary protein estimates should be made prior to initiation of therapy, every month for the first 9 months of therapy and at periodic intervals thereafter (USP DI). Proteinuria may occur, particularly in patients with renal disease.

PHARMACOKINETICS

Approximately 60–75% of captopril is rapidly absorbed from the gastrointestinal tract. Absorption is reduced by food. Thus, the drug should be given one hour before meals. Forty to 50% of captopril is excreted in the urine unchanged, and the remainder is eliminated by metabolism, primarily via formation of a disulfide dimer and cysteine disulfide in the liver. The half-life of captopril is approximately 2 hours but is increased during renal impairment. The antihypertensive action of captopril is not correlated with plasma half-life but with inhibition of tissue-converting enzyme. The onset of action is approximately 30 minutes after the initial dose, with a time to peak effect of 60–90 minutes. The duration of action is approximately 6–12 hours and is dose related. Full therapeutic effect may not be seen until several weeks after the initiation of therapy.

DOSAGE FORMS AND STRENGTHS AVAILABLE

Tablets: 12.5, 25, 50, and 100 mg

DOSAGES

Adult: Mild to moderate hypertension — initially, 12.5 mg 2 or 3 times daily; severe hypertension — initially, 25 mg 2 or 3 times daily; may be increased to 50 mg 2 or 3 times daily after 1 or 2 weeks. If required, dosage may be increased further at 1–2 week intervals to a maximum of 150 mg 2 or 3 times daily. Maximal daily dose should not exceed 450 mg. Generally, doses more than 150 mg daily are rarely needed. In patients who are salt- and water-depleted as a result of diuretic therapy, or who have congestive heart disease, an initial dose of 6.25–12.5 mg 2 or 3 times daily should be used.

Children: initially, 0.36 mg/kg 3 times daily, increased as needed in increments of 0.36 mg/kg at intervals of 8–24 hours to the minimum effective dose.

Enalapril

Enalapril is a prodrug that is hydrolyzed to the active dicarboxylic acid compound, enalaprilate. In addition, enalapril lacks the sulfhydryl group that characterizes captopril. Thus, enalapril differs from captopril pharmacokinetically, having a longer time period to onset, and, possibly, in the incidence of side effects thought to be associated with a sulfhydryl group (see above).

ADVERSE EFFECTS

Enalapril may cause a marked fall in blood pressure in patients who are either Na^+- and water-depleted and/or have congestive heart disease. Lower doses of enalapril should be used initially in these patients. The incidence of rash, taste disturbance, neutropenia, and proteinuria is less with enalapril than with captopril, which may be due to the lack of a sulfhydryl group on the enalapril molecule.

Additional adverse reactions include headache, dizziness, nausea, diarrhea, and hyperkalemia.

PHARMACOKINETICS

Approximately 60% of enalapril is absorbed from the gastrointestinal tract, with approximately 40% bioavailable as enalaprilate. Both the parent and active compound are eliminated unchanged, by renal excretion. Peak concentration of enalaprilate occurs at approximately 4 hours but takes longer to be achieved in patients with renal failure. Converting enzyme inhibition by enalapril is almost complete for at least 10 hours after a single 10-mg dose, is still depressed at 24 hours, and does not return to baseline by 72 hours.

DOSAGE FORMS AND STRENGTHS AVAILABLE

Tablets: 5, 10, and 20 mg.

DOSAGES

Adults: initially, 2.5 mg for patients receiving a diuretic and those whose renal function is moderately to severely impaired (creatinine clearance equal to or less than 30 ml/min). An initial dose of 5 mg daily may be given to those who are not taking a diuretic and whose renal function is normal. Maintenance: 10–40 mg daily.

Angiotensin-Converting Enzyme Inhibitors—Drug Interactions

CAPTOPRIL PLUS ASPIRIN

Aspirin decreases the antihypertensive effect of captopril. This may be due to aspirin-induced inhibition of the synthesis of a vasodilator prostaglandin. The blood pressure should be monitored during combined therapy, and it may be necessary to discontinue the aspirin.

CAPTOPRIL PLUS CHLORPROMAZINE

Chlorpromazine intensifies the blood pressure lowering effect of captopril, possibly leading to marked hypotension. Patients receiving the combination should have their blood pressure monitored, and, if hypotension occurs, one or both of the agents may need to be discontinued.

CAPTOPRIL PLUS FUROSEMIDE AND OTHER LOOP DIURETICS

The interaction of captopril and furosemide and other loop diuretics may occur upon the initiation of captopril therapy if the patient is significantly Na^+-depleted. In this case, the patient may experience a precipitous fall in blood pressure. In those cases in which hypotension occurs, the patient may be placed in a supine position and may be given an infusion of normal saline, if required to control the hypotension. The interaction may also be avoided by discontinuing the diuretic or increasing Na^+ intake one week before starting captopril therapy.

Calcium (Ca^{2+}) Channel Antagonists

The Ca^{2+} channel antagonists are effective as antianginal, antiarrhythmic, and antihypertensive agents. They act by inhibiting the entry of Ca^{2+} into both cardiac and vascular smooth muscle cells via voltage-dependent Ca^{2+} channels. The three prototype Ca^{2+} antagonists are diltiazem, nifedipine, and verapamil. While these agents all act by inhibiting Ca^{2+} channels, there are important differences in their effectiveness at different sites. For example, nifedipine blocks Ca^{2+} channels in vascular smooth muscle at concentrations approximately 10 times below those necessary to block Ca^{2+} channels in cardiac muscle. Thus, the most predominant effect of this agent in therapeutic concentrations is vasodilation. On the other hand, verapamil blocks Ca^{2+} channels in heart and vascular smooth muscle at the same concentrations. Diltiazem is intermediate between verapamil and nifedipine, tending to more closely resemble verapamil.

EFFECTS OF CA^{2+} CHANNEL BLOCKADE IN THE HEART

Diltiazem and verapamil block the voltage dependent Ca^{2+} channels of cardiac muscle, pacemaker tissue, and conducting tissue. Thus, they reduce the intracellular Ca^{2+} concentration and may decrease cardiac contractility, although this would not be clinically significant, except in cases of preexisting depressed cardiac function. The Ca^{2+} channel blockers may also decrease heart rate by decreasing the rate of entry of Ca^{2+} during the 0 phase of the Ca^{2+}-dependent action potential in the sinoatrial node. This effect is also modest in healthy subjects. The most dramatic and clinically significant effect of the Ca^{2+} channel blockers is on the AV node, where the rate of rise of the 0 phase of the action potential is slowed, resulting in decreased AV nodal conduction and increased duration of the effective refractory period. Thus, conduction through the AV node is slowed, and diltiazem and verapamil may also produce partial AV block. This is a major component of the therapeutic use of these agents in the treatment of arrhythmias (see Chap. 2).

In contrast to diltiazem and verapamil, nifedipine causes reflex tachycardia secondary to its vasodilating action. While nifedipine has the potential to block calcium channels in the heart such action does not occur.

EFFECTS OF CA^{2+} ANTAGONISTS IN BLOOD VESSELS

An elevation in the cytosolic concentration of Ca^{2+} mediates subsequent events, leading to vascular smooth muscle contraction. The cytosolic calcium concentration is increased by two mechanisms: entry of Ca^{2+} via voltage dependent Ca^+ channels and release of Ca^{2+} from intracellular storage pools. The calcium antagonists, diltiazem, nifedipine, and verapamil, reduce cytosolic Ca^{2+} concentration by inhibiting the voltage-dependent Ca^{2+} channels, and this leads to vasodilation of coronary and systemic resistance vessels. The Ca^{2+} antagonists have little or no effect on most venous beds. The antihypertensive effect of the Ca^{2+} antagonists results from a reduction in total peripheral resistance.

THERAPEUTIC USE

The Ca^{2+} channel antagonists possess a high level of antihypertensive efficacy. They are particularly effective in the elderly, black, and other hypertensive subgroups characterized by low plasma renin levels.

All three Ca^{2+} antagonists appear to be equieffective in antihypertensive potency and will control hypertension in about two-thirds of patients with mild to moderate hypertension.

The Ca^{2+} channel antagonists are also effective as step 2 in stepped-care therapy. Not only is the antihypertensive effect of these agents additive with that of the diuretic, their use instead of a beta blocker avoids important side effects in patients with asthma or chronic obstructive airway disease.

The Ca^{2+} channel antagonists are also effective as step 3 of the stepped-care approach as alternatives to hydralazine or other vasodilators. The combination of a diuretic (step 1), a beta blocker (step 2), and nifedipine (step 3) is highly efficacious, since three different parameters affecting blood pressure are reduced, namely, plasma volume, cardiac output, and peripheral resistance, respectively. Diltiazem and verapamil may also be used as step 3 agents. However, caution must be used if the step 2 agent is a beta blocker, since the combination of a beta blocker and a Ca^{2+} channel antagonist could cause excessive depression of cardiac function.

PHARMACOKINETICS

Diltiazem

Diltiazem is rapidly and nearly completely absorbed after oral administration. However, it undergoes extensive first pass metabolism, reducing bioavailability to 40% initially. However, after continuous therapy, the bioavailability increases to 90%, indicating saturation of liver metabolism. Blood levels of diltiazem decline biphasically, with a half-life of 20–30 minutes in the first phase and approximately 3–4 hours in the second phase. Diltiazem undergoes extensive metabolism, and the half-life of the compound is increased in hepatic dysfunction. Diltiazem is 70–80% plasma-protein bound. The major metabolite of diltiazem, desacetyl diltiazem, has between 25% and 50% of the Ca^{2+} channel blocking activity of diltiazem.

Nifedipine

Nifedipine is rapidly absorbed but undergoes significant first-pass metabolism, which reduces the bioavailability of nifedipine to 65–70%. Nifedipine is also eliminated from the blood by biphasic pharmacokinetics. The half-life of the first phase is 2.5–3 hours, and that of the longer phase is 5 hours. Since nifedipine is also eliminated almost exclusively by metabolism, the half-life is increased in hepatic dysfunction.

Verapamil

Verapamil is rapidly and nearly completely absorbed from the gastrointestinal tract. However, it undergoes marked first-pass metabolism, reducing the oral bioavailability to 10–35%. Verapamil is eliminated by hepatic metabolism. The major metabolite, norverapamil, has about 20% of the Ca^{2+} channel blocking activity of verapamil. The initial half-life of verapamil is 3–7 hours. However, it increases to 7–13 hours with continuous therapy and may be markedly prolonged in patients with hepatic dysfunction. Verapamil is 90% plasma-protein bound.

ADVERSE EFFECTS

The major adverse effects of diltiazem and verapamil relate to their cardiac effects and are generally observed only in patients with pre-existing disease of the pacemaker, conducting, or contractile tissues. These effects include second or third AV block, possibly leading to bradycardia; hypotension due to severe reduction in cardiac contractility plus peripheral vasodilation; and severe arrhythmias in patients with WPW syndrome. Nifedipine generally exhibits little or no adverse effects on the heart. However, it can cause severe hypotension (systolic pressure less than 90 mm Hg).

Additional adverse effects of the Ca^{2+} channel antagonists include constipation; dizziness or lightheadedness; headache; nausea; and swelling of ankles, feet, or lower legs (peripheral edema). Tachycardia may also occur. In patients receiving either verapamil or diltiazem, atrial flutter or fibrillation may occur involving an accessory AV pathway such as Wolff-Parkinson-White syndrome. Reflex tachycardia is seen in patients receiving nifedipine because of its vasodilator effect.

Individual Calcium (Ca^{2+}) Channel Antagonists

Diltiazem: Cardizem

DOSAGE FORMS AND STRENGTHS AVAILABLE
Tablets: 30 and 60 mg.

DOSAGES
Adult: 60–120 mg 3 times daily.

Nifedipine: Adalat, Procardia

DOSAGE FORMS AND STRENGTHS AVAILABLE
Capsules: 10 mg.

DOSAGES

Adult: initially, 10 mg 3 times daily; may be increased to 20 mg 3 times daily.

Verapamil Hydrochloride: Calan, Isoptin

DOSAGE FORMS AND STRENGTHS AVAILABLE

Tablets: 80 and 120 mg.
Injection: 2.5 mg/ml.

DOSAGES

Adult: 80–120 mg 3 times daily.

References

1. Amery, A., et al. Efficacy of antihypertensive drug treatment according to age, sex, blood pressure and previous cardiovascular disease in patients over the age of 60. *Lancet* 2(8507):589, 1986.
2. Croog, S. H., et al. The effects of antihypertensive therapy on the quality of life. *N. Engl. J. Med.* 314:1657, 1986.
3. Dannenberg, A. L., and Kannel, W. B. Remission of hypertension: The natural history of blood pressure treatment in the Framingham study. *J.A.M.A.* 257:1477, 1987.
4. Dustan, H. P. Atherosclerosis complicating chronic hypertension. George Lyman Duff Memorial Lecture. *Circulation* 50:871, 1974.
5. Ferguson, R. K., and Vlasses, P. H. Hypertensive emergencies and urgencies. *J.A.M.A.* 255:1607, 1986.
6. Guyton, A. C., et al. Blood pressure regulation: Basic concepts. *Fed. Proc.* 40:2252, 1981.
7. Laragh, J. A. Vasoconstriction-volume analysis for understanding and treating hypertension: The use of renin and aldosterone profiles. *Am. J. Med.* 55:261, 1973.
8. Leenen, F. H. H. et al. Vasodilators and regression of left ventricular hypertrophy. Hydralazine versus prazosin in hypertensive humans. *Am. J. Med.* 82:969, 1987.
9. Lewis, P. The essential action of propranolol in hypertension. *Am. J. Med.* 60:837, 1976.
10. McLenachan, J. M. Ventricular arrhythmias in patients with hypertensive left ventricular hypertrophy. *N. Engl. J. Med.* 317:787, 1987.
11. McMahon, F. G. *Hypertension: The New Low-Dose Era* (2nd ed.). Mount Kisco, NY: Futura, 1984. P. 23.
12. Prichard, B. N. C., and Gillam, P. M. S. Treatment of hypertension with propranolol. *Br. Med. J.* [*Clin. res.*] 1:7, 1969.
13. Resnick, L. M., et al. Divalent cations in essential hypertension. Relations between serum ionized calcium, magnesium and plasma renin activity. *N. Engl. J. Med.* 309:888, 1983.
14. Stamler, R. Nutritional therapy for high blood pressure. *J.A.M.A.* 257:1484, 1987.
15. Tarazi, R. C. Management of the patient with resistant hypertension. *Hosp. Pract.* [*Off.*] 16:49, 1981.

16. Tarazi, R. C., et al. Can the heart initiate some forms of hypertension? *Fed. Proc.* 42:2691, 1983.
17. Thier, S. O. Potassium physiology. *Am. J. Med.* 80:3, 1986.
18. Trimarco, B., et al. Participation of endogenous catecholamines in the regulation of left ventricular mass in progeny of hypertensive parents. *Circulation* 72:38, 1985.
19. Veterans Administration Cooperative Study Group on Antihypertensive Agents. *J.A.M.A.* 202:1028, 1967.
20. Wagner, H. P., and Keith, N. M. Diffuse arteriolar disease with hypertension and associated retinal lesions. *Medicine (Baltimore)* 18:317, 1939.
21. Wikstrand, J., et al. Antihypertensive treatment with metoprolol or hydrochlorothiazide in patients aged 60 to 75 years. *J.A.M.A.* 255:1304, 1986.

Selected Reading

ARTICLES

Conway, J. Hemodynamic aspects of essential hypertension in humans. *Physiol. Rev.* 74:617, 1984.

Frohlich, E. D. Antihypertensive therapy: Newer concepts and agents. *Cardiology* 72:349, 1985.

Hollenberg, N. K. The kidney and effective antihypertensive therapy. *Am. J. Cardiol.* 56:52H. 1985.

Kirkendall, W. M. Treatment of hypertension in the elderly. *Am. J. Cardiol.* 57:63C, 1986.

Laragh, J. H. Modification of stepped care approach to antihypertensive therapy. *Am. J. Med.* 77:78, 1984.

Perry, H. M. The evolution of antihypertensive therapy. *Am. J. Cardiol.* 56:75H, 1985.

Rinke, C. M. Hypertensive emergencies and urgencies. *J.A.M.A.* 255:1607, 1986.

Weber M. A., and Drayer J. I. Central and peripheral blockade of the sympathetic nervous system. *Am. J. Med.* 77:110, 1984.

BOOKS

Kaplan, N. M. *Clinical Hypertension* (4th ed.). Baltimore: Wilkins & Wilkins, 1986.

McMahon, F. G. *Management of Essential Hypertension: The New Low-Dose Era* (2nd ed.). Mount Kisco, NY: Futura, 1984.

Angina, Ischemia, and Myocardial Injury and Infarction

Angina pectoris (angina) is an imbalance, between myocardial oxygen supply and demand that may or may not be overtly perceived as pain by the patient. Classic effort angina reflects an inability of diseased coronary arteries to deliver sufficient blood to meet the oxygen requirements of the myocardium. However, the imbalance may be asymptomatic and, in this form, is silent. Another form of angina, variant angina (or Prinzmetal's) is not effort-related and comes about because of inappropriate contraction of large-sized coronary arteries. Some patients experience all three forms of angina — effort, noneffort, and silent.

The heart is unique in its ability to extract oxygen (O_2) from the coronary capillary blood, even under basal conditions. A near maximal O_2 extraction (75%) takes place with each passage of blood through the coronary bed, as contrasted to 20–25% O_2 extraction as blood passes through other vascular beds. Increases in O_2 demand by the heart muscle must, therefore, be met by a proportional increase in the blood transport capacity of the coronary arterial bed brought about by mobilizing capillaries from a reserve pool.

A myocardial O_2 ($M\dot{V}O_2$) consumption rate at rest of approximately 9 ml/100 gm/min supports contractile activities (60%), the basic metabolic requirements (20%), and electrical activity (20%), maintaining the steady-state levels of sodium (Na^+) and potassium (K^+) within the cell and the ionic gradients that are involved in the generation of action potentials on changes in sarcolemmal membrane conductance and supporting the calcium (Ca^{2+}) pump which moves Ca^{2+} into the sarcoplasmic reticulum.

Anatomic Considerations of Coronary Artery Blood Flow

The coronary arterial bed has the potential for doubling or quadrupling the O_2-carrying blood flow via an instantaneous recruitment of capillaries from the capillary reserve. For example, at rest, an estimated 900 functional capillaries can be increased to more than 2000 capillaries/mm^2 with exercise or emotional tension.

At rest, the anatomy favors blood flow and O_2 exchange in the subendocardial regions of the left ventricle, as evidenced by the greater capillary density (1100 vs. 750/mm^2) and a shorter intercapillary distance (16.5 vs. 20.5 μm) when comparing subendocardial with subepicardial regions. Furthermore, blood flowing through the subepicardial region is carried by numerous branch arteries that are largely unaffected by the systolic intramyocardial compression, whereas blood flowing to the subendocardial region is interrupted by compression of long and unbranched "straight" arteries passing through the full thickness of the left ventricle. As the intramyocardial pressure exceeds the intraluminal pressure, these unbranched intramural arteries become compressed. When the intraluminal pressure falls below a critical level, the functional lumen becomes exceedingly unstable and ultimately is obliterated in some vessels. The obliterating or closing pressure sharply rises as blood flow reduction through the "straight" intramural arteries approaches 75%.

The precompressed intraluminal pressure is a major determinant of vessel collapse. Reduction in the precompression intraluminal pressure of the "straight" arteries, as with obstruction or critical narrowing of the upstream supplier epicardial artery, favors critical closure of intramyocardial branch arteries supplying the subendocardial region. Recognition of the vulnerability for critical closure of intramyocardial "straight" arteries in patients with significant stenosis of the large parent epicardial coronary artery is important when considering therapeutic choices in patients with subendocardial ischemia/infarction.

Physiologic Considerations of Coronary Artery Blood Flow

In addition to anatomic factors, the tissue oxygen tension (tpO_2) influences blood flow to the epicardial and endocardial regions of the left ventricle, since tpO_2 is a powerful stimulus for autoregulation of coronary resistance arterioles. The net tpO_2 (balance between the arterial pO_2 and $M\dot{V}O_2$) is sensed by endothelial cells in resistance arterioles, metarterioles, and precapillary sphincters. A relatively low tpO_2, as in the subendocardial area, is the probable basis for a lower resistance to blood flow and a preferential blood flow to the subendocardium when compared to flow in the subepicardial region during diastolic relaxation of the left ventricle.

ENDOTHELIAL CELLS

Recently, the striking influence of endothelial cells on the physiology of vascular smooth muscle cells was discovered. Now it is known that some smooth muscle relaxants operate through endothelial cells; others do not. Smooth muscle relaxation operating through endothelial cells is mediated by an endothelial cell-derived relaxation factor (EDRF) [8]. Endothelium-dependent and independent smooth muscle relaxations in response to various substances (including drugs) are summarized in Table 4-1.

Mechanism of EDRF Action

EDRF activates guanylate cyclase, which converts guanosine triphosphate into 3′, 5′-cyclic guanosine monophosphate (cGMP), which, in turn, activates a cGMP-dependent protein kinase. Changes in phosphorylation of specific proteins of the contractile apparatus and of the Ca^{2+} regulatory systems by the protein kinase then causes relaxation. Recent evidence suggests that EDRF is nitric oxide (NO). Some drugs, such as sodium nitroprusside, release NO and directly activate guanylate cyclase,

Table 4-1. Factors affecting arterial smooth muscle relaxation

Relaxation mediated through EDRF	Relaxation independent of endothelium
Endogenous substances	
ATP, ADP	Adenosine, AMP
Thrombin	Prostacyclin
Bradykinin	Atrial natriuretic factor
Peptides	Histamine (H_2-receptor)
Substance P	Norepinephrine (β-receptor)
Arachidonic acid	
Platelet-activating factor	
Drugs	
Ca^{2+} Ionophore A23187	Nitrovasodilators
Clonidine	Isoproterenol
	Hydralazine

Key: EDRF = endothelial cell-derived relaxation factor; ATP = adenosine triphosphate; ADP = adenosine diphosphate; AMP = adenosine monophosphate.

relaxing vascular smooth muscle in the absence of the endothelium (see below under nitrates).

Physiologic Significance of EDRF

EDRF is released from the endothelium of all vascular tissues; the stability and duration of its action is inversely related to arterial pO_2. EDRF may be the prime mediator of vasodilation to hypoxia. Release of EDRF maintains a "fourth power" relationship between diameter and flow so that the pressure gradient in each vessel approaches a constant value as high flow rates [11].

EDRF, by activating the guanylate cyclase in platelets, inhibits platelet aggregation and actually promotes platelet disaggregation. Aggregated platelets release serotonin and ADP, which stimulate the release of EDRF from the endothelium and induce vasodilation. Adherence of platelets onto vessel walls is counteracted by the production and release of EDRF.

EDRF is complementary to the action of prostacyclin (PGI_2) in regulating vascular reactivity. PGI_2 functions by activating the adenylate cyclase system and relaxes smooth muscle contraction, and, in platelets, antagonizes platelet aggregation. EDRF affects the same target cells, but by a different mechanism, that is, by activating guanylate cyclase. Interestingly, EDRF and PGI_2 evoke opposite responses to changes in pO_2 and pH.

Role of the Autonomic Nervous System

Stimulation of the sympathetic nerves to the heart increases the resistance in large-sized coronary arteries, while decreasing the resistance in small-sized vessels. The resistance response in the large vessels is abolished by α-adrenergic receptor blockade.

Powerful vasoconstrictor nerve fibers superimpose their effects on the basic tone of vascular smooth muscle cells. Generally, the

Table 4-2. Vasoreactive modifiers

Humoral substances		Local environment or metabolite	
Agent	Response	Agent	Response
Catecholamines			
Epinephrine	VCR, VDIL	Hypoxia	VDIL
Norepinephrine	VCR	Adenosine and adenosine nucleotides	VCR, VDIL
Dopamine	VCR, VDIL		
Other amines			
Serotonin	VCR, VDIL	H^+	VDIL
Histamine	VDIL	K^+	VDIL
Acetylcholine	VDIL	Inorganic phosphate	VDIL
Polypeptides			
Angiotensin	VCR	Hypercapnia	VDIL
Kinins	VDIL	Prostaglandins	VCR, VDIL mdf
Vasopressin	VCR mdf	Hyperosmolarity	VDIL
Oxytocin	VCR, VDIL mdf		
Glucagon	VDIL		
Androgens	Modifiers		
Estrogens	Modifiers		

Key: VCR = vasoconstriction; VDIL = vasodilation; mdf = modifier.

density of vasoconstrictor fibers is inversely related to the basal tone, and the effects of vasoconstrictor-mediated stimuli are more apparent in the epicardial right than in the left anterior descending coronary artery. Intramural coronary arteries have relatively few constrictor fibers.

Receptors for agonists of smooth muscle contraction exhibit various degrees of sensitivity in different vascular areas. These variations include responses to locally produced or released vasoactive compounds — histamine, serotonin, and norepinephrine.

A summary of autonomic nervous system mediators as well as other coronary artery autoregulation determinants is presented in Table 4-2.

CONTRIBUTIONS OF PROSTAGLANDINS

Prostaglandins (PGs) are members of a family of oxygenated 20-carbon fatty acids that control platelet activity and modulate arterial wall tone. Prostaglandins are metabolites of cell membrane arachidonic acid (Fig. 4-1) and are synthesized in and around blood vessels, especially by endothelial cells. Particular species of PGs dilate (prostacyclin, PGI_2, PGE_2) or constrict (thromboxane A_2, leukotrienes) blood vessels. The PGs influence norepinephrine release from sympathetic nerve endings and can

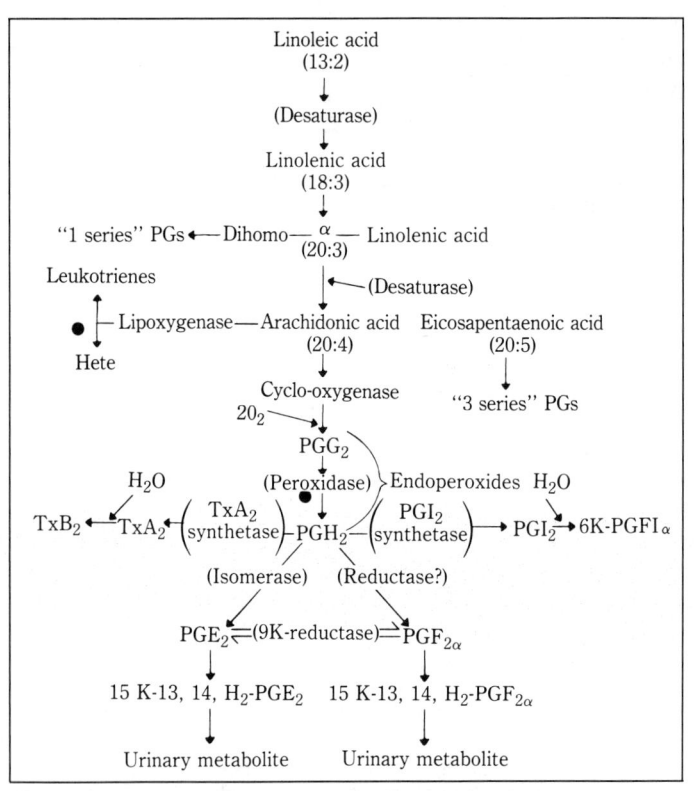

```
                    Linoleic acid
                       (13:2)
                         ↓
                    (Desaturase)
                         ↓
                   Linolenic acid
                       (18:3)
                         ↓
"1 series" PGs ← Dihomo—α—Linolenic acid
                       (20:3)
Leukotrienes             ↓ ← (Desaturase)
  ↑
  •—Lipoxygenase—Arachidonic acid   Eicosapentaenoic acid
Hete                   (20:4)              (20:5)
                  Cyclo-oxygenase
                  20₂ ↓                "3 series" PGs
                       PGG₂
   H₂O          (Peroxidase) • ⟩Endoperoxides  H₂O
TxB₂ ← TxA₂ ← TxA₂ synthetase ⎞-PGH₂-⎛ PGI₂ synthetase → PGI₂ → 6K-PGFI_α
              (Isomerase)      (Reductase?)
                  PGE₂ ⇌ (9K-reductase) ⇌ PGF_{2α}
                    ↓                        ↓
              15 K-13, 14, H₂-PGE₂    15 K-13, 14, H₂-PGF_{2α}
                    ↓                        ↓
              Urinary metabolite       Urinary metabolite
```

Fig. 4-1. Dietary essential fatty acids, linoleic, and alpha linolenic conversion to the cell membrane arachidonic acid and the subsequent prostaglandin (PG) biosynthesis and metabolism. Sites of free radical generation are indicated by large dot (•). (From M. Karmazyn and N. S. Dhalla. Physiological and pathophysiological aspects of cardiac prostaglandins. *Can. J. Physiol. Pharmacol.* 61:1208, 1983.)

induce a reflex modulation of arterial blood pressure. Other PG sources are blood platelets and neutrophils.

Vasoactive PGs synthesized and released by endothelial cells, platelets, and neutrophils may alter coronary artery blood flow by acting directly on vascular smooth muscle, by affecting synthesis and release of vasoactive endothelium-derived factors, and/or by influencing norepinephrine release from nerve endings.

Adaptation to Coronary Artery Stenosis-Subendocardial Region Vulnerability

Development of stenosing lesions in the epicardial coronary arteries causes relaxation of resistance metarterioles and precapillary sphincters and recruitment from the capillary bed reserve

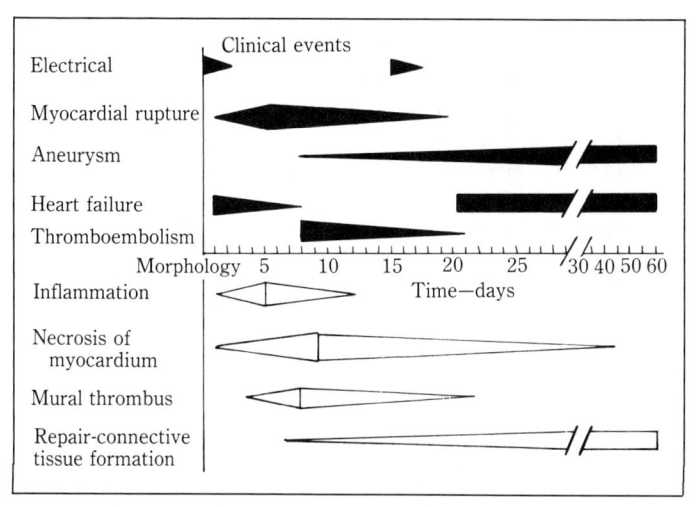

Fig. 4-2. Pathophysiology of clinical complications of myocardial infarction. The clinical events (upper panel) are related temporally to the post-myocardial infarction morphologic changes of inflammation, necrosis, thrombogenesis, and tissue repair.

pool to meet the $M\dot{V}O_2$. Predictably, the subendocardial region is most vulnerable to a recruitment from the capillary bed reserve. As discussed above, with patent coronary arteries, intermittent systolic compression of the "straight" intramural arteries supplying the subendocardium leads to a near-maximum recruitment of the capillary bed in that region. However, with coronary artery stenosis and recruitment of intramural capillary beds, competition is set up between low resistance capillary beds of the subendocardial area and low resistance beds of the newly recruited capillary reserve. In such competition, the subendocardium suffers and becomes edematous, ischemic, or infarcted.

Myocardial Ischemia and Reperfusion

PATHOPHYSIOLOGY OF MYOCARDIAL INFARCTION

After 30–60 minutes of ischemia, irreversible myocardial cellular changes lead to cell death. Within the initial 2–4 hours, a waxing and waning of ischemic injury occurs, as suggested by electrocardiogram (ECG) changes and by angiographic and visual (surgery) evidence of thrombosis and spontaneous thrombolysis in some obstructed arteries. The waxing and waning appears to be influenced by the extent of coronary collateral circulation to the ischemic region. Such waxing and waning of tissue ischemia is associated with nonhomogeneous oxygenation of myocardial tissue, a condition that temporally relates to the electrical instability during the initial hours of a myocardial infarction (MI) (Fig. 4-2). Additionally, prolonged myocardial ischemia leads to tissue injury and an activation of kinin, complement, and thrombogenesis processes, all of which converge in initiating an inflammatory reaction (see Fig. 6-4). The inflammatory reaction and subsequent myocardial necrosis intensify over 5–7 days, during which time the left ventricle is vulnerable to myocardial rupture. However, the inflammatory reaction is essential since its attenuation by corticosteriods or nonsteroidal drugs increases the risk of myocardial rupture following MI [29].

Activation of the extrinsic and intrinsic coagulation factors by myocardial injury and infarction (see Fig. 6-1) may initiate a mural thrombus, most commonly with anteroseptal MI (see Fig. 4-2). From the third to the seventh days, the frequency and size of the mural thrombus increases. Those assuming a sessile configuration are most likely to embolize. The likelihood of thromboembolism is greatest from the seventh to the fourteenth days after MI.

ALTERATION OF PROSTAGLANDIN PRODUCTION WITH ISCHEMIA/INFARCTION

Transient myocardial ischemia initiates prostaglandin production, as evidenced by thromboxane A_2 (TxA_2) release into the coronary venous blood [13, 28]. In the conscious dog model, PG synthesis blockade prevents a decrease in coronary vascular resistance and an increase in collateral blood flow an hour after coronary occlusion [17]. Patients with coronary artery disease have significant increases in coronary artery resistance and decreases in coronary blood flow after pharmacologic inhibition of cyclo-oxygenase (PG production) with indomethacin [9]. A TxA_2 receptor antagonist, administered to anesthetized cats 30 minutes after ligation of the left anterior descending coronary artery, results in significant reduction of the ECG injury current and in plasma myocardial creatine kinase activity, suggesting a role for TxA_2 in extending ischemic damage [4]. PGI_2 and TxA_2 production is increased during the development of MI in humans, as measured by urinary metabolites of the two compounds [12].

Within minutes after myocardial ischemia, circulating polymorphonuclear leukocytes (PMN) adhere to and migrate through the endothelial lining [24]. Interactions between PMNs and endothelial cells can promote increases in vascular resistance (vasospasm) or capillary blockade (capillary "shut down"). Reperfusion results in more PMN adherence to endothelial cells and subsequent invasion into the myocardium. PMNs in the myocardium exacerbate tissue injury (release of PGs, including lipoxygenase-mediated metabolites and oxygen-derived free radicals [see below]) and favor the development of arrhythmias.

The inflammatory response and myocardial necrosis with macrophage removal of tissue debris initiates the connective tissue repair processes by fibroblasts (invasion commences around the fifth to the seventh day). Fibroblast invasion and the formation of connective tissue repair are completed during the tenth to the twenty-first days of the post-MI period. Collagen deposition, remodeling, and contraction (which influences left ventricular size and ejection fraction) is, however, not completed until 60–90 days after the MI.

Heart failure may appear early (within 24 hours) as acute pulmonary edema (see Chap. 1) or as mild left ventricular dysfunction. Evidence of mild left ventricle failure usually subsides over the third to the fifth day after the MI. In some patients, late heart failure develops after 21 days (see Fig. 4-2).

PATHOPHYSIOLOGY OF REPERFUSION MYOCARDIAL INJURY

In the early minutes and the initial few hours following coronary artery occlusion by thrombus, the left ventricle is alternately totally deprived of O_2 or exposed to intermittent reperfusion of O_2-carrying blood. The reperfusion may be spontaneous or may be intensified by successful pharmacologic thrombolysis (heparin, thrombolytics—see Chap. 6) or by an effective angioplasty (percutaneous transluminal coronary angioplasty [PTCA]).

What is the mechanism underlying reperfusion tissue injury? Myocardial cells, more than other cells of the body, are aerobic. Although O_2 is necessary for life, many of the biochemical reactions in which it participates generate O_2-containing free radicals as by-products. By definition, the survival of aerobic cells in an O_2 environment implies successful management of the generation and the control of these highly reactive chemical species (Fig. 4-3). A free radical is an atom, group of atoms, or a molecule with one unpaired electron occupying an outer orbital.

These intermediates are too reactive to be liberated into tissues; therefore, protective and controlling enzymatic mechanisms have evolved as part of the cytochrome oxidase complex in the mitochondria. The $O_2^{\cdot-}$ flux in aerobic cells is managed by enzyme systems, such as superoxide dismutase (SOD), catalase (CAT), and peroxidases, and by compounds, such as reduced glutathione. These enzymes and compounds catalytically scavenge $O_2^{\cdot-}$ and reduce H_2O_2 (CAT and peroxidases).

Transient ischemic injury of myocardial cells is accompanied by a drop in the cellular SOD, glutathione peroxidase, and glutathione and makes possible a free radical-mediated destructive reaction when molecular O_2 is restored to the tissue as part of the reperfusion phenomenon.

Reperfusion injury refers to additional cell damage or death with the introduction of O_2-carrying blood. A sudden and massive reduction of myocardial blood flow reduces the availability of O_2 and sets in motion, within seconds, the formation of metabolic by-products, protons, lactate, inorganic phosphate, and free rad-

Fig. 4-3. **Biological control of O_2.** The complete reduction of O_2 involves the addition of four electrons and the formation of two highly reactive intermediates, hydrogen peroxide and the hydroxyl radical.

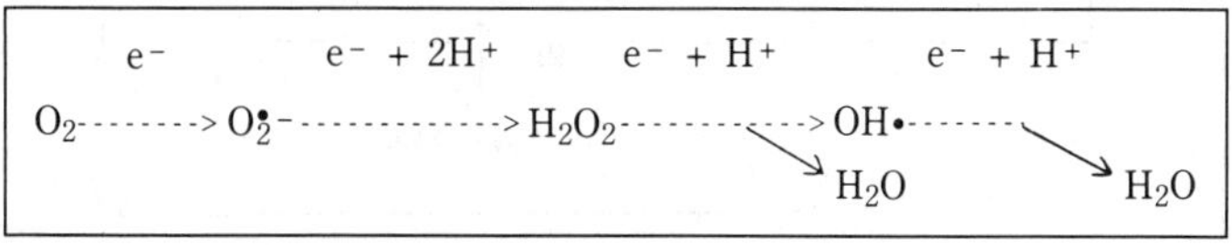

$$O_2 \xrightarrow{e^-} O_2^{\cdot-} \xrightarrow{e^- + 2H^+} H_2O_2 \xrightarrow{e^- + H^+} OH\cdot \xrightarrow{e^- + H^+} H_2O$$
$$\searrow H_2O \qquad \searrow H_2O$$

icals. Within a few minutes, adenosine triphosphate (ATP) and phosphocreatinine (PC) are severely depleted, contractility is reduced or lost, K^+ leaks from the intracellular to the extracellular spaces, and Na^+ moves intracellularly [25].

Should the restoration of O_2-carrying blood flow be delayed beyond 20 minutes, the levels of the adenine nucleotide pool approach zero and the terminal products inosine and hypoxanthine become available as enzyme substrates that generate free radicals (Fig. 4-4). Continued increases in ammonium ions and phosphate increase tissue osmolarity, and fluid accumulates beneath the cell membrane sarcolemma (SL) and mitochondria become swollen. Accumulation impairs the sarcoplasmic teticulum (SR) activity and cytosolic Ca^{2+} levels rise.

An ischemia extending beyond 30 minutes results in sarcolemma degradation. Tissue xanthine oxidase activity increases, and the activities of the endogenous free-radical scavengers decrease. The superoxide radicals favor lipid peroxidation, leading to further breakdown of the sarcolemma. Reperfusion, if carried out early (within minutes), promptly restores cell function. Reperfusion within the initial 20 minutes of ischemia may accelerate cell death, and contribute to the "washout" of intracellular enzymes (creatine kinase), a rapid accumulation of Ca^{2+}, and the generation of free radicals. Ca^{2+} accumulation activates a number of intracellular pathways, leading to the loss of energy stores, generation of thromboxane, platelet aggregation, and thrombus formation, with consequent further reduction of coronary blood flow.

Fig. 4-4. The endothelial cell–myocyte connection in the generation of free radicals ($\cdot O_2^-$) and production of reperfusion (reoxygenation) injury. Ischemia reduces myocyte levels of adenosine triphosphate (ATP) and raises the adenosine levels. Adenosine is reduced enzymatically to inosine, hypoxanthine, and xanthine. Ischemia favors the conversion of xanthine dehydrogenase to xanthine oxidase, which, in turn, converts hypoxanthine and xanthine to uric acid and generates free radicals ($\cdot O_2^-$). (From B. R. Lucchesi, et al. Interaction of the formed elements of blood with the coronary vasculature in vivo. *Fed. Proc.* 46:63, 1987.)

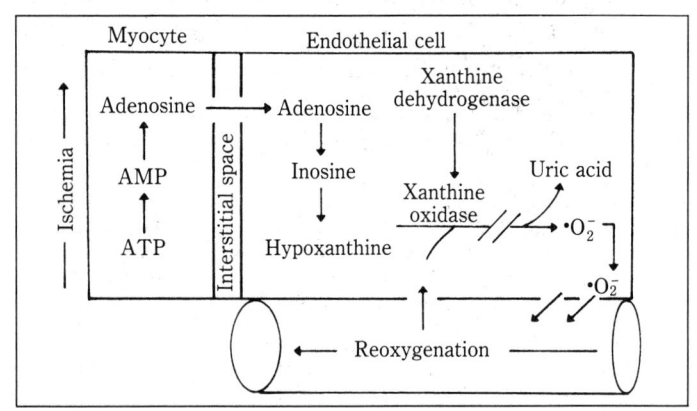

White blood cell aggregation along the endothelial surface leads to the activation of PMNs, owing to the presence of NADPH oxidase on the cell surface, which reduces O_2 to O_2^- (see Fig. 4-5), with concomitant oxidation of cytosolic NADPH. This reaction allows PMNs to generate oxidizing agents O_2^-, H_2O_2, ·OH, hypochlorous acid (HOCl), and N-substituted chloramines (R-NHCl). PMNs contain an additional enzyme, myeloperoxidase, which is required for R-NHCl production. The O_2^- of activated PMNs serves to activate a latent chemotactic factor in extracellular fluids that serves as a "chemical beacon" [27] to nearby inactive PMNs. McCord [20] proposed that exogenously administered SOD prevents the activation of the O_2^--dependent chemoattractant and thereby acts as an anti–inflammatory agent.

The free radicals, O_2^- and OH-mediated cell injury, may be operative in postischemic myocardial reperfusion injury. Free radicals generated during the formation of PGs (see Fig. 4-1), by activation of PMNs (see Fig. 4-5), or after reperfusion (see Fig. 4-4) and the release of norepinephrine (see below) act in concert to produce severe vasoconstriction. Such vasoconstriction, coupled with PMN-plugging of capillaries, serves to extend or amplify myocar-

Fig. 4-5. NADPH oxidase, a surface-bound enzyme on polymorphonuclear leukocytes (PMN), reduces O_2 to O_2^- using NADPH as the electron donor. A proportion of the O_2 generated is released into the extracellular space, and H_2O_2 formation results from spontaneous dismutation. Extracellular OH· and O_2^- formation may result from an interaction of H_2O_2 and O_2^-·. Myeloperoxidase (MP) using H_2O_2 and Cl^- as substrates can generate hypochlorite (OCl^-), which can interact with amino acids to form other radical species with exceedingly long half-lives that are capable of inducing lipid peroxidation of membranes and causing irreversible tissue injury. (From B. R. Lucchesi, et al. Interaction of the formed elements of blood with the coronary vasculature in vivo. *Fed. Proc.* 46:63, 1987.)

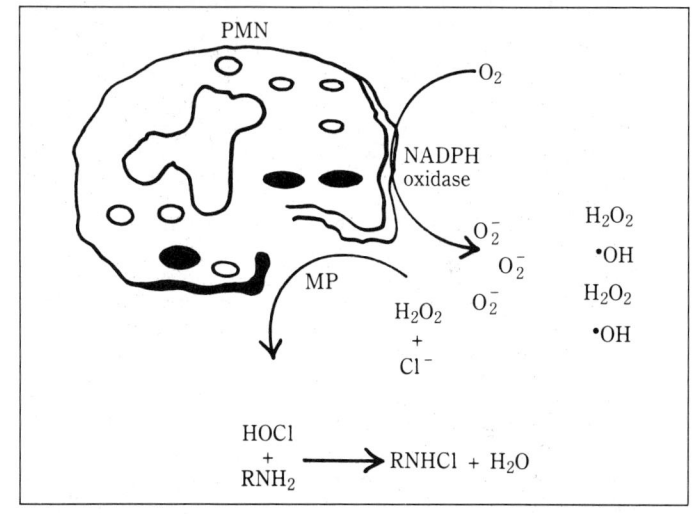

dial injury and cell death. As summarized by Simpson and colleagues [30], the endogenous antioxidant defense mechanisms (ascorbate, α-tocopherol, glutathione peroxidase, catalase, and superoxide dismutase) are rapidly overmatched by free radical generation secondary to reperfusion myocardial injury.

An endothelial/myocyte, cell to cell interaction is a potent coupling during reperfusion injury (see Fig. 4-4). According to McCord [22], a modification of endothelial cells during reperfusion (reoxygenation) increases cytosolic Ca^{2+} and activates a protease (calpain), which converts xanthine dehydrogenase to xanthine oxidase. Xanthine oxidase is found in capillary endothelial cells [16]. Concomitantly, cellular ATP is converted to adenosine monophosphate (AMP), which is subsequently catabolized to adenosine, inosine, and hypoxanthine. Hypoxanthine, as well as xanthine, serve as substrates for xanthine oxidase (E_o). Molecular O_2 supplied by reperfusion, along with hypoxanthine and xanthine, serve as substrate for E_o to produce O_2^-.

The O_2^--mediated injury secondary to reperfusion injury can be summarized as follows: Peroxidation of membranes, activation of phospholipases, release of arachidonic acid, prostaglandin formation, the xanthine oxidase reaction, complement activation, and the chemotaxis of neutrophils are phenomena that generate free radicals with myocardial ischemia and reperfusion. Within the myocardium, the endothelial cells of the vascular bed, rather than the myocytes, are the principal source of the free radicals [35].

MYOCARDIAL ISCHEMIA, INFARCTION, AND SYMPATHETIC DISCHARGE

Myocardial ischemia rapidly enhances adrenergic receptor expression, and, following an acute coronary occlusion and MI, the infarct size appears to be influenced by the extent of β-adrenergic stimulation. High levels of plasma norepinephrine and urinary catecholamine excretion are documented largely in patients with complicated MI, but in experimental unanesthetized animals, an early rise of norepinephrine (within 2 minutes) develops in anterior wall myocardial infarction. Myocardial adrenoceptor activity with ischemia can be summarized as follows:

Myocardial ischemia (15, 30, 60, 90 min) → progressive externalization of α- and β-adrenoceptors from intracellular light vesicles to sarcolemma. One hour duration → increased numbers of β-adrenoceptors in the left ventricle, which persist for 8 hours (dog) [14, 15].
No change in the muscarinic cholinergic receptors.
Adrenoceptors can activate physiologic responses.

Infarct size (small, medium, and large) is linearly related to plasma levels of epinephrine and norepinephrine. Furthermore, transmural infarctions may produce areas of myocardium that are denervated of sympathetic and afferent responses in infarcted as well as noninfarcted myocardium, and the afferent denervation is not homogeneous. Such inhomogeneity of denervation affects the electrical stability of the myocardium.

Release of myocardial norepinephrine, while influenced by ischemia, is profoundly affected by reperfusion of the ischemic myocardium.

Ischemia of less than 10 minutes is not associated with increased overflow of catecholamines (or metabolites).

Longer ischemic periods cause rapid increases in catecholamines. Norepinephrine release is highest during the initial minute of reperfusion.

Interesting, in this regard, is the observation that myocardial ischemia during coronary occlusion (angioplasty) in patients with coronary artery disease can be prevented, delayed in onset, or diminished in magnitude by beta blockers [16, 17]. Furthermore, myocardial damage during the process of dying may be related to endogenous catecholamine release and may influence the early failure in a donor heart following cardiac transplantation [18].

RATIONALE FOR CLINICAL INVESTIGATION OF REPERFUSION THERAPY

As the number of patients with clinically inducible myocardial ischemia (after thrombolytic therapy, percutaneous transluminal coronary angioplasty [PCAT], or coronary artery bypass surgery), and unstable angina pectoris increases, and as the number of cardiac transplantation candidates increases, there arises a growing need for understanding the pathophysiology of reperfusion myocardial ischemia. What is clear is that the injury process involves CA^{2+} overloading, altered adenine nucleotide metabolism, impaired cell volume regulation, and, very likely, the generation of free radicals.

Presently, applications of anti-free radical approaches are appearing in cardiovascular surgery:

Plasma H_2O_2 levels have been shown to be significantly elevated in 15 patients undergoing cardiopulmonary bypass for myocardial revascularization. Concurrently, the complement (C3a) pathway was activated and neutrophils were sequestered in the pulmonary vessels [5].

O_2-derived free radical generation associated with cardiopulmonary bypass was suppressed by pretreatment with free radical antioxidants (mannitol or allopurinol) in 25 patients when compared with values for 20 untreated patients serving as controls [6].

Disturbed Myocardial Physiology with Ischemia

Within seconds after the onset of severe ischemia, the rate of diastolic relaxation slows, and, a minute or so later, the rate of contraction declines. Coincident in time is a rapid rise in extracellular K^+ due to a leak across the sarcolemma. The process of Ca^{2+} sequestration occurs during the initial minutes of ischemia. These mechanical and ionic disturbances develop long before cellular ATP declines. The last system to fail is the Na^+-K^+ pump, which may continue to function for 20–25 minutes in a total anaerobic state.

The sequence of altered contractility and electrocardiographic abnormalities with myocardial ischemia is documented clinically by echoelectrocardiographic studies immediately before, during, and following PTCA. Transiently altered contractility (segmental asynergy) develops within 8–12 seconds after balloon inflation and returns to baseline within 19–43 seconds after balloon deflation. ECG changes do not develop in more than 50% of the cases and, when present, appear many seconds after the mechanical changes [2, 35]. A temporally late manifestation of PTCA-induced ischemia is angina pectoris.

Impaired diastolic relaxation, an early contractile dysfunction with ischemia, has been attributed to a reduction of the sarcoplasmic reticulum to remove Ca^{2+} from the cytoplasm. With progression of the ischemia, the incomplete diastolic relaxation gives way to contraction, which is caused by further disturbances in intracellular Ca^{2+} (increased amounts of free Ca^{2+} in the vicinity of myofilaments) or by ATP depletion.

While ECG changes are delayed after PTCA-induced myocardial ischemia, ECG abnormalities predisposing to lethal arrhythmias manifest themselves (in the experimental laboratory) within seconds after the onset of ischemia. The lethal arrhythmias following transient myocardial ischemia in humans depend largely on the inhomogeneity of the cellular environment of ischemic and normally perfused myocardium. Some clinically relevant factors contributing to ECG abnormalities during acute myocardial ischemia include:

Inhomogeneity of myocardial O_2 and autonomic nervous tissue function
Elevated extracellular K^+ concentration
Intracellular acidosis and lactate accumulation
Catecholamine release
Fatty acid ester accumulation (free fatty acid accumulation)
Generation of free radicals

These factors lead to cellular depolarization, decreased excitability, depression of the action potential upstroke velocity, shortening of the action potential duration, and altered refractoriness. The net effect clinically is a pronounced slowing of conduction and unidirectional conduction block within the ischemic zone, which favors reentrant arrhythmias (see Chap. 2).

Drug Treatment of Myocardial Ischemia and Infarction

Drugs used in the treatment of angina are directed towards increasing blood flow to the ischemic myocardium, reducing myocardial wall tension and O_2 requirements, limiting ischemic injury secondary to local catecholamine release, or reducing intracellular Ca^{2+} accumulation. The available drugs are nitrates, β-adrenergic receptor antagonists, and Ca^{2+} channel blocking drugs.

NITRATES

Uses and/or Actions

Nitrates are direct-acting vasodilators that conserve myocardial O_2 requirements by reducing venous tone and pooling blood in the peripheral veins, thereby decreasing myocardial preloading. The resultant ventricular volume and tension reduction lowers $M\dot{V}O_2$. At high doses, nitrates moderately reduce peripheral arteriolar resistance and conserve myocardial O_2 requirements by lowering left ventricular afterload.

Nitrates increase the myocardial O_2 supply by dilating large epicardial arteries without affecting the intramyocardial resistance arterioles. Nitrates dilate both normal and diseased coronary arteries, as well as the collateral vessels, and thereby improve regional myocardial blood flow to ischemic areas. Nitrates relieve spasms of angiographically normal and diseased arteries.

It is not clear how nitrates induce vasodilation, though some suggest nitrate receptors on vascular smooth muscle cells. A sulfhydryl group (-SH) on the receptor is purported to undergo oxidation in the presence of nitrates. In support of this idea is the potentiation of nitrate vasodilation by prior administration of N-acetylcysteine, an agent that increases the availability of -SH groups. Others suggest that the nitrate enters the smooth muscle cell and is either converted into a nitrosothiol or is denitrated by a glutathione-organic nitrate reductase to release free nitric oxide, both of which activate intracellular guanylate cyclase and raise the level of cyclic guanine monophosphate. Raising the intracellular cGMP levels is believed to cause smooth muscle relaxation.

A large arterial-venous nitroglycerin gradient between the systemic arterial and venous circulation suggests a rapid uptake of nitrates by blood vessels. Veins have a particularly high affinity for nitrates, as evidenced by venodilation occurring at much lower plasma nitrate concentrations than arterial vasodilation. Arteriolar or resistance vessel dilation is seen only with high plasma nitrate concentrations. Plasma nitrate levels may represent only 1% of the total body nitrate stores.

Pharmacologic Properties

The basic function of nitrites and nitrates is to relax smooth muscle in general, irrespective of its innervation or response to adrenergic, cholinergic, or other types of agonists. Nitrites and nitrates do not prevent cells from responding to an appropriate stimulus, although nitrates can antagonize norepinephrine, acetylcholine, histamine, and other receptor-mediated vasoconstrictors.

Pharmacokinetics of Organic Nitrates

Absorption and Distribution

Organic nitrates are absorbed from the gastrointestinal tract, buccal mucosa, and skin. The majority of nitrites and nitrates are taken up and metabolized by veins and arteries.

Metabolism

Regardless of the administration route, nitrates are rapidly converted to two inactive metabolites, the isomeric 1, 2 and 1, 3 glyceryl dinitrates, which are excreted in the urine. The half-life of the nitrates is less than 5 minutes.

Isosorbide dinitrate, particularly when taken orally, is metabolized by the glutathione organic nitrate reductase system of the liver. Two metabolites are produced, 2-isosorbide mononitrate (2-ISMN) and 5-isosorbide mononitrate (5-ISMN). The 5-ISMN has potent vasodilatory action, while 2-ISMN appears to be less active. Isosorbide dinitrate is metabolized and cleared more rapidly than the two metabolites. The concentration of 5-ISMN rises over time and remains elevated for hours after an oral dose (half-life of 4–4.5 hours). Only 20–25% of the oral isosorbide dinitrate is systemically bioavailable; 5-ISMN has a 90% bioavailability. Some believe that the clinical effects of isosorbide dinitrate come from the nitrate and that the protracted effect comes from 5-ISMN.

Other organic nitrates, pentaerythritol tetranitrate and erythritol tetranitrate, are also degraded by the hepatic enzyme glutathione organic nitrate reductase. Pentaerythritol tetranitrate is effective at doses of at least 40 mg.

Adverse Effects

Headache, flushing, and dizziness are often noted early in treatment, but these symptoms can be minimized by using small initial doses of the drug. Because of the pronounced action of nitrates on capacitance vessels, the therapeutic effect is enhanced, but adverse effects are also increased when the patient is in an upright position. Marked orthostatic hypotension and, occasionally, syncope can be avoided by instructing the patient to sit down after taking the nitrate. Rarely, generalized vasodilation may produce severe hypotension and reflex tachycardia, and the resultant drop in coronary artery perfusion pressure may worsen angina. Indeed, syncope and the sweating (plus angina) may simulate an acute MI.

Bradycardia

Severe bradycardia is occasionally associated with hypotension and, in part, is vagally mediated, since it responds to atropine.

Cerebral Ischemia

Rarely nitrates cause transient ischemic attacks.

Miscellaneous

Allergic contact dermatitis may occur with topical nitrates. Anaphylactoid reactions have rarely occurred. An aggravation of peripheral edema has been noted.

Precautions

Tolerance

Tolerance is defined as a condition in which increasing nitrate doses are required to induce a given hemodynamic or antianginal effect. Nitrate tolerance may be due to changes in pharmacokinetics or involve depletion of the free vascular -SH groups, since it may be reversed by dithiothreitol, a -SH-regenerating agent or N-acetylcysteine, a -SH-donor compound. Vascular tolerance to organic nitrates becomes apparent within 24 hours for intravenous infusion or after a few days and may reach a severe magnitude within a 2-week period with transcutaneous or oral routes of administration. Each of the available nitrate formulations have varying propensities to induce tolerance.

SHORT-ACTING NITROGLYCERIN AND ISOSORBIDE DINITRATE (ISDN). Sublingual nitroglycerin (NTG) and ISDN have not been reported to induce tolerance.

ORAL NITROGLYCERIN. Tolerance has been documented with long-term dosing of NTG. Tolerance to the hypotensive actions may develop, even though the antiangina effect persists.

OINTMENT. Tolerance has been reported.

INTRAVENOUS NITROGLYCERIN. Tolerance usually is not a concern for IV NTG because of the short duration of its use; however, sustained infusion can result in vascular tolerance within 24 hours.

BUCCAL NITROGLYCERIN. It is difficult to induce tolerance with buccal NTG.

TRANSDERMAL NITROGLYCERIN. The unusual pharmacokinetics of transdermal NTG appears to be intimately related to tolerance. In many well-controlled studies in patients with angina or congestive heart failure, attenuation or disappearance of nitrate actions may develop within 24 hours, in spite of large doses of nitrates (120 mg/24 hours). The attenuation of action is not caused by decreased NTG availability or a decline in the plasma NTG concentrations. A similar tolerance is reported for long-acting ISDN cream and sustained release oral isosorbide, 5-mononitrate.

Abrams [1] suggests nitrate tolerance is related to continuous nitrate release over 24 hours. Others suggest transdermal NTG or sustained action ISDN creams lose their antianginal effects after 1–2 weeks of daily use. According to Abrams, removal of nitrates rapidly restores responsiveness to the drug. The length of the nitrate-free interval is presently unsettled; some say 24 hours, others suggest shorter intervals. Nitrate tolerance may be prevented by using longer dosing intervals, a shorter-acting nitrate, or both. Transdermal patches or creams should perhaps be removed each day after 10 or 12 hours.

Dependence

Workers exposed to high levels of NTG over months or years (as in a munitions plant) may develop angina attacks or suffer an MI and sudden death with job changes or retirement. Rebound vasoconstriction upon sudden withdrawal of nitrates may occur as a manifestation of dependence.

Cardioversion

NTG patches may contribute to electrical arcing during cardioversion. Cardioversion paddles or ECG electrodes should not touch skin areas containing NTG ointment.

Hypertrophic Cardiomyopathy

Nitrates, by reducing peripheral resistance, may increase the left ventricular outflow gradient in this condition and should be avoided.

Methemoglobinemia

NADH-methemoglobin reductase deficiency may be exacerbated by nitrates (development of additional methemoglobin). Asymptomatic methemoglobinemia may occur without the enzyme deficiency.

Drug Interactions

Hypotension secondary to nitrates may be potentiated by alcohol, beta blockers, Ca^{2+} channel blockers, and tricyclic antidepressants.

Nitroglycerin Storage Requirements

Conventional NTG tablets gradually lose potency through volatilization and exposure to ultraviolet (UV) light. The drug is packaged in a UV-shielded glass container with a tightly fitted metal screw cap. Loss of potency is reduced by refrigerating the stock bottle of 100 and parceling 6 or 12 tablets in a UV-shielded carrying bottle for daily needs. After the carrying NTG are used or after 2 weeks, the tablets are discarded and replaced by tablets from the stock bottle. Stabilized tablets retain potency for longer periods than conventional tablets.

Sublingual Nitroglycerin

One tablet is dissolved under the tongue or in the buccal pouch at the first sign of an acute anginal attack. Additional or larger doses may be taken at 5-minute intervals, but no more than 3 tablets should be taken within a 15-minute period. The dosage must be individualized in each patient to relieve symptoms with minimal adverse effects.

DOSAGE AND ADMINISTRATION

Dose: 0.3–0.8 mg.
Onset of action: 2–5 minutes.
Peak action: 4–8 minutes.
Duration: 10–30 minutes.

DOSAGE FORMS AND STRENGTHS AVAILABLE

Nitrostat (stabilized) (Parke-Davis) and **generic tablets:** 0.15, 0.3, 0.4, and 0.6 mg.

Isosorbide Dinitrate

Dose: 2.5–10 mg.
Onset of action: 5–20 minutes.

Peak action: 15–60 minutes.
Duration: 45–120 minutes (or longer—3 hrs).

DOSAGE FORMS AND STRENGTHS AVAILABLE

Isordil (Ives), **Sorbitrate** (Stuart), and **generic tablets:** 2.5, 5, and 10 mg.

Erythrityl Tetranitrate

DOSAGE FORMS AND STRENGTHS AVAILABLE

Cardilate (Burroughs Wellcome) **tablets:** 5 and 10 mg.
  Dose: Oral, sublingual, or buccal, 5–10 mg 3–4 times daily.
Cardilate (Burroughs Wellcome) **chewable tablets:** 10 mg.
  Dose: Oral, 10 mg 3–4 times daily.

Lingual Nitroglycerin Aerosol

DOSAGES

Adult: One or two sprays into mouth may be repeated every 3–5 minutes, but no more than 3 doses in a 15-minute period.

DOSAGE FORMS AND STRENGTHS AVAILABLE

Nitrolingual (Rorer) **aerosol spray** 0.4 mg per metered dose.

Buccal Nitroglycerin

The pill is placed in the buccal pouch between the upper lip and the teeth. A seal or gel forms rapidly and the tablet adheres to the mucous membrane. NTG is immediately released and absorbed and the onset of the nitrite effect is as rapid as the sublingual NTG. The NTG is absorbed at a relatively constant rate over 3–6 hours.

Dose: 1–3 mg.
Onset of action: 2–5 minutes.
Peak action: 4–10 minutes.
Duration: 30–300 minutes.

Oral Nitroglycerin

Oral NTG was originally believed to be relatively ineffective or useless due to hepatic nitrate degradation, but recent evidence clearly indicates a bioactivity and clinical effectiveness that may last for hours. The peak plasma concentration is related to the dose and absorption as well as plasma levels, which vary widely and in an unpredictable fashion. Consequently, large doses (larger than pharmaceutical literature lists) may be required to obtain the desired clinical effects. Patients not relieved by sublingual NTG are unlikely to benefit from another nitrate.

Dose: 6.5–19.5 mg.
Onset of action: 20–45 minutes.
Peak action: 45–120 minutes.
Duration: 2–6 hours (or longer—8 hours).

DOSAGE FORMS AND STRENGTHS AVAILABLE

Generic plain, timed-release capsules: 2.5, 6.5, and 9 mg.
Nitro-Bid (Marion) **timed-release capsules:** 2.5, 6.5, and 9 mg.
Nitroglyn (Key) **timed-release capsules:** 2.5, 6.5, and 9 mg.
Nitro-Stat SR (Parke-Davis) **timed-release capsules:** 2.5, 6.5, and 9 mg.
Nitrospan (USV) **timed-release capsules:** 2.5 and 6.5 mg.
Nitrong (Wharton) **timed-release tablets:** 2.6, 6.5, and 10 mg.

Isosorbide Dinitrate

Dose: 10–60 mg.
Onset of action: 15–45 minutes.
Peak action: 45–120 minutes.
Duration: 2–6 hours (or longer—8 hours).

DOSAGE FORMS AND STRENGTHS AVAILABLE

Generic plain, timed-release capsules: 40 mg.
Generic tablets: 5, 10, 20, 30, and 40 mg.
Generic timed-release tablets: 40 mg.
Dilatrate-SR (Reed & Carnrick) **timed-release capsules:** 40 mg.
Isordil (Ives) **tablets:** 5, 10, 20, 30, and 40 mg.
Isordil timed-release capsules and tablets: 40 mg.
Isordil chewable tablets: 10 mg.
Onset (Bock) **chewable tablets:** 5 and 10 mg.
Sorbitrate (Stuart) **tablets:** 5, 10, 20, 30, and 40 mg.
Sorbitrate timed-release tablets: 40 mg.
Sorbitrate chewable tablets: 5 and 10 mg.

Pentaerythritol Tetranitrate

Dose: 40–80 mg.
Onset of action: 60 minutes.
Peak action: 60–120 minutes.
Duration: 3–6 hours.

DOSAGE FORMS AND STRENGTHS AVAILABLE

Generic timed-release capsules: 30 and 80 mg.
Generic tablets: 10, 20, 40, and 80 mg.
Generic timed-release tablets: 80 mg.
Pentritol (USV) **timed-release capsules:** 30 and 60 mg.
Peritrate (Parke-Davis) **tablets:** 10, 20, and 40 mg.
Peritrate timed-release tablets: 80 mg (Peritrate SA).

Topical Nitroglycerin

NITROGLYCERIN OINTMENT (2%) 15 MG/IN.

Dose: ½–2 in. (rarely 4–5 in.) every 4–8 hours.
Onset of action: 15–60 minutes.
Peak action: 30–120 minutes.
Duration: 3–8 hours.

DOSAGE FORMS AND STRENGTHS AVAILABLE

Generic ointment 2%: 20, 30, and 60 gm containers.
Nitro-Bid (Marion) **ointment 2%:** 1, 20, and 60 gm containers.
Nitrol (Rorer) **ointment 2%:** 3, 30, and 60 gm containers.
Nitrong (Wharton) **ointment 2%:** 30 and 60 gm containers.
Nitrostat (Parke-Davis) **ointment 2%:** 30 and 60 gm containers.

Nitroglycerin-Containing Discs or Patches

Discs should be applied to a site free of hair and not on distal parts of an extremity and should be removed after 10–12 hours. Discs release ½ mg of NTG/cm^2/disc area. Plasma NTG concentration with 5–10 mg/24 hours is well below 0.5 ng/ml. Efficacy of discs or patches at the 5–10 mg/24 hours dose as an antiangina regimen is inconsistently demonstrated. Larger doses consistently demonstrate antianginal effects and improve exercise tolerance. Doses of 15–120 mg/24 hours produce beneficial hemodynamic responses (left ventricular filling pressure and right heart pressure) in patients with chronic congestive heart failure. The major concern of discs and patches is the phenomenon of acute tachyphylaxis or tolerance that may appear within 12–24 hours.

Dose: 10–20 mg.
Onset of action: 30–60 minutes.
Peak action: 60–180 minutes.
Duration: possibly 24 hours.

A comparison of available NTG discs or patches is given in Table 4-3.

Intravenous Nitroglycerin

Intravenous NTG represents a major advance in treatment of the acutely ill patient. IV NTG is useful therapy for acute pulmonary edema and severe congestive heart failure (see Chap. 1), acute and recurrent chest pain during MI, systemic hypertension (see Chap. 3) with acute MI or immediately following aorto-coronary bypass grafting, and control of arterial pressure during neurosurgical procedures and abdominal aortic aneurysm repair. The action of IV NTG is infuenced by blood concentration levels. At high concentrations, the action is on the arteries and arterioles, and peripheral resistance falls. With lower concentrations (infusion rates), the action is on the venous system.

Manufacturers differ in concentration and/or volume per vial, and the literature must be consulted for dilution instructions. Care must be exercised in substituting one preparation for another. NTG should be diluted with a dextrose (5%) or sodium chloride (0.9%) injection and should not be mixed with other drugs. Glass containers should be used for dilution and storage. A solution of 100 µg/ml may be used for initial dosage titration. A more concentrated solution may be substituted if fluid restriction is required.

DOSAGES

Adult: 5 µg/min of dilute solution is infused and may be increased gradually by 5 µg/min every 3–5 minutes, until a response is noted. If no response is achieved with 20 µg/min, increments of 10 µg/min, and later 20 µg/min, may be necessary. Rarely infusion rates of 200 µg/min or more are necessary to relieve chest pain or lower pulmonary artery wedge pressure while maintaining near-normal arterial perfusion pressure. Blood pressure and heart rate must be monitored continuously.

DOSAGE FORMS AND STRENGTHS AVAILABLE

Nitroglycerin injection (Abbott)—**sterile solution:** 5 mg/ml in 5 ml containers (alcohol 50%).

Nitro-Bid IV (Marion)—**sterile solution:** 5 mg/ml in 1, 5, and 10 ml containers (alcohol 50%).

Nitrostat IV (Parke-Davis)—**sterile solution:** 0.8 mg/ml in 10 ml containers (alcohol 5%) and 5 mg/ml in 10 ml containers (alcohol 30%) with or without delivery set.

Tridil (American Critical Care)—**sterile solution:** 5 mg/ml in 5 and 10 ml containers (alcohol 30%) with or without delivery set (Tridilset).

Table 4-3. Transcutaneous nitroglycerin compounds

Trade name	Release rate (mg/24 hr)	Surface area (cm^2)	Nitroglycerin content (mg/unit)
Nitrodisc	5	8	16
(Searle)	10	16	32
Nitro-Dur	2.5	5	26
(Key)	5	10	51
	7.5	15	77
	10	20	104
Nitro-Dur II	2.5	5	20
(Key)	5	10	40
	7.5	15	60
	10	20	80
	15	30	120
Transderm-Nitro	2.5	5	12.5
(CIBA)	5	10	25
	10	20	50
	15	30	75

Beta-Adrenergic Receptor Antagonists: Beta Blockers

Beta blockers reversibly inhibit the effects of catecholamines at beta-adrenergic receptor (adrenoceptor) sites. Beta adrenoceptors are located predominantly in the heart, arteries, and arterioles of skeletal muscle and in the bronchi, where they mediate cardiac excitation, peripheral vasodilation, and bronchial relaxation.

Beta adrenoceptors are classified into β_1 and β_2 subtypes: β_1-adrenoceptors are located in the heart and mediate increases in heart rate and myocardial contractility: β_2 are found in smooth muscle of bronchi and peripheral arteries (see Chaps. 2 and 3 for full description of beta blockers). Blockade of β_1 adrenoceptors reduces heart rate, myocardial contractility, and cardiac output; prolongs AV conduction time; and suppresses automaticity.

PHARMACOLOGIC AND PHARMACOKINETIC PROPERTIES

(See Chaps. 2 and 3).

Use in Angina Pectoris

The beneficial effect of beta blockers in angina is due to a decrease in heart rate, myocardial contractility, and arterial pressure, the major determinants of $M\dot{V}O_2$. Reduction of heart rate prolongs the diastolic interval during which the left ventricle receives its major flow of coronary blood. Beta blockers attenuate the cardiovascular response to exercise and prevent reflex increases in heart rate and the rate of contractility produced by nitrates or Ca^{2+} channel blocking drugs that elicit a reflex response (nifedipine).

Beta blockers plus nitrates may be viewed as first-line drugs for the treatment of angina. Both classes of drugs reduce myocardial oxygen demand by different and, perhaps, additive mechanisms. Beta blockers attenuate the reflex tachycardia secondary to the nitrates, and the nitrates counteract the increase in heart size and prolongation of ventricular diastole associated with the beta blocker. The response of beta blockers in vasospastic angina, variant or Prinzmetal's, is not always predictable. Since beneficial, as well as detrimental, effects are reported, beta blockers as the sole therapy in vasospastic angina should be avoided.

Patient age alters the pharmacokinetics of beta blockers; consequently, their use in the elderly as an antianginal agent is open to question. The age-associated reduced hepatic blood flow lowers the "first pass" metabolism and results in an accumulation of beta blockers in the blood and raises the possibility of serious central nervous system side effects. Additionally, malnourishment and its attendant lowering of plasma proteins would raise blood levels of plasma-bound beta blockers (propranolol, oxprenolol, alprenolol, and pindolol). Additionally, β-adrenoceptor density is decreased with age.

Use in Acute Myocardial Infarction

The IV administration of a beta blocker during the acute phase of MI decreases O_2 requirements of the left ventricle by reducing cardiac output, arterial pressure, and heart rate. The beta blocker narrows the arterial-coronary sinus O_2 difference, decreases myocardial lactate production, and may shift the balance to lactate extraction.

Prospective epidemiologic studies have identified subsets of patients who survived MI with high, intermediate, or low mortality risk. The high-risk subset (15%) had a mortality ranging from 20–40% in the first year following hospital discharge. This group had cardiac symptoms prior to infarct, frequent ventricular ectopy, and depressed left ventricular function. Geriatric-age (> 65 years) patients with acute MI are among high-risk patients. The low-risk subset (30%), with 2% mortality in the first year, had no cardiac symptoms before and no ventricular ectopy during infarction and a negative submaximal exercise test prior to hospital discharge. The remaining 55% had one or two characteristics of the high-risk group and a 10% mortality during the initial post-infarction year.

Objective evidence of beneficial effects of beta blockers in acute MI include:

Reduced chest pain
Decreased ST segment elevation in transmural infarction
Improved regional wall motion (pindolol)
Significantly lower creatine kinase levels (peak, calculated release, and cumulative values) (propranolol 0.1 mg/kg IV followed by 320 mg PO for next 17 hours). Similar results with IV atenolol and timolol were reported in two randomized double-blind studies.

Use of beta blockers in the setting of an acute MI requires hemodynamic monitoring of the cardiac output, pulmonary wedge pressure (Swan-Ganz catheter), and arterial pressure (arterial line) if the patient has an acute sympathetic syndrome or there is a suggestion of heart failure (mild). (Beta blockers are contraindicated with frank heart failure.) Cardiac output should not fall below 2.2 liters/min/m^2 body surface area, and the wedge pressure should not exceed 15–18 mm Hg. Beta blockers used to control chest pain or limiting the infarct size also require cardiac output and wedge pressure monitoring. Cardiac index will drop approximately 15–20% with the beta blockers. Beta blockers should be withdrawn (or withheld) if the systolic pressure drops below 90 mm Hg and if the heart rate drops below 50–55 beats/min. If lidocaine hydrochloride is in use, the dose may be reduced by one-third upon starting the beta blocker.

The question of a reduced short-term mortality (e.g., first two weeks following an acute MI) in patients receiving a beta blocker was addressed by the Metoprolol in Acute Myocardial Infarction (MIAMI) trial carried out in Sweden [14]. A large number of patients (5778) who were not on beta blockers or Ca^{2+} channel blockers prior to the infarction were randomized (within 7 hours after chest pain, 20% had normal electrocardiograms and 70% showed signs of acute MI, predominantly anterior wall in location) to placebo (2901) and metoprolol (2877). Use of cardiac supportive drugs (cardiac glycosides, diuretics, atropine) was equivalent in the two groups.

The findings regarding mortality rate showed:

No effect in patients with low and median risk infarctions
Significant reduction (39%) in the high risk groups

The beneficial effects in acute MI are seen only when the beta blockers are given early (4–6 hours) after the onset of pain in high-risk patients, particularly those with anterior wall infarction. Beta blockers started 12 hours after the onset of pain show no consistent beneficial effects.

Use After Acute Myocardial Infarction

Three reported large scale and well-designed studies of beta blocker therapy following MI provided remarkably similar findings (a reduction in total mortality ranging from 26–39%):

1. A multicenter, double-blind randomized study of the effect of timolol on mortality and reinfarction in patients surviving acute MI (1884 patients) [32].
2. Effect on mortality of metoprolol in acute MI: a double-blind randomized trial [15].
3. Beta Blocker Heart Attack Trial (BHAT) Research Group: A randomized trial of propranolol in patients with acute MI (3837 patients) [3].

Follow-up reports from the Timolol-Norwegian study, which initiated beta blocker therapy (10 mg twice daily) 7–28 days after confirmed MI in men and women and continued for at least 12 months, with patient follow-up for 12–33 months, provides the following information [33]:

1. Mortality and reinfarction rates of patients with new and unequivocal Q waves were significantly lower (39%) in the treated than in the untreated groups (10.1 vs. 15.4%, $p < 0.01$); for the no-Q-wave patients, the rates of reinfarction as well as mortality were similar for the two groups.
2. In patients without angina prior to the MI a beta blocker reduced mortality by 61% and the occurrence of the first nonfatal reinfarction was decreased by 16.9% when compared to the placebo group. Patients with angina prior to the MI had a 21.8% reduction in mortality and a 48.6% reduction in the first nonfatal reinfarction. Similar benefits of beta blocker therapy were documented for patients with post-infarction angina. Thus, the use of beta blockers after MI should not depend on pre-infarction and post-infarction angina.
3. In high risk patients—that is, those who are 65–75 years of age, those with cardiomegaly and compensated heart failure, and those with stable diabetes mellitus—the number of cardiac deaths and reinfarction prevented by beta blockers was twice as high as that of patients below 65 years of age.
4. A 72-month (6-year) follow-up showed a significantly lower cumulative mortality rate of 32.3% (placebo) and 26.4% (beta blocker).
5. The beta blocker heart attack trial (BHAT) was a randomized

and double-blind placebo controlled trial of propranolol hydrochloride administered to men and women with at least one MI. The drug was started 5–21 days after infarction. The drug dose (180–240 mg/day given in divided doses) was controlled by serum levels; however, no correlation was found between the plasma propranolol levels and a beneficial effect. Both arteriosclerosis-related mortality and sudden death were reduced significantly (26%) over a 27-month follow-up period.

Unlike the Norwegian and the BHAT studies, the MIAMI trial used the β_1 selective blocker, metoprolol. The drug started within 12 hours of the initial chest pain (15 mg IV followed by 100 mg PO twice daily), showed a significant reduction in mortality (approximately 36%) for all age groups at 3 months after the MI and a 25% reduction after 3 years of follow-up [15].

Mechanism of Benefit

The cause of the reduced mortality with the beta blocker initiated after an acute MI is due to a lower incidence rate of cardiovascular deaths. Prevention of sudden death appears to be one factor in the analysis of benefits.

Beta blockers, by attenuating cardiac stimulation from the sympathetic nervous system and by lowering the level of stress-induced rise in plasma free fatty acids (arrhythmia-promoting factor) through inhibition of lipolysis may decrease the potential for reentrant ventricular arrhythmias and sudden death. Beta blockers raise the ventricular fibrillation threshold in the ischemic myocardium. In the BHAT trial propranolol reduced the incidence rate of total and complex ventricular arrhythmias, as indicated by 24-hour ambulatory monitoring.

Reduction of cardiac stimulation by endogenous catecholamines as the result of beta blockade may reduce chronic ischemic responses in the myocardium. The anti-ischemic effect may also be due to reduced myocardial O_2 demand (secondary to lowering afterload, heart rate, and myocardial contractility at rest and with exercise and to increasing the diastolic interval, thereby enhancing coronary blood flow).

Not all series of patients with MI treated with other beta blockers show long-term improvement in survival or reinfarction rates. Beta blockers with intrinsic sympathomimetic activity, oxyprenolol and pindolol, appear to be less beneficial. The most favorable effects on mortality in all subgroups of patients are reported in series using timolol, metoprolol, and propranolol. Selection of the beta blocker should be determined by the systemic and cardiopulmonary side effects. When using beta blockers in patients requiring an intact sympathetic nervous system, **caution must be exercised** to insure optimum myocardial and bronchial function. This is particularly germane to patients with the greatest potential for benefiting from long-term beta blockers—the geriatric-aged, MI patient.

With the benefit of the MIAMI (Sweden), the timolol (Norwegian), the BHAT (United States), and the metoprolol (Sweden) trials, the indications for beta blockers in managing the acute and the post-MI patient are clarified. Timing following the onset of chest pain and risk stratification of the MI are essential for identifying patients with the greatest prospects of benefits from beta blockers. Beta blockers given within 5 hours are of benefit in high-risk patients with uncomplicated MI as long as the following guidelines are followed:

Angina (or equivalent) prior to infarction
Anterior wall infarction
Cardiomegaly, but fully compensated heart failure
Depressed left ventricular function
65–75 years of age

How long beta blockers should be continued is unclear, but in the absence of hard data, the consensus view is 1–3 years.

ADVERSE EFFECTS

(See Chaps. 2 and 3.)

Individual Beta Blockers

The dosage interval for beta blockers should be increased with the creatinine clearance in an inverse manner. For example, with a one-a-day beta blocker (long-acting propranolol or nadolol):

Creatinine clearance (ml/min/1.73 m^2)	Dosage interval (hours)
> 50	24
31–50	24–36
10–30	24–48
< 10	40–60

Propranolol Hydrochloride

Propranolol hydrochloride is a nonselective β_1 and β_2 adrenoceptor antagonist.

Propranolol is often combined with nitrates and/or Ca^{2+} channel blocking drugs to control angina (for information on pharmacokinetics, see Chaps. 2 and 3).

DOSAGES

Adult: *Oral*—for angina, initially 10–20 mg 3 or 4 times daily, with a gradual increase as required to control symptoms. Most patients require 160–240 mg daily, and some may need 400 mg (usually in 4 divided doses). Geriatric-age (> 65 years) patients do not tolerate doses greater than 80–160 mg daily because of neurologic, psychiatric, and/or neuromuscular side effects.
Long-lasting—initially, 80 mg daily, increasing to 160 mg daily.

DOSAGE FORMS AND STRENGTHS AVAILABLE

Inderal (Ayerst) **tablets:** 10, 20, 40, 60, 80, and 90 mg.
Inderal LA (Ayerst) **timed-release capsules:** 80, 120, and 160 mg.

Acebutolol Hydrochloride

Acebutolol hydrochloride is a cardioselective beta blocker with partial agonist activity that may be useful in patients with rest angina or severe angina of effort. This drug may be associated with an increased incidence of antinuclear antibody formation, hypersensitivity pneumonitis, pleurisy, and pulmonary granulomas.

DOSAGES

Adult: *Oral*—for angina, initially 400 mg daily in 2 divided doses. Dosage may be increased gradually as needed.

DOSAGE FORMS AND STRENGTHS AVAILABLE

Sectral (Wyeth) **capsules:** 200 and 400 mg.

Atenolol

Atenolol is a relatively cardioselective long-acting beta blocker. This drug is a hydrophilic compound that does not cross the blood-brain barrier as readily as the lipophilic compounds.

DOSAGES

Adult: *Oral*—for angina, 50, 100, or 200 mg once daily. Dosage may need to be increased in patients with impaired renal function.

DOSAGE FORMS AND STRENGTHS AVAILABLE

Tenormin (Stuart) **tablets:** 50 and 100 mg.

Metoprolol Tartrate

Metoprolol tartrate is a relatively cardioselective long-acting beta blocker that may be a drug of choice in asthmatics and diabetics.

DOSAGES

Oral: for angina, 50 mg 3 or 4 times daily; in long-term prophylaxis after acute MI, 100 mg twice daily.
IV: for acute MI, initially three bolus injections of 5 mg at two-minute intervals. Blood pressure, heart rate, and electrocardiogram should be monitored. Oral therapy is instituted 15 minutes after the last IV dose, initially 25 or 50 mg every 6

hours for 48 hours followed by maintenance therapy (100 mg twice daily).

DOSAGE FORMS AND STRENGTHS AVAILABLE
Lopressor (Geigy) **tablets:** 50 and 100 mg.
Lopressor IV solution: 1 mg/ml in 5 ml containers (for early treatment of acute MI).

Nadolol

Nadolol is a nonselective beta blocker.

DOSAGES
Oral: for angina, initially 40 mg once daily with gradual increases in 40–80 mg increments at 3- to 7-day intervals, until desired effect is obtained. Maintenance dose is usually 40–80 mg daily. (See page 243 for renally impaired patients.)

DOSAGE FORMS AND STRENGTHS AVAILABLE
Corgard (Squibb) **tablets:** 40, 80, 120, and 160 mg.

Pindolol

This drug may not be a drug of choice for angina because of the partial agonist activity. If bradycardia is a problem with other beta blockers, then pindolol may be useful in angina.

DOSAGES
Oral: for angina, 10 mg twice daily; long-term post-MI, 10 mg twice daily.

DOSAGE FORMS AND STRENGTHS AVAILABLE
Visken (Sandoz) **tablets:** 5 and 10 mg.

Timolol Maleate

The antianginal actions of timolol maleate appear to be comparable to propranolol. Timolol reduces mortality and myocardial reinfarction when used on a long-term basis (Norwegian Multicenter Study Group [25]). Timolol is a nonselective β_1- and β_2-adrenoceptor antagonist.

DOSAGES
Adult: *Oral*—for angina, 10–30 mg twice daily. Sublingual and long-acting nitrates should be continued as needed. For long-term prophylaxis after acute MI, 10 mg twice daily.

DOSAGE FORMS AND STRENGTHS AVAILABLE

Blocadren (Merck, Sharp & Dohme) **tablets:** 5, 10, and 20 mg.

Ca^{2+} Channel Blockers in the Treatment of Ischemic Heart Disease

The anti-ischemic effectiveness of Ca^{2+} channel blockers is mediated by an alteration of the major determinants of myocardial O_2 supply and demand (preloads and afterloads, myocardial contractility, and, to a limited degree, heart rate).

STABLE ANGINA PECTORIS

Many cross-over, placebo-controlled, randomized studies involving nifedipine demonstrate a decrease in the frequency of angina and increases in exercise tolerance. The duration of exercise stress electrocardiographic testing is prolonged before ST-T segment changes develop or angina appears.

UNSTABLE ANGINA PECTORIS

Unstable angina pectoris, a clinical syndrome of an increase in symptomatic manifestations of myocardial ischemia (angina) with pain occurring at rest and after rest, accompanied by reversible electrocardiographic changes, is associated with substantial morbidity and mortality. Most recent studies show that unstable angina has fixed coronary artery lesions that are obstructing. The unstable angina is probably due to a destabilization of the atherosclerotic plaque (fissures resulting, in many instances, from intramural hemorrhage within or below the plaque, endothelial cell dysfunction, platelet aggregation, and thrombus formation). Presently, the detailed recognition of the pathophysiology of unstable angina is required before a proper therapeutic strategy can be arranged. At the root of such studies should be a coronary arteriogram.

Success with beta blockers alone or in combination provides a false sense of success in the management of unstable angina, since the results of a number of studies point to the high incidence rates of MI and death in this subset of angina patients. Present evidence strongly supports an aggressive approach initiated with coronary arteriography followed by the institution of antiplatelet and plasminogen activators (heparin, tissue-type plasminogen activator, t-PA [see Chap. 6]) and, if indicated, coronary angioplasty and bypass surgery. Such aggressiveness is particularly necessary in the setting of a critical narrowed left anterior descending artery.

VARIANT OR PRINZMETAL'S ANGINA PECTORIS

Variant or Prinzmetal's angina pectoris occurs most commonly in patients with a fixed obstructive lesion in the coronary artery. It is seen in patients with angina at rest, with cyclical attacks occurring at the same time of the day and often at night; with unstable angina; and as the forerunner of sudden death. The cause of variant angina is a reversible narrowing of a large epicardial coronary artery due to an inappropriate constriction of the arterial smooth muscle cells. The constriction or spasm occurs in the more proximal segments of the epicardial coronary arteries and may develop without underlying obstructive atherosclerosis (43%) or associated with an atherosclerotic lesion (57%).

The vasospastic site exhibits hypersensitivity to vasoconstrictor stimuli such as norepinephrine, serotonin, and/or histamine. Numerous studies implicate an involvement of α-adrenoceptors, and an apparent synergism for provoking coronary artery spasm between norepinephrine and serotonin. Aberrant contraction of medial smooth muscle cells in coronary arteries appears to be precipitated by conditions surrounding the already-compromised vessel lumen. For example, an altered endothelial cell metabolism would promote platelet aggregation and the release of thromboxane A_2, serotonin, histamine, and epinephrine.

Nitrates are particularly effective in reversing coronary artery spasm and represent first-line therapy. When variant angina occurs in the setting of normal or near-normal coronary arteries, the Ca^{2+} slow channel blockers may be effective in more than 90% of patients. In patients with underlying coronary artery stenotic lesions and variant angina, the effectiveness of the Ca^{2+} channel blockers is reduced to approximately 82%. The reported efficacy rates of nifedipine, diltiazem, and verapamil with variant angina is 94%, 91%, and 86%, respectively.

SILENT OR ASYMPTOMATIC MYOCARDIAL ISCHEMIA (SILENT ANGINA)

It is estimated that 4–5 million individuals in the United States have recurring silent myocardial ischemia. The estimate includes 50,000 patients without symptoms following MI, 3 million with overt angina, and 1–2 million without a history of previous MI or angina. Asymptomatic ST-T depression or elevation is a common occurrence in the postmyocardial infarct period, in spite of anti-ischemic medications. Recognition of patients with silent myocardial ischemia requires some form of continuous monitoring such as electrocardiographic recordings of ST-T segment changes. Continuous ambulatory ECG monitoring of patients with ischemic heart disease indicates "that in both unstable and chronic stable angina, over two-thirds of myocardial ischemic episodes are clinically silent." In addition, "most symptomatic and asymptomatic episodes are not triggered by increases in the determinants of oxygen demand" [31]. These silent ischemic periods may persist for 10–20 minutes.

Approximately 80% of ischemic episodes in unstable angina are silent. A documentation of silent myocardial ischemia is of prognostic significance in patients with coronary artery disease that is independent of the coronary angiographic findings.

Clinical clues to the presence of silent ischemia can be summarized as follows:

Post-myocardial infarct patients with angina or with a positive exercise stress test

Positive exercise stress test in asymptomatic, high risk individuals (history of MI or documented coronary artery disease)

Transient left ventricular wall motion abnormality at rest or during exercise (echocardiography)

ECG evidence of old MI with no history of prolonged chest pain

Transient ST segment elevation or depression ($\geq$ 1 mm) on random or ambulatory monitoring

Among patients with variant angina and unstable angina, episodes of silent ischemia appear to be as frequent as episodes of angina: Ca^{2+} channel blockers decrease the frequency of silent ischemic episodes. Persistence of silent ischemic episodes in the face of therapy in patients with unstable angina identify patients at high risk for an unfavorable outcome. Patients with stable angina may have episodes of silent ischemia that are 5 times as frequent as the episodes of angina.

Treatment of silent myocardial ischemia is presently not settled, but the combination of nifedipine and beta blocker reportedly eliminates 95% of the ECG abnormalities.

ANGINA-LIKE DISTRESS WITH "CLEAN" CORONARY ARTERIES

Precordial chest distress responsive to nitrates but without critical narrowing of the large-sized epicardial coronary arteries has been thought to be due to disease in "small-vessel"-intramural coronary arteries. Intramural coronary arteries are allegedly "protected" from atherosclerotic disease. However, morphologic changes in these arteries may accompany or occur independently of atherosclerotic stenosis of the epicardial coronary arteries. Even in hearts with minimal nonstenosing atherosclerotic disease of the epicardial coronary arteries, thickening and hyalinization of the media and adventitia; a reorientation, proliferation, and migration of pleomorphic smooth muscle cells; and new elastin and collagen as part of intimal hyperplasia in intramural arteries may appear.

The intramural arteries and the arterioles and precapillary sphincters are the ultimate regulators of myocardial perfusion. The prevailing explanation for the mechanism of atypical chest pain responsive to nitrates and angiographically normal coronary arteries is an inappropriate coronary arteriolar vasodilatory reserve. Patients with the presumed aberrant vasodilatory reserve respond to Ca^{2+} channel blockers with alleviation of the angina and improved exercise tolerance. Furthermore, the intramural arteries and arterioles may undergo spastic episodes that are terminated by Ca^{2+} channel blockers.

ACUTE MYOCARDIAL INFARCTION

In spite of favorable effects of Ca^{2+} channel blockers in protecting the myocardium in animal models of acute MI, studies of nifedipine in humans show no, or even deleterious, effects.

USE IN NON-Q-WAVE MYOCARDIAL INFARCTION

Patients experiencing a non-Q-wave MI are at high risk for early reinfarction. The multicenter studies showing a reduced reinfarction incidence rate and post-MI mortality with beta blocker therapy dealt with patients with Q-wave infarctions. Now, the report of a multicenter study using diltiazem offers an effective long-term treatment for patients with non-Q-wave MI by reducing the incidence rate of angina (verapamil gave mixed results and nifedipine may be harmful) [10]. The rationale of long-term diltiazem for the non-Q-wave MI patient was: (1) reduce $M\dot{V}O_2$ via effects on afterload, contractility, and heart rate; (2) augment coronary flow to ischemic zones; and (3) interfere with Ca^{2+} entry into myocardial cells. An entry of 576 patients with non-Q-wave myocardial infarction was randomized to placebo or diltiazem (24–72 hours post-MI) and followed for the primary endpoint, that is, reinfarction, and the secondary endpoint of angina, effort-related and silent angina. The results of the study are as follows:

A 51% reduction in reinfarction rate (9.3% placebo and 5.2% drug)

Cardioprotection was recognized after the fourth day post-MI.

Post-MI angina was twice as frequent with non-Q-wave as with Q-wave infarctions. Angina with ECG changes occurred in 24% of the placebo-control compared with 15.7% of the diltiazem-treated patients. Appearance of refractory angina was 6.9% for controls and 3.5% for the diltiazem group.

The 2-week reinfarction rate was 20% with angina and ECG changes, and 5.3% in those without ECG changes. Mortality rate was 11.3% for the angina and ECG changes, as compared to 1.5% for angina without ECG changes.

These protective findings with diltiazem stand in sharp contrast to the lack of benefit from nifedipine in six multicenter studies (7590 patients).

USE IN CORONARY ARTERY BYPASS SURGERY AND IN ANGIOPLASTY

Myocardial injury is followed by an accumulation of Ca^{2+} in the mitochondria and in the sarcoplasmic reticulum. Such intracellular accumulations of Ca^{2+} can be blocked in ischemic and reperfused experimental animal hearts by perfusing the coronary arteries with a solution containing nifedipine.

In open heart surgery in humans, nifedipine inclusion in the cardioplegia solution may improve the hemodynamic function following bypass surgery and reduce myocardial damage (myocardial enzyme release and pyrophosphate scan). These impressions were subsequently confirmed by a study of 205 patients that included 35 randomized controls and 39 nifedipine-treated patients. The nifedipine group showed a twofold improvement in cardiac index and stroke volume, left ventricular stroke work index, and pulmonary vascular resistance immediately after bypass surgery when compared to the control group. The mortality rate due to acute low cardiac output was 4% for the nifedipine group and 11% for the control group. Similar results are reported with verapamil addition to the cardioplegia solution.

Intracoronary nifedipine administered immediately before angioplasty (0.2 mg into the left main coronary artery) reduces the mechanical function of the left ventricle and nearly suppresses the lactate production (coronary sinus blood) following a 15-second occlusion of the left anterior descending artery.

A similarly protective effect is reported for diltiazem.

Individual Ca^{2+} Channel Blockers

Nifedipine

The mechanism of nifedipine action is in offering some improvement of coronary blood flow, but it predominantly acts by decreasing myocardial O_2 demand. The effect on myocardial O_2 demand is the result of reduced systemic resistance (afterload).

Dose requirements with nifedipine require careful titration. Some patients are rendered asymptomatic with 10 mg 3 times per day and deteriorate after higher doses. Others are refractory to any size dose of nifedipine. Therefore, each patient with stable angina, particularly geriatric-age patients, require careful titration of doses beginning with the lowest dose (10 mg 3 times per day).

Some patients receiving nifedipine will note an aggravation of angina (10%). The mechanism for this paradoxic effect may be (1) reflex increase in myocardial contractility, (2) increase in heart rate secondary to sympathetic activation from a drop in blood pressure, (3) reduction in coronary artery perfusion pressure due to a blood pressure reduction, (4) "coronary steal" phenomenon (diversion of blood from ischemic areas to normal areas), and (5) alteration in the transmural distribution of myocardial perfusion with increased flow to the subepicardial area and a reduced flow to the subendocardial area.

Nifedipine reduces the frequency of anginal attacks, enhances the effect of oral nitrates, and improves exercise tolerance. In general, the efficacy of nifedipine in the management of stable angina is comparable to that of isosorbide dinitrate. Nifedipine is an effective substitute for beta blockers in patients experiencing troublesome side effects, such as lethargy, fatigue, and male impotence. When beta blockers, half-dose beta blocker plus nifedipine, and nifedipine alone were compared in a 12-week sequential one-month phase study, the antianginal effects were significantly greater with half-dose beta blocker plus nifedipine and nifedipine alone than with the beta blockers alone. In addition, the adverse side effects of beta blockers were reduced with the half-dose beta blocker plus nifedipine when compared to the full-dose beta blocker regimen.

Nifedipine may provide an additional benefit when maximum doses of nitrates and/or beta blockers are ineffective in controlling angina. However, a slow and well monitored initiation (for hypotension, heart failure, and aggravated myocardial ischemia) of nifedipine and beta blockers is necessary. The combination of nifedipine and beta blockers are reported to (1) increase work tolerance, (2) increase exercise tolerance before angina or ST-T depression appears, (3) reduce ST-T depression with exercise, and (4) increase mean left ventricular ejection fraction with exercise (assessed by gated radionuclide ventriculography) beyond changes noted with beta blockers alone.

USES AND/OR ACTIONS

The drug has potent peripheral arterial vasodilator properties, with little or no depressant effect on SA or AV nodal function. It usually relieves myocardial ischemia but promotes angina in some by reducing the coronary filling pressure (arterial pressure) and/or promoting coronary steal. By reducing arterial pressure, nifedipine may cause a reflex tachycardia.

Nifedipine is most effective in relief of angina, secondary to coronary spasm. Nifedipine also relieves effort-related stable angina when used alone or in conjunction with nitrates and/or beta blockers.

ADVERSE EFFECTS

(See Chap. 3.)

DOSAGES

Adult: *Oral*—initially, 10 mg 3 times per day, increased to 20 mg, if needed. Variant angina patients may require 30 mg 3 times per day.

DOSAGE FORMS AND STRENGTHS AVAILABLE

Adalat (Miles) **capsules:** 10 and 20 mg.
Procardia (Pfizer) **capsules:** 10 mg.

Verapamil Hydrochloride

Verapamil hydrochloride is not as active as nifedipine on vascular smooth muscle and therefore causes less pronounced effects on the systemic arterial pressure.

Verapamil reduces myocardial oxygen demand by decreasing heart rate and reducing the afterload of the left ventricle. It reduces the frequency of attacks in stable angina and improves exercise tolerance and, in this respect, is comparable to, or greater than, nifedipine and is as effective as a beta blocker drug. Verapamil has an advantage over beta blockers in that verapamil does not reduce left ventricular function (cardiac output). Verapamil plus beta blockade may have a greater antianginal effect than either drug alone. As with diltiazem, the combination of verapamil and a beta blocker is useful only in patients without antecedent conduction system disease (SA or AV nodal dysfunction) and without severe left ventricular depression (low ejection fraction) or clinical congestive failure. Drug tolerance has not been shown even after a 5-year period of therapy.

USES AND/OR ACTIONS

Verapamil has antiarrhythmic, antianginal, and antihypertensive properties. It depresses SA and AV nodal functions. Verapamil increases myocardial oxygen supply by reducing coronary artery spasm and reduces myocardial oxygen demand by decreasing heart rate and reducing afterload.

ADVERSE EFFECTS

Constipation is the most common side effect. Headache, vertigo, weakness, nervousness, pruritus, flushing, rash, and gastric disturbances may occur.

PRECAUTIONS

Orthostatic hypotension, AV block and dissociation, pedal edema, pulmonary edema, and congestive heart failure may develop. Rebound angina may follow sudden withdrawal. Hyperprolactinemia and galactorrhea have been observed.

INTERACTIONS

When given IV, verapamil may cause severe hypotension, bradycardia, or cardiac failure. Heart block may develop with verapamil plus a beta blocker (including timolol eye drops). Verapamil should be avoided in sick sinus syndrome or in second or third degree AV block. Verapamil increases serum digoxin levels, and serious hypotension may occur when combined with quinidine.

Elevated transaminase and alkaline phosphate levels and hepatitis have developed rarely.

DOSAGES

Adult: *Oral*—for angina, 240–480 mg daily in 3 or 4 divided doses. Patients with impaired hepatic function should receive approximately 30% of this dose.

DOSAGE FORMS AND STRENGTHS AVAILABLE

Calan (Searle) **tablets:** 80 and 120 mg.
Isoptin (Knoll) **tablets:** 80 and 120 mg.

Diltiazem

Diltiazem has cardiovascular effects similar to those of verapamil. It dilates peripheral arteries and arterioles, depresses the sinoatrial (SA) and atrioventricular (AV) nodal function, and prevents spasm of normal and diseased coronary arteries. It improves exercise performance and reduces the frequency of anginal attacks in patients with stable angina. It has an efficacy comparable to that of propranolol in stable angina and, like nifedipine, has an additive beneficial effect with propranolol.

USES AND/OR ACTIONS

Diltiazem is used in patients with different forms of angina, as described above.

The cardiovascular effects are similar to those of verapamil. Diltiazem reduces heart rate to a lesser extent than verapamil.

ADVERSE EFFECTS

Adverse effects experienced with diltiazem are similar to verapamil, but the incidence rate is lower. Hypersensitivity reactions, such as rash and pruritus, and shoulder and elbow pain, as well as akinesia, have been reported.

DOSAGES

Adult: *Oral*—initially, 30 mg 4 times per day before meals, with gradual increases to a maximum of 360 mg daily.

DOSAGE FORMS AND STRENGTHS AVAILABLE

Cardizem (Marion) **tablets:** 30 and 60 mg.
Cardizem tablets: 30 and 60 mg.

Table 4-4 offers a summary of the Ca^{2+} channel blockers:

Prostaglandin-Related Agents

As reviewed above, the prostaglandin system modulates vascular tone and platelet aggregation. Two of the PGs, prostacyclin (PGI_2) and thromboxane A_2 (TxA_2), have opposing pharmacologic actions on vascular smooth muscle and platelet function. PGI_2, synthesized largely by endothelial cells, dilates coronary resistance arteriolar vessels and inhibits platelet aggregation. TxA_2, on the other hand, potentiates platelet aggregation and causes coronary arteriolar constriction. However, all circumstantial evidence suggests a reactive, rather than a causative, role for PGI_2 and TxA_2 in angina pectoris and in MI. In some patients with intractable angina or with angina in the post-MI period, PG-related agents may make an important contribution.

Dipyridamole

The interesting compound dipyridamole is a coronary vasodilator and platelet aggregation inhibitor. Although it acts on the coronary resistance vessels, conclusive evidence of an antianginal action is not recorded. In fact, by dilating coronary resistance vessels, dipyridamole may worsen angina by causing coronary artery steal.

ADVERSE EFFECTS

Dizziness, headache, syncope, gastrointestinal disturbances, and rash may occur.

Table 4-4. Summary of Ca^{2+} channel blockers

Pharmacokinetics	Nifedipine	Verapamil	Diltiazem
Onset of action	Oral: < 20 min	Oral: < 30 min	Oral: < 30 min
	Ling: 3 min	IV: 1–2 min	IV: 1–2 min
Plasma level	25–100 ng/ml	200–600 ng/ml	50–200 ng/ml
Metabolism	Liver	Liver	Liver
Elimination	80% renal	Renal 70%; liver 30%	Renal 35%, GI 60%
Clinical effects			
Peripheral vasodilation	+ + +	+ +	+
Myocardial contractility	Reflex	Reflex	–
Heart rate	Reflex (20%)	Reflex (10% IV) (± 5% oral)	7–10%
AV nodal conduction	–		
A. Fib-Flutter	Rare	Rare	Rare
Adverse effects			
Hypotension	+ + +	+ +	+
Headache	+ + +	+ +	Rare
Peripheral edema	+ + +	+ +	±
Constipation	–	+ +	–
Congestive heart failure	–	+	–
AV Block	–	+ + +	+ +
Drug interactions			
Beta blockers	Use with safety	Caution	Caution
Digoxin (Reduce digoxin by 50%)	Digoxin levels elevated	Digoxin levels elevated	Unknown

Key: – = effect absent; + = small effect; + + = moderate effect; + + + = marked effect.

DOSAGES

Since its efficacy is uncertain, no effective dosage can be given.

DOSAGE FORMS AND STRENGTHS AVAILABLE

Persantine (Boehringer Ingelheim) **tablets:** 25, 50 and 75 mg.
Generic tablets: 25, 50, and 75 mg.

Epoprostenol Sodium

Epoprostenol is a potent coronary vasodilator and inhibitor of platelet aggregation that, because of a short half-life, must be infused (IV) continuously for a pharmacologic effect. The effectiveness of the compound in angina is variable, and infusion during acute MI does not appear to reduce infarct size.

ADVERSE EFFECTS

The compound may cause flushing, headaches, restlessness, anxiety, nausea, vomiting, hypotension, and reflex tachycardia.

DOSAGES

No dosage can be recommended because of insufficient data as to its benefits.

DOSAGE FORMS AND STRENGTHS AVAILABLE

Cyclo-Prostin (IV) (Upjohn) **powder** (investigational drug)

References

1. Abrams, J., et al. Tolerance to organic nitrates. *Circulation* 74:1181, 1986.
2. Alam, M., et al. Echocardiographic evaluation of left ventricular function during coronary artery angioplasty. *Am. J. Cardiol.* 57:20, 1986.
3. Beta Blocker Heart Attack Trial (BHAT). A randomized trial of propranolol in patients with acute myocardial infarction. *J.A.M.A.* 247:1707, 1982.
4. Brezinski, M. E., et al. Anti-ischemic actions of a new thromboxane receptor antagonist during acute myocardial ischemia in cats. *Am. Heart J.* 110:1161, 1985.
5. Cavarocchi, N. C., et al. Oxygen free radical generation during cardiopulmonary bypass: Correlation with complement activation. *Circulation* 74(Suppl. 3):111, 1986.
6. England, M. D., et al. Infuence of antioxidants (mannitol and allopurinol) on oxygen free radical generation during and after cardiopulmonary bypass. *Circulation* 74(Suppl. 3):111, 1986.
7. Feldman, R. , et al. Effect of propranolol on myocardial ischemia occurring during acute coronary occlusion. *Circulation* 73:727, 1986.
8. Fridovich, I., et al. Endothelium-derived relaxing factor: In

search of the endogenous nitroglycerin. *News in Physiolog. Sci.* 2:61, 1987.
9. Friedman, P. L., et al. Coronary vasoconstrictor effect of indomethacin in patients with coronary artery disease. *N. Engl. J. Med.* 305:1171, 1981.
10. Gibson, R. S., et al. Diltiazem and reinfarction in patients with non-Q-wave myocardial infarction. Results of a double-blind, randomized, multicenter trial. *N. Engl. J. Med.* 315:423, 1985.
11. Griffith, T. M., et al. EDRF coordinates the behavior of vascular resistance vessels. *Nature* 329:442, 1987.
12. Henriksson, P., et al. In vivo production of prostacyclin and thromboxane in patients with acute myocardial infarction. *Br. Heart J.* 55:543, 1986.
13. Hirsch, P. D., et al. Prostaglandins and ischemic heart disease. *Am. J. Med.* 71:1009, 1981.
14. Hjalmarson, A., et al. The MIAMI Study: Effect on mortality of metoprolol in acute myocardial infarction. *Lancet* 2(8251):823, 1981.
15. Hjalmarson, A., et al. The use of beta blockers after myocardial infarction. In K. Engleman (ed.), *Acute Myocardial Infarction: The Post-Hospital Phase. MIAMI.* Atlanta: Med-Ed, 1982, Pp. 1–8.
16. Jarasch, E. D., et al. Significance of xanthine oxidase on capillary endothelial cells. *Acta Physiol. Scand.* 548:39, 1986.
17. Jugdutt, B., et al. Effect of prostaglandin inhibition on collateral blood after coronary artery occlusion in conscious dogs. *Circulation* 55, 56(Suppl. 3):111, 1977.
18. Lucchesi, B. R., et al. Interaction of the formed elements of blood with the coronary vasculature in vivo. *Fed. Proc.* 46:63, 1987.
19. Maisel, A. S., et al. Externalization of β-adrenergic receptors promoted by myocardial ischemia. *Science* 230:183, 1985.
20. McCord, J. M., et al. A mechanism for the anti-inflammatory activity of superoxide dismutase. In A.P. Autor, *Pathology of Oxygen.* New York: Academic, 1982, P. 75.
21. McCord, J. M. Oxygen-derived free radicals in postischemic tissue injury. *N. Engl. J. Med.* 312:159, 1985.
22. McCord, J. M. Oxygen-derived radicals: A link between reperfusion injury and inflammation. *Fed. Proc.* 46:2402, 1987.
23. Mukherjee, A., et al. Relationship between β-adrenergic receptor numbers and physiological responses during experimental canine myocardial ischemia. *Circ. Res.* 50:735, 1982.
24. Mullane, K. M., et al. Leukocyte-derived metabolites of arachidonic acid in ischemia-induced myocardial injury. *Fed. Proc.* 46:2422, 1987.
25. Nayler, W. G., and Elz, J. S. Reperfusion injury: Laboratory artifact or clinical dilemma? *Circulation* 74:215, 1986.
26. Novitzky, D., et al. Prevention of myocardial injury during brain death by total cardiac sympathectomy in the Chacma Baboon. *Ann. Thorac. Surg.* 41:520, 1986.
27. Petrone, W. F., et al. Free radicals and inflammation: Superoxide-dependent activation of a neutrophil chemotactic factor in plasma. *Proc. Natl. Acad. Sci. USA* 77:1159, 1980.
28. Robertson, R. M., et al. Thromboxane A_2 in vasotonic angina pectoris. *N. Engl. J. Med.* 304:998, 1981.
29. Silverman, H. S., and Pfeifer, M. P. Relation between use of anti-inflammation agents and left ventricular free wall rupture during acute myocardial infarction. *Am. J. Cardiol.* 59:363, 1987.

30. Simpson, P. J., et al. Free radical scavengers in myocardial ischemia. *Fed. Proc.* 46:2413, 1987.
31. Singh, B. N., et al. Hemodynamic and electrocardiographic correlates of symptomatic and silent myocardial ischemia: Pathophysiologic and therapeutic implications. *Am. J. Cardiol.* 58:3B, 1986.
32. The Norwegian Multicenter Study Group. Timolol-induced reduction in mortality and reinfarction in patients surviving acute myocardial infarction. *N. Engl. J. Med.* 304:801, 1981.
33. Pedersen, T. R. The Norwegian Multicenter Study Group. Six-year follow-up after acute myocardial infarction. *N. Engl. J. Med.* 313:1055, 1985.
34. Visser, C. A., et al. Two-dimensional echocardiography during percutaneous transluminal coronary angioplasty. *Am. Heart J.* 111:1035, 1986.
35. Werns, S. W., et al. Free radicals and myocardial injury: Pharmacologic implications. *Circulation* 74:1, 1986.
36. Zalewski, A., et al. Myocardial protection during transient coronary artery occlusion in man: Beneficial effects of regional β-adrenergic blockade. *Circulation* 73:734, 1986.

5

Hyperlipidemia and Hypercholesterolemia

According to the Lipid Research Clinics Coronary Primary Prevention Trial (LRC-CPPT) [20], a multicenter 10-year study in hyperlipidemic men (35–59 years of age with cholesterol levels $\geq$ 265 mg/dl and triglyceride levels $\leq$ 300 mg/dl), every 1% reduction in serum cholesterol is associated with a 2% reduction in the risk of atherosclerosis-related coronary artery disease death. Whether elderly adults (> 65 years) or adults or children with low to normal levels of serum cholesterol should be "treated" with a "prudent diet" or with drugs aimed at lowering serum cholesterol levels in the expectation of retarding the development of atherosclerosis is presently uncertain.

Atherosclerosis-related artery wall disease is the leading cause of death in the western world. Deaths from cardiac, cerebral, and peripheral atherosclerotic arterial disease account for approximately half of the mortalities in industrial countries. Atherosclerosis "is not merely a change or transformation attending the process of aging, it is not a mere 'infirmity' of old age, but rather a disease of the vessels manifesting itself mainly during senescence" [3]. No artery is immune to the process, but none is more commonly involved than the coronary artery.

Theories of Atherosclerosis Pathogenesis

ENDOTHELIAL CELLS AND FIBRIN DEPOSITION

Current theories into the initiating mechanism(s) of atherosclerosis are but extensions of seminal observations made by pathologists and experimental physiologists of the nineteenth and early twentieth centuries, with but one exception. Publications such as those by Von Rokitansky (1844–1852) suggested that the generation of the fibrous plaque commences with an excessive deposition of the blood material identified as fibrin; contemporary views suggest that endothelial cell modification leads to blood platelet aggregation and subsequent conversion of plasma fibrinogen to fibrin on the endothelial surface.

Fibrin is deposited on endothelial surfaces after interactions between altered endothelial cells, blood cells, platelets, and plasma prothrombin (see Chap. 6). In this interaction, prothrombin is converted to thrombin and thrombin binds to the platelet surface and causes platelet aggregation, the release of serotonin, histamine, adenine nucleotides, proteolytic enzymes, polypeptide cell growth stimulating hormones, and synthesis of a prostaglandin, thromboxane A_2 (TxA_2). Thrombin also binds to receptors on endothelial cells and stimulates the synthesis and release of another prostaglandin, prostacyclin (PGI_2). The local net balance between the synthesis of TxA_2 by platelets and PGI_2 by endothelial cells determines, to a large extent, whether additional platelets aggregate and bind to the endothelial cell surface.

Although, on the average, endothelial cells are metabolically highly stable and undergo extremely slow turnover, they may become metabolically altered locally and synthesize mediators or signals for anatomic and physiologic remodeling of underlying arterial tissue. As examples, altered blood flow patterns (pulse-pressure-volume aberrancies or turbulences) or reduced partial pressure of oxygen may stimulate endothelial cells to produce hormones (autocoids), which, in turn, influence a migration and phenotypic change of some medially located smooth muscle cells. Of importance to considerations of this chapter, metabolic activities of endothelial cells can be influenced by hyperlipidemic blood serum.

INSPISSATION OF BLOOD-BORNE MATERIAL THROUGH ENDOTHELIAL CELLS

A somewhat different paradigm for atherosclerosis pathogenesis was introduced by R. Virchow in 1856 and centered around the inspissation of blood-borne material through endothelial cells to loosen and initiate an almost neoplastic proliferation of subendothelial cells. Contemporary expression involves the passage of serum lipid and protein (lipoprotein) aggregates through or between endothelial cells to initiate a subendothelially-located fatty streak. The inspissated lipoprotein, in turn, stimulates the invasion of blood-borne monocytes and possibly influences the production and activities of proteases such as elastase, which, in turn, become involved in local remodeling processes of the artery wall.

INJURY AND REPAIR: FOCAL HEMODYNAMIC-MEDIATED REMODELING

Virchow suggested that serum lipoproteins were inspissated at sites of tearing and stretching of the intimal coat due to mechanical factors (hemodynamic-related, for the most part). Hemodynamic forces are generally expressed as analogs of hydrodynamic terms. Liquid flowing through a tube, according to Hagan, is determined largely by the exponent of the radius (r) (found to be 4). Poiseuille noted that the volume discharged per unit time through a tube was proportional to the pressure head (P) and r^4, and inversely proportional to the tube length. It turns out that for arterial blood flow, r^4 ("fourth power") and the length of the stenotic segment are the main determinants.

Poiseuille noted that the relationship between pressure and flow passed from linear to turbulent at high flow rates. Reynolds derived a formula to express turbulent flow with distinct vortices and noted the appearance of turbulence when the Reynolds number (Re) exceeds 2000. For arteries, the critical Re was greater than 2000 for S-shaped curves and for wide- or right-angled bifurcations. Stehbens [25], a contemporary experimental pathologist, summarized the hemodynamic considerations of intimal thickening (the precursor arterial remodeling of the fibrous plaque) as follows:

> Jets, wakes and separated boundary layers are prone to be unstable at relatively low Re ($<$ 200 for wakes and jets), and their periodic shedding of vortices could induce vibrations in

neighboring walls. The energy involved in these sinusoidal pressure fluctuations is difficult to assess, for the complex geometry of the vascular tree and the viscoelastic properties of its walls cannot be incorporated satisfactorily in mathematical analyses.

Stehbens suggested that arterial tissues are injured and undergo reparative changes in response to vibrational energies. Persistence (chronicity) of vibrational-energy-mediated injury could result in mechanical fatigue and expand the native fenestrae of elastic membranes. Expansion of the fenestrae and/or fragmentation of elastic membranes in the internal elastic membrane may result in the generation of elastin peptides that are chemotactic for local and circulating cells.

Coalescences of Von Rokitansky's and Virchow's paradigms would integrate hemodynamic forces, metabolic activity of endothelial cells as influenced by the "fourth power" (see Chap. 4), platelet adherence, production of local autocoids, synthesis and release of proteases (including elastase), elastic lamellar disruption, generation of elastin peptides, and chemotaxis of blood borne monocytes and medial smooth muscle cells into the subendothelial space. Extracellular connective tissue is then synthesized by modified smooth muscle cells and retained as intimal hyperplasia. An intensified process at selected and predictable sites in human arteries progresses into the fibrous plaque, which ultimately is modified by macrophages and lipoprotein inspissation (see below) into an atherosclerotic lesion.

SERUM CHOLESTEROL

A number of so-called risk factors seem to predispose the artery to fibrous plaque formation and the subsequent process of atherosclerosis. These include male sex, strong family history, and hypercholesterolemia. The clinical significance of hypercholesterolemia depends on the absolute level of cholesterol; the higher the cholesterol, the greater the risk for coronary or cerebral complications of atherosclerosis. Hypercholesterolemia as a risk factor is increased by the use of cigarettes and the presence of hypertension or diabetes mellitus. The hypercholesterolemia effect is modified by the genetic characteristics of the individual.

Hypercholesterolemia and atherosclerosis were first associated by Anitschkov's observation in 1913 that cholesterol feeding in rabbits produces fatty streaks and atheromatouslike lesions in the aorta. Since the cholesterol-atherosclerosis linkage made by Anitschkov, numerous epidemiologic surveys associate high serum cholesterol levels (hypercholesterolemia) with increased incidence rates of coronary artery disease.

Cholesterol is a four-ring structure delivered as part of the diet or synthesized from two-carbon fragments (acetate) through the action of at least 30 enzymes. The primary sites of synthesis are the liver and intestines and the scheme for cholesterol synthesis is outlined in Fig. 5-1.

Importantly, HMG-Coa reductase was identified as an early rate-limiting enzyme in cholesterol biosynthesis.

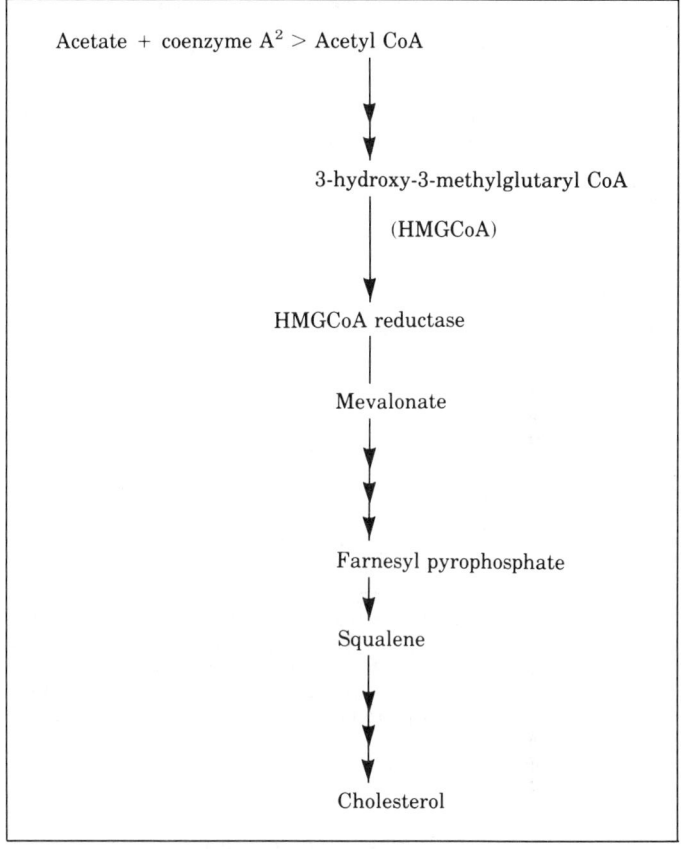

```
Acetate + coenzyme A² > Acetyl CoA
                    │
                    ▼
      3-hydroxy-3-methylglutaryl CoA
                  (HMGCoA)
                    │
                    ▼
             HMGCoA reductase
                    │
                 Mevalonate
                    │
                    ▼
           Farnesyl pyrophosphate
                    │
                    ▼
                 Squalene
                    │
                    ▼
                Cholesterol
```

Fig. 5-1. Conversion of acetate to cholesterol—an abbreviated scheme. (From E. L. Bierman. *Current Concepts: Hyperlipoproteinemia.* Kalamazoo, MI: The Upjohn Co., 1986.)

Plasma Lipoproteins

In humans, cholesterol is derived from the diet (200–400 mg/day) and from endogenous synthesis (750–1000 mg/day). As cholesterol and triglycerides (fatty acids) are water insoluble, they must circulate in the aqueous blood as soluble lipoprotein aggregates consisting of apoproteins, phospholipids, triglycerides, and cholesterol. Lipoprotein consists of an inner core of nonpolar lipids (cholesterol ester and triglycerides) surrounded by a surface coat of hydrophilic water-soluble components that include protein and polar lipids (phospholipids). Unesterified cholesterol is also located in the surface coat. The lipoprotein aggregates vary in size and density and may be separated and quantified by gravimetric (ultracentrifuge) techniques. The nomenclature, composition and size of the major lipoproteins are summarized in Table 5-1.

Table 5-1. Composition and size of the plasma lipoproteins

Lipoproteins	Triglyceride (%)	Cholesterol (%)	Protein (%)	Size (Å)
Chylomicrons	86	5	2	750–12,000
Very low density (VLDL)	55	19	8	300–700
Intermediate (IDL)	23	38	19	
Low density (LDL)	6	50	22	180–300
High density (HDL_2)	5	22	40	50–120
High density (HDL_3)	3	17	55	50–120

Exploiting differences in apoprotein composition and electrical charges, the lipoproteins are separable by paper electrophoresis as well. After lipid staining, three lipoprotein bands migrating in alpha (α), pre-beta (β), and β-globulin regions are recognized. The high density lipoproteins (HDLs), in general, travel to the α, very low density lipoproteins (VLDL) to the pre-β, and the low density lipoproteins (LDL) to the β-globulin fractions. The electrophoretic properties of the lipoproteins, as well as their apoproteins, are summarized in Table 5-2.

Table 5-2. Electrophoretic mobility and apoproteins of plasma lipoproteins

Lipoprotein	Electrophoretic mobility	Major apoproteins	Minor apoproteins
Chylomicrons	Origin (cathode)	A-I, A-IV, B-48, C-I, C-II, C-III	A-II, E
VLDL	Pre-beta	B-100, E, C-I, C-II, C-III	A-I, A-II, A-III (or D), A-IV (trace)
LDL	Beta	B-100	Trace of C-I, C-II, C-III, D
HDL	Alpha	A-I, A-II	A-IV, B-48, B-100, C-I, C-II, C-III, D, E

Key: VLDL = very low density lipoproteins; LDL = low density lipoproteins; HDL = high density lipoproteins.

METABOLIC PATHWAYS OF PLASMA LIPOPROTEINS

Dietary cholesterol and triglycerides are transported in plasma to adipose tissue, and to skeletal muscle as chylomicrons (Fig. 5-2). The chylomicrons are reduced in size by lipoprotein lipase (found in plasma and endothelial cells) into chylomicron "remnants," that transport dietary cholesterol and triglycerides to the liver. Under normal conditions, chylomicrons are rapidly catabolized and essentially disappear from the plasma after 12–14 hours.

The very low density lipoproteins (smaller in size and containing less triglycerides and relatively more cholesterol than chylomicrons) are produced primarily in the liver from free fatty acids (FFA). Plasma VLDL levels are not independently atherogenic

Fig. 5-2. Scheme for the absorption from the gut and transport of fats and cholesterol as lipoproteins (L), chylomicrons, and very low density (VLDL), intermediate density (ID), low density (LDL) and high density (HDL) cholesterols. Location of lipoprotein lipase and the transport of lipids and cholesterol into adipose tissue is indicated by the broken lines.

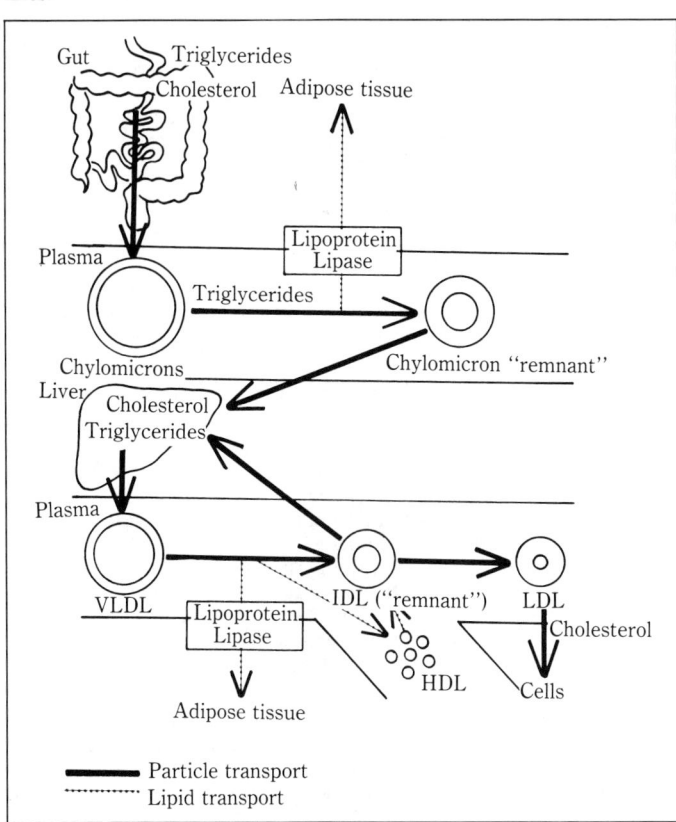

and can be elevated by any condition that raises FFA, such as large carbohydrate intake, high caloric intake, alcohol ingestion, stress, and exercise.

VLDL that has been modified by lipoprotein lipase to form the intermediate density lipoprotein (IDL) contains relatively less triglyceride and more cholesterol and protein than VLDL. IDL is not present in large concentrations in the plasma.

Breakdown of IDL produces the low density lipoproteins (LDL) containing 50% cholesterol, only 6% triglycerides, and 22% protein (see Table 5-1). LDL transports about 75% of circulating cholesterol in the blood to cells. High plasma LDL levels are associated with excessive atherosclerosis.

The IDLs also give rise to high density lipoproteins (HDLs), which, by weight, are made up of 40–55% protein, 17–22% cholesterol, and 3–5% triglycerides.

HDLs are subdivided into lipid-rich HDL_2 and protein-rich, lipid-poor HDL_3. Males and females have approximately the same plasma HDL levels until puberty, when the concentration decreases in males and thereafter remains about 20% lower in males than in females. In adult life, the HDL concentrations are approximately 45 mg/dl in males and 54 mg/dl in females. Low concentrations of HDL-cholesterol may be inherited as a dominant trait and may be associated with precocious atherosclerosis, may be a part of poorly controlled diabetes mellitus, or may be developed secondary to steroids. High HDL-cholesterol levels are seen in familial hyperalphalipoproteinemia that develops secondary to hepatic toxins, after alcohol ingestion, or strenuous exercise.

Function of Apoproteins

Apoproteins play a role in maintaining the structure of lipoproteins. Apoproteins serve as binding ligands for cell-surface receptors that facilitate cell uptake and catabolism and act as cofactors to enzymes (lipoprotein lipases [LPL], lecithin/ cholesterol acyltransferase [LCAT]) involved in lipoprotein metabolism.

HORMONE MODULATION OF LIPOPROTEINS

Hormones influence lipid and lipoprotein metabolism in adipocytes by affecting their ability to hydrolyze and store triglycerides and to subsequently release triglycerides as free fatty acids [27]. Hormones affecting these processes exert a reciprocal action on the activity of LPL and lipase by acting intracellularly to hydrolyze triglycerides into FFA and glycerol. Hormones that stimulate LPL include insulin, thyroxine, glucocorticoids, and progestogens, while estrogens, prolactin, and beta blockers inhibit the enzyme. Lipase, on the other hand, is stimulated by glucagon, growth hormone, corticosteroids, and catecholamines and is inhibited by insulin and beta blockers.

Major hormone-sensitive control mechanisms are: (1) in the adipocyte, the LPL and the lipase; (2) in the hepatocyte, the branch point for FFA metabolism, the synthesis of hepatic lipase, the HDLs, and the LDL receptor; and (3) in the peripheral cells, the LPL activity and the synthesis and expression of LDL receptors.

Perhaps the most overt manifestations of hormone modulation of lipoproteins are the events that accompany the loss of ovarian estrogen secretion in menopause and the decreases in hepatic synthesis of triglycerides and HDL and LDL receptors. At that time, the unopposed actions of adrenal androgenic steroids are associated with a slight increase in hepatic lipase activity and a decreased output of VLDLs, even with a slightly increased peripheral lipolysis. As a result, plasma triglyceride levels are low; however, with an increased peripheral conversion of VLDLs to LDLs and a reduced LDL clearance (decreased cellular LDL receptors), plasma cholesterol levels increase to hypercholesterolemia levels. These lipid abnormalities are promptly reversed by estrogen supplementation and, to a lesser extent, by estrogen plus progestogens.

Adrenergic receptor antagonists modulate the adrenergic hormone effect on lipid metabolism. Briefly, beta blockers raise plasma triglyceride levels and lower HDL levels; alpha blockers (prazosin) increase HDL levels (see Chap. 3). β_1-selective antagonists cause smaller plasma lipid changes than β_2-blockers. Beta blockers appear to inhibit the peripheral action of lipoprotein lipase and thereby retard the catabolism of VLDLs. Beta blockers with intrinsic sympathomimetic activity, such as pindolol, apparently do not affect serum lipids [24]. In fact, chronic pindolol therapy significantly lowers triglyceride and raises HDL-cholesterol when compared to the effects of long-term propranolol.

Lipoproteins and Atherosclerosis

During the early 1970s, clinical associations between plasma lipoprotein levels and expressions of atherosclerosis suggested that elevated concentrations of LDL cholesterol and reduced levels of HDL cholesterol were independent risk factors that accelerate progression of atherosclerosis and its complications. In addition, in the early 1980s, it was reported that dietary reduction of plasma lipids delayed the development of atherosclerosis and its clinical manifestations.

In hypercholesterolemic males (type II patients), 2-year changes in levels of intermediate density lipoproteins (IDL) (analytical ultra centrifugation separation of lipoproteins based on mass-fraction with flotation rate 12–20) were strongly **predictive** of coronary artery disease (CAD) progression at 5 years. Levels of the other lipoproteins (LDL, VLDL, HDL_2, and HDL_3) were similar in men with and without definite CAD progression [17].

LOW DENSITY LIPOPROTEIN AND INTRACELLULAR CHOLESTEROL HOMEOSTASIS

Plasma levels of LDL are regulated by the LDL receptor, a cell surface glycoprotein. Defects in the gene encoding the LDL receptor occurs in patients with familial hypercholesterolemia. In these patients, plasma LDL levels are extremely elevated and premature and precocious coronary atherosclerosis develops. The physiologically important LDL receptors are located in the liver.

LDL is attracted and bound to apo B and apo E surface receptors that are located in regions called *coated pits* [6]. Once bound, the cell membrane engulfs the receptor plus the LDLs by endocytosis. The internalized vesicle fuses with the intracellular lysosomes, where the LDL is broken down by enzymes (e.g., acid cholesterol esterase and proteases) and cholesterol is released intracellularly. The released intracellular cholesterol reduces cholesterol biosynthesis by inhibiting HMGCoA reductase and increasing esterification (stimulating acyl-cholesterol acyltransferase [ACAT]) and decreases the formation of LDL receptors. The sequential steps in the LDL receptor pathway in which intracellular cholesterol levels serve as a second message in regulating cholesterol synthesis and esterification are shown in Fig. 5-3. Approximately two-thirds of LDL clearance from the serum may be mediated through the LDL receptor pathway; the other third is cleared by a less efficient nonreceptor mechanism.

A less efficient LDL removal process is carried out by macrophages when the plasma concentration rises. The LDL or modified LDL is taken up by a low-affinity non-receptor-mediated, non-saturable pathway related to the plasma lipoprotein level and is referred to as the scavenger receptor pathway [7]. The scavenger pathway is present in macrophages and endothelial cells and takes up LDL that is modified by various means. The pathway is not down-regulated by high cellular cholesterol levels and macrophages become filled with lipid droplets and acquire the morphologic appearance of the classical foam cell. Lipid-laden foam cells are a characteristic feature of fatty streaks and atherosclerotic plaques.

Fig. 5-3. Sequestral steps in the LDL uptake via receptors, internalization, and liposome fusion into endosomes and breakdown into cholesterol and amino acids. Intracellular cholesterol serves as a second messenger that suppresses the transcription of an early rate-limiting enzyme of cholesterol biosynthesis (HMG-CoA reductase) and accelerates the degradation of the enzyme; cholesterol activates a cholesterol-esterifying enzyme, acyl-CoA: cholesterol acyltransferase (ACAT) for cholesterol storage as cholesterol oleate (ester droplets) and lowers the concentration of LDL-receptor messenger RNA, thereby adjusting the numbers of LDL receptors to provide sufficient cholesterol for the metabolic needs of the cell. (From M. S. Brown and J. L. Goldstein. A receptor-mediated pathway for cholesterol homeostasis. *Science* 232:34, 1986. © The Nobel Foundation 1986.

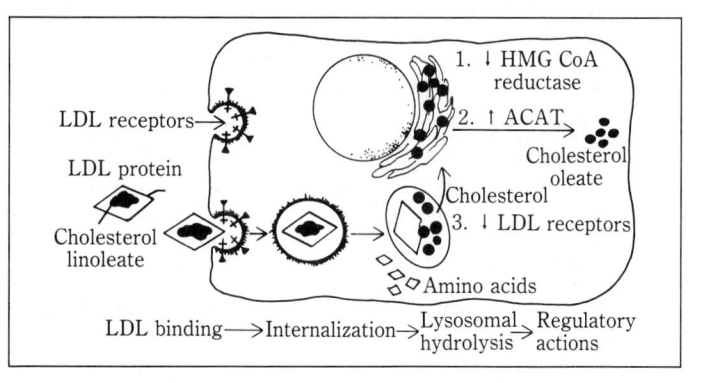

Lipid and Cholesterol Removal from Cells

Once cholesterol is delivered and released into the cell interior, cholesterol esters are resynthesized into lipid droplets by the enzyme ACAT. The lipid droplets are, in turn, acted on by the enzyme cholesterol ester hydrolase. Cholesterol ester hydrolase continually acts to turn over cholesterol esters and to release free cholesterol. Free cholesterol may recycle via ACAT into cholesterol esters and limited amounts may migrate to and through the cell membrane, while larger amounts are removed from the membrane by HDL bound to the membrane by apo A-1 protein of the lipoprotein.

An enzyme of HDL, lecithin-cholesterol acyltransferase (LCAT), renders the cholesterol esters hydrophobic and favors their migration to the core of the lipoprotein particle. Esterification and migration of cholesterol frees up the apo A-1 and facilitates additional binding of free cholesterol. Thereafter, the apo A-1, along with the cholesterol ester exchanged protein, transfers cholesterol esters from the core of the HDL particle to other particles. By internalization and exchange, the cholesterol-binding sites on apo A-1 are prevented from becoming saturated. Any removal of cholesterol from atherosclerotic plaques is accomplished by the action of apo A-1 and activation of LCAT.

Comparing plasma levels of the apoproteins for HDL and LDL as discriminators of coronary artery disease shows superiority of A-1 followed by A-11 and apo B-100. All plasma levels of the three apoproteins are better indicators of coronary artery disease severity than HDL-cholesterol (HDL-C), HDL-C/total cholesterol, or total triglycerides. A recently reported study of 43 patients (331 males, 10 females) with coronary artery disease [15] concluded that in this patient group with low HDL-cholesterol: (1) HDL_3-cholesterol is more informative than HDL_2-cholesterol for **severity** of coronary artery disease, and (2) levels of apo-A-1 or apo-A-11 of HDL_3-cholesterol are independent of coronary artery disease **severity** or myocardial infarction in correlating positively with the left ventricular ejection fraction (LVEF).

LIPOPROTEIN UPTAKE BY ENDOTHELIAL AND ATHEROMATOUS LESIONS

Endothelial cells certainly have VLDL-like receptors and possibly have LDL-like receptors. The classic LDL receptor is not found in layers of contact-inhibited cultured endothelial cells: An LDL receptor exists, but the LDL is not internalized. However, modified LDL, as with interaction with oxygen radicals (derived from platelet-related or endothelial cell prostaglandin production [see Fig. 4-1]), oxidation of lipids, action by lipoprotein lipase is subsequently taken up by endothelial cells. LDL passes through arterial endothelial cells (monolayer culture) without undergoing degradation [13].

While the mechanism of LDL passage through endothelial cells remains unclear, LDL is recovered in the subendothelial areas in regions where the endothelium is actively regenerating following injury (experimental animal-rabbit models) [23] and appears to concentrate in atheromatous lesions (technetium-labeled LDL

[Tc-99mLDL]) in humans [19]. Positive scintigrams following Tc-99mLDL uptake by atheromatous lesions appear to be inversely related to the chronicity of the lesion.

VLDL (and possibly chylomicrons) are taken up by endothelial cells on specific receptors. Once bound, lipoproteins become associated with the LPL. Triglycerides and FFA are removed from the lipoprotein, causing the release of remnants and the transfer of peptides from VLDL to HDL.

Genetic Basis for Atherosclerosis

A contemporary paradigm of the pathogenesis of atherosclerosis centers around genetic considerations of the disease. A genetic basis for a rare form of precocious atherosclerosis, familial hypercholesterolemia (FH), was well accepted, but recognition of a genetic basis for the more common forms of atherosclerosis is less certain.

Genes coding for the eight apolipoproteins, A-I, A-II, A-IV, B, C-I, C-II, C-III, and E (Table 5-2), have been described [5]. However, gene polymorphism may have clinical importance in this regard. For example, apoprotein B levels of LDL show polymorphism in B-gene restriction-fragment-length (RFLP) analyses; some RFLP fragments are uniquely elevated in patients with myocardial infarctions as compared with matched controls. [14]. Available evidence strongly associates genetic variation at the chromosome II locus with lipoprotein abnormalities and at the chromosome 19 locus for the LDL receptor gene with increases in the susceptibility to atherosclerosis.

While five major phenotypes of hyperlipoproteinemia are described (Table 5-3), the lipoprotein levels may change with age, weight, or diet and, as mentioned above, with hormones and sex. Primary hyperlipoproteinemias are genetically determined or sporadic. Secondary hyperlipoproteinemias may be associated with poorly controlled diabetes mellitus, alcoholism, hyperthyroidism, obstructive liver disease, nephrotic syndrome, uremia, and other less common diseases associated with dysproteinemias. The phenotypes and the abnormal lipoproteins and nomenclature most commonly associated with atherosclerosis are summarized in Tables 5-3 and 5-4.

Approximately 20% of patients with coronary artery disease may have a monogenic form of hyperlipidemia that is recognized by (1) elevated levels of serum cholesterol, (2) elevated levels of serum triglycerides, and (3) an abnormal profile of lipoproteins, as determined by electrophoresis or density gradient ultracentrifugation separation.

Identifying High Risk Factors for Coronary Artery Disease

Members of families with a high incidence rate of atherosclerosis-related diseases (myocardial infarction, stroke, or peripheral

Table 5-3. Lipoprotein phenotypes

Lipoprotein phenotypes	Autosomal mode of inheritance	Elevation in plasma lipoprotein concentration	Coronary disease
Type I	Recessive	Chylomicrons	No Increase
Types IIA, IIB (familial Hypercholesterolemia)	Dominant	LDL	Increase (threefold)
Types IIA, IIB, IV, V (familial combined)	Dominant	LDL	Increased by age 60 (males)
Types IIA, IIB	Polygenic	VLDL/LDL	Increased by age 60
Type III	Dominant	IDL	Increased
Types IV, V (familial hypertriglyceridemia)	Dominant	Chylomicrons, VLDL	No increase
Types IV, V (sporadic hypertriglyceridemia)	Nongenetic	Chylomicrons, VLDL	No increase

Key: LDL = low density lipoprotein; VLDL = very low density lipoprotein; IDL = intermediate density lipoprotein.

Table 5-4. Atherosclerosis and lipoprotein phenotypes

Pattern	Lipoprotein	Elevated lab values	Nomenclatures
IIA	LDL	Cholesterol	Familial hypercholesterolemia Polygenic hypercholesterolemia
IIB	LDL, VLDL	Cholesterol and slight triglyceride	Familial combined hyperlipoproteinemia Multiple lipoprotein Hyperlipidemia
IV	VLDL, LDL	Triglyceride and slight cholesterol	"Mixed" hyperlipidemia

Key: LDL = low density lipoprotein; VLDL = very low density lipoprotein.

arterial insufficiency) who are less than 60 years of age should be screened by measuring the fasting level of serum cholesterol and refrigerating the remaining sera overnight. Less dense, lipid-rich chylomicrons float to the top while the serum clarifies; failure of the serum to clarify indicates a lactescence due to hyperlipidemia. Elevated serum cholesterol levels without lactescent serum suggests type IIA or type IIB phenotypes of hyperlipoproteinemia. Slightly elevated serum cholesterol levels with lactescent serum suggest familial combined hyperlipoproteinemia of the type IV variety. Serum cholesterol values requiring treatment are listed in Table 5-5.

MODIFYING RISK FACTORS FOR CORONARY ARTERY DISEASE

Prevention of coronary artery disease is, of course, the long-range goal in managing high-risk patients and their families. In addition to the LRC-CPPT (see above), there are a number of reports on the results of primary prevention of coronary artery disease and its sequelae. The results of four such studies are summarized as follows:

1. The incidence rate of nonfatal and fatal MI and sudden death was reduced by approximately 25% in 19,409 men (40–59

Table 5-5. Serum cholesterol values requiring treatment (high risk for cardiovascular events)

Age (years)	Moderate risk (75th to 90th percentile)	High risk (> 90th percentile)
2–19	> 170 (4.4 mmol/L)	> 185 (4.8 mmol/L)
20–29	> 200 (5.2 mmol/L)	> 220 (5.7 mmol/L)
30–39	> 220 (5.7 mmol/L)	> 240 (6.2 mmol/L)
40 and over	> 240 (6.2 mmol/L)	> 260 (6.7 mmol/L)

years of age) by health education, a cholesterol-lowering diet, discontinuance of cigarette smoking, weight control, physical activity, and treatment of arterial hypertension [16].
2. A vegetarian diet with a polyunsaturated to saturated ratio greater than or equal to 2 and less than 100 mg of cholesterol given to 39 patients (< 60 years of age: 35 men and 4 women) with coronary angiogram-established coronary artery disease (at least 50% obstruction of one vessel) resulted in a significant lowering of body weight, systolic arterial pressure, serum cholesterol, and the ratio of total/HDL-cholesterol. Angiogram assessment was visual (with blinding) and computer-assisted image analysis and these assessments showed regression in 21 patients. No lesion growth could be documented in 18 patients. Coronary lesion growth correlated with total/HDL-cholesterol (> 6.9) but not with blood pressure, smoking status, alcohol intake, weight, or drug treatment [2].
3. The Helsinki Heart Study was a randomized, double-blind, placebo-controlled primary prevention analysis of 4,081 middle-aged men with a five-year follow-up to test the effect of plasma lipid lowering by the drug gemfibrozil. To qualify, participants were required to have LDL and VLDL cholesterol values ≥ 200 mg/dl. Almost two thirds had elevated LDL cholesterol (type IIA); most of the remaining were type IIB, and a small number were type IV. The results indicate a marked reduction in the combined incidence of fatal or nonfatal myocardial infarction and cardiac death. The findings were in accord with previous reports on beneficial effects using clofibrate or niacin [10].
4. Drugs and diet favorably affected coronary artery and aortocoronary venous bypass grafts as assessed by angiography [4].

Elevated Levels of Plasma Cholesterol and/or Triglyceride

Just how should one proceed once elevated levels of plasma cholesterol and/or triglycerides are recognized? A directional flow chart in Fig. 5-4 is provided as an answer to the question.

A major criterion for treatment is an elevated LDL level (Fig. 5-5).

In high-risk families, two or more first-degree relatives have (or have had) complications of coronary or cerebral atherosclerosis. In approximately one-fourth of high-risk families, cigarette smoking or hypertension represent concordant risk factors.

Whether diet or drugs are used, an initial goal is to reach an ideal body weight. For women, allow 100 pounds for 5 feet of height and 5 pounds for each additional inch. For men, allow 106 pounds for 5 feet of height and 6 pounds for each additional inch.

The 24-hour caloric requirements for weight reduction can be estimated by multiplying ideal weight by 10.

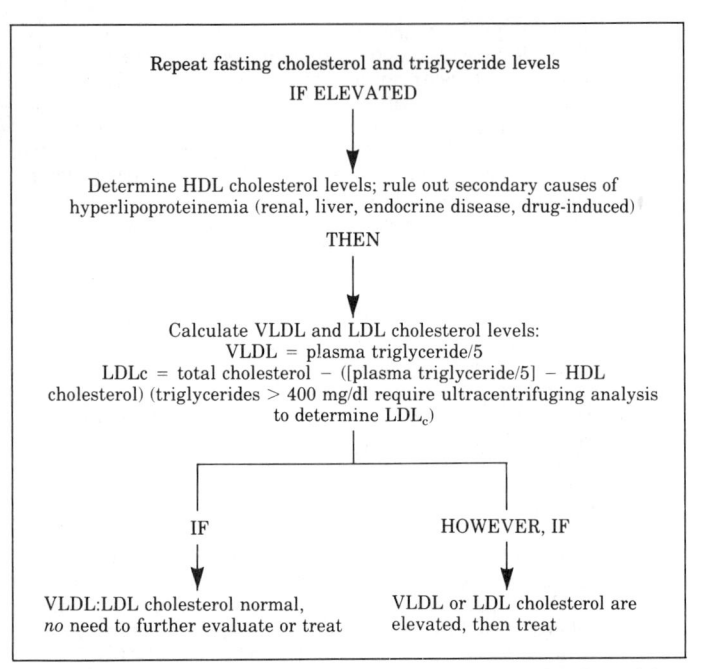

```
          Repeat fasting cholesterol and triglyceride levels
                          IF ELEVATED
                               ↓
   Determine HDL cholesterol levels; rule out secondary causes of
    hyperlipoproteinemia (renal, liver, endocrine disease, drug-induced)
                              THEN
                               ↓
         Calculate VLDL and LDL cholesterol levels:
               VLDL = plasma triglyceride/5
    LDLc = total cholesterol − ([plasma triglyceride/5] − HDL
    cholesterol) (triglycerides > 400 mg/dl require ultracentrifuging analysis
                    to determine LDL_c)
                    ↓                              ↓
                    IF                        HOWEVER, IF
                    ↓                              ↓
   VLDL:LDL cholesterol normal,           VLDL or LDL cholesterol are
   no need to further evaluate or treat   elevated, then treat
```

Fig. 5-4. Procedures to follow with an elevated cholesterol and/or triglyceride plasma level.

Dietary Modulation of Hyperlipoproteinemia

A lipid-lowering diet with reduced amounts of cholesterol and saturated and fatty acids, and increased amounts of monounsaturated and polyunsaturated fatty acids is a mainstay of treatment for hyperlipoproteinemias. Even in children of high-risk parents, a dietary reduction of fat (from 35% to 24% of total caloric energy) and an increase in the ratio of polyunsaturated: saturated fats from 0.18 to 0.61 will reduce serum cholesterol level 15% and increase the HDL level [26].

Dietary modulation of hypercholesterolemia is particularly germane for the primary prevention of atherosclerosis. The value of dietary modulation of hypercholesterolemia for patients with established ischemic heart disease remains an open question, but its usefulness following coronary artery bypass surgery appears to be generally accepted.

Table 5-6 provides an outline of general dietary restrictions of the five lipoprotein phenotypes.

DIETARY CHOLESTEROL

Cholesterol is supplied only by foods of animal origin. Egg yolk and organ meats are very high in cholesterol. Any food containing meat or meat fat, including poultry, contains cholesterol. Foods of plant origin contain no cholesterol.

```
┌─────────────────────────────────────────────────────────────────┐
│ If calculated LDL levels are elevated (with or without triglyceride and VLDL) │
│                 (Types IIA, IIB, and III hyperlipoproteinemia)                │
│                                                                 │
│                        THEN PATIENT IS AT:                      │
│        ┌──────────────────┬──────────────────┐                  │
│        ▼                  ▼                  ▼                  │
│  Very high risk if   High risk if total   Moderate risk if total│
│  plasma LDL > 600    cholesterol and LDL  cholesterol and LDL are│
│  mg/dL               are in upper 10% for in 75–90% range for   │
│                      age & sex (e.g., >175 age and sex (e.g., >100│
│                      mg/dl)               mg/dl)                │
│        │                  │                  │                  │
│        ▼                  ▼                  ▼                  │
│  Aggressively treat  Treat with diet      Treat with diet       │
│  with combination    │                    │                     │
│  diet and drugs      ▼                    ▼                     │
│                      IF                   IF                    │
│                      │                    │                     │
│                      ▼                    ▼                     │
│                 Total cholesterol and  Total cholesterol and    │
│                 LDL inadequately       LDL inadequately         │
│                 controlled by diet, go controlled by diet and   │
│                 to drug treatment      family is H_x positive   │
│                                        for CVD, consider drug   │
│                                        treatment                │
└─────────────────────────────────────────────────────────────────┘
```

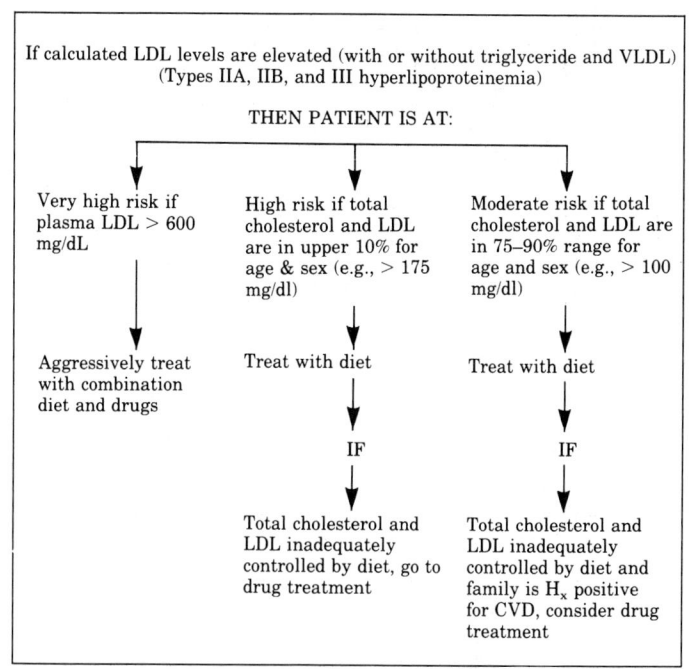

Fig. 5-5. Directional scheme for an elevated plasma low-density lipoprotein level.

SATURATED FAT

Usually a fat of animal origin that is solid or hard at room temperature tends to raise blood cholesterol. Saturated fat is present in such foods as lunch meat, sausage, hot dogs (or processed meats), butter, cream, whole milk, and cheese made from whole milk or cream. Among the few vegetable fats that are saturated are coconut oil and palm oil (used in nondairy cream substitutes, some frozen desserts, and so forth) and cocoa butter (the fat in chocolate). Other vegetable oils, unsaturated by nature, may be made saturated by hardening or hydrogenation. The amount of saturation is indicated by the degree of hardness. For example, a tub margarine is less saturated than a stick margarine.

Mounting evidence supports a unique advantage for dietary monounsaturated fats as opposed to polyunsaturated fats. The Second International Colloquium on Monounsaturated Fats sponsored by the Heart, Lung and Blood Institute of the United States National Institutes of Health and by the International Olive Oil Council [4] brought out the following research results:

1. Replacement of saturated fats with oleic acid (a monounsaturated fat making up more than 70% of the total fats in olive oil) significantly lowers serum cholesterol levels.
2. Unlike polyunsaturated fats, such as vegetable oils, which

Table 5-6. Dietary measures to lower hyperlipoproteinemia

	Type I	Type IIA	Type IIB	Type III	Type IV	Type V
General R_x	Low fat: supplement with medium-chain triglycerides and high carbohydrates	Low cholesterol: low saturated fat; supplement with unsaturated fats	Low cholesterol: low saturated fat; supplement with unsaturated fats	Low cholesterol: balanced, modified fat and carbohydrates, low alcohol	Controlled carbohydrate, modified fat, low alcohol	High protein, moderate fat and carbohydrate reduction, no alcohol
Calories	Unrestricted: weight difficult to maintain with high energy needs	Unrestricted	Restricted to maintain ideal weight	Restricted to maintain ideal body weight	Restricted to maintain ideal body weight	Restricted to maintain ideal body weight
Protein	Unrestricted: 15–20% (50–100 gm/day)	Unrestricted: 15–20% (50–100 gm/day)		Moderate: 18–21% (75–125 gm/day)	Moderate: 18–21% (75–125 gm/day)	High: 21–24% (90–145 gm/day)
Fat	Adult: < 25 gm/day Child 6–12: < 15 gm/day saturated or unsaturated fat supplements with medium-chain triglycerides according to caloric intake	Restricted to 30% or less/day; low saturated fat (< 5% of calories), supplemented w/unsaturated fats to increase P/S ratio to > 1.1		Restricted: 30%/day with substituted unsaturated fats for a portion of saturated fats	Restricted: Unsaturated substituted fats for portion of saturated fats	Restricted: 20% or less/day with unsaturated fats substituted for portion saturated fats
Cholesterol	Unrestricted	Low: Adult, < 300 mg/day; Child, < 200 mg/day		Low: < 300 mg/day	Moderate: < 500 mg/day	Moderate: < 500 mg/day
Carbohydrate	Unrestricted (substitute for fat)	Unrestricted		40%/day	40%/day	< 50%/day
Alcohol	None allowed	Unrestricted		2 servings/day (substitute for carbohydrate)	2 servings/day (substitute for carbohydrate)	None allowed
Remarks	Diet should reduce chylomicrons to normal	Diet should lower LDL 15–30%				

Key: LDL = low density lipoprotein.
Source: Modified from American Medical Association, *Drug Evaluations* (6th ed.). Chicago: American Medical Association, 1986.

also lower serum cholesterol levels including HDL-cholesterol, olive oil raised the HDL-cholesterol level.
3. Olive oil (20% of the caloric intake) exercises a favorable effect on the catabolism of LDL-cholesterol, and patients fed low fat and low cholesterol diets and diets rich in monounsaturated fats show similar drops in total cholesterol and LDL-cholesterol levels.
4. Decreases in serum cholesterol levels were comparable in diets rich in complex carbohydrates and diets containing olive oil. However, the carbohydrate-rich diet lowers, while the olive oil diet raises, the HDL-cholesterol levels. These findings are of particular importance in the management of patients with diabetes mellitus.

Presently, the dietary recommendations of the American Heart Association are that the dietary intake of polyunsaturated fats should not exceed 10%, and of saturated fats should not exceed 10%. The remaining fat content should be made up of monounsaturated fats.

These changes in eating habits are recommended:

1. Control cholesterol intake.
2. Omit egg yolks and organ meats.
3. Restrict all fats, particularly saturated fats, and substitute monounsaturated and polyunsaturated fats by using olive or hi-oleic safflower oil and, to a limited degree, corn oil or a soft (tub) safflower margarine. Use one teaspoon of monounsaturated fat for each ounce of cooked meat.
4. Include fish, chicken, turkey, and veal as part of the weekly menus. Veal has more cholesterol than fish, chicken, and turkey. Limit beef and pork to 3 ounces, 3 times per week.
5. Choose skim milk and skim milk products rather than whole milk, cream, ice cream, and cheese. When baking, use skim milk or evaporated skim milk and use egg whites rather than whole eggs to replace commercial goods containing egg yolks, whole milk, and butter or other saturated fat.

To restrict saturated fat, it is necessary to limit the meat in the diet and to use foods other than meat. Specific amounts of monounsaturated or polyunsaturated blends (oil or margarine), in proportion to saturated fat (meat in the diet), must be included. Recommended proportions are as follows:

1. Limit all meat, including fish and poultry, to less than 9 ounces of cooked meat per day.
2. Limit beef, lamb, ham, and pork to a 3-ounce portion 3 times per week.

Fish are naturally lower in fat and should be used in place of meat as often as possible.

If it is not possible or practical to limit the beef, lamb, ham, and pork, the desired polyunsaturated to saturated fat ratio may be achieved with this alternate plan:

1. Limit all meat to less than 9 ounces of cooked meat per day.
2. Consume, in some fashion, 6 teaspoons of monounsaturated or polyunsaturated fat for each 3 ounces of cooked meat.

The recommended monounsaturated or polyunsaturated fat (olive oil, margarine, or corn oil) does not have to be used with the meat. It may be used as desired and need not be limited to this amount. However, for weight reduction, the amounts of monounsaturated or polyunsaturated fats need to be limited as well.

WAYS OF USING MONOUNSATURATED AND POLYUNSATURATED OILS

Monounsaturated and polyunsaturated oils may be used in food preparation in the following ways:

Broiling, baking, or frying meats, fish, and poultry
Popping corn

They may be used as an ingredient in the following foods:

Salad dressings
Barbecue sauces
Cream sauces made with skim milk
Marinades
Pie crusts
Cakes and cookies made with skim milk and egg whites
Cooked vegetable seasonings (add spices, herbs, and so forth)

ESTIMATING MEAT, FISH, AND POULTRY PORTIONS

There are 16 ounces to a pound. Raw meat, fish, or poultry lose weight when they are cooked. Three oz of cooked meat equals:

4 oz of raw meat or fish without bone
¾ cup cooked, flaked, or chopped meat, poultry or fish
A ground beef patty, 3 in. diameter × 1 in. thick, cooked
½ large chicken breast, cooked
One chicken thigh plus one drumstick, cooked

FISH OIL-DERIVED FATTY ACIDS IN THE TREATMENT OF HYPERLIPOPROTEINEMIA

Fish oils, highly unsaturated but nonessential fatty acids (omega-3), and vegetable oils (omega-6) containing large amounts of linoleic acid are hypocholesterolemic agents in humans, but there are differences in the effects of omega-3 and omega-6 oils on plasma lipids and lipoproteins [12]. Furthermore, the low death rate from coronary artery disease among the Greenland Eskimos has been ascribed to their high fish consumption. The average fish consumption of Eskimos is estimated to be about 13 oz/day. In Japan, death rates from coronary artery disease are significantly lower in fishing villages than in farming villages. Studies from the University of Leiden, Holland, suggest that the consumption of as little as one or two fish dishes per week may reduce the mortality from coronary artery disease [18]. Fish oils, given as a dietary supplement to healthy human volunteers (8.2 gm of omega-3 fatty acids daily for 4 weeks) significantly decreases serum triglycerides and VLDL levels without consistently lowering the total cholesterol or HDL-cholesterol and with variable changes in LDL-cholesterol levels. Large daily supplements of salmon oil reduces plasma total cholesterol and the lipoproteins VLDL, LDL, and HDL cholesterol.

Type IIB hyperlipoproteinemia patients may experience a sizeable reduction in plasma cholesterol levels (> 25%) after a low-cholesterol (150 mg), low-fat (20–30% of total calories) diet followed by a 4-week fish-oil diet (where the fat came from salmon oil or commercially available fish). The fish-oil diet decreases plasma cholesterol by reducing VLDL, LDL, and HDL cholesterol, and reduces plasma triglyceride levels as well. Highly polyunsaturated vegetable-oil containing diets led to less remarkable decreases in plasma cholesterol and triglycerides due to a limited effect on VLDL, no effect on LDL, and increased levels of HDL.

The effects of a fish-oil diet on type V hyperlipoproteinemia are more striking than those seen with the IIB phenotype. There is a virtual disappearance of chylomicrons; total plasma triglyceride values drop by nearly 80%; the VLDL-triglyceride level decreases in a parallel manner; and plasma cholesterol levels drop to the normal range, accounted for largely by the fall in VLDL cholesterol.

Dietary fish oils significantly lower the rate of LDL synthesis in normolipidemic individuals. The fact that LDL apolipoprotein B is derived from VLDL apoprotein B is indirect evidence that dietary fish oil inhibits VLDL synthesis [22]. Fish oils increase the removal of VLDL by peripheral tissues or by the liver (VLDL remnants), perhaps by increasing lipoprotein lipase. Diets rich in marine fatty acids or marine fatty acid supplements reduce cell membrane arachidonic acid. Arachidonic acid is metabolized into various cyclo-oxygenase products (prostaglandins, PG, and thromboxane (TxA_2) as well as lipoxygenase products (monohydroxy) and leukotrienes (LTs). Fish oils are rich in eicosopentaenoic acid (EPA) and EPA is also metabolized into cyclooxygenase and lipoxygenase products in various tissues. Diets containing animal and vegetable fats result in arachidonic acid conversion to the cyclooxygenase-mediated prostacyclin (PGI_2) by endothelial cells and TxA_2 by blood platelets. Diets rich in EPA, on the other hand, lead to the production of a biologically weaker prostacyclin (PGI_3) by endothelial cells and to the synthesis of TxA_2 by blood platelets. Decreases in blood platelet counts are even recorded after diets rich in EPA. Observed decreases in thrombogeneity is probably due to the production of PGI_3, a platelet anti-aggregation factor and to reduced TxA_2 formation. Consequently, bleeding may complicate the rise of supplemental dietary fish oils in the management of hyperlipoproteinemia.

Drug Management of Hyperlipoproteinemia

In at least one-third of patients, dietary restriction lowers serum cholesterol. Exercise facilitates maintenance of ideal body weight and, if intense enough, may reduce LDL-cholesterol and raise HDL-cholesterol. While alcohol may increase HDL-cholesterol, triglyceride-rich lipoproteins and caloric intake are increased with alcohol. Consequently, alcohol should be reduced or eliminated from the diet. Success with the dietary approach might reduce total and LDL cholesterol levels by 25–35%. Target plasma cholesterol values for patients below 60 years of age is 180–200 mg/dl, according to the National Institutes of Health (NIH) Consensus Development Conference. However, even more modest serum cholesterol reduction may reduce the appearance of atherosclerosis-related angina pectoris, heart attack, and stroke, particularly in patients < 60 years of age.

Not all patients with dietary refractory hyperlipoproteinemia require drug therapy. Oster and Epstein [21], in an important contribution, considered the cost-effectiveness of drug therapy using cholestyramine as a model in the primary prevention of coronary heart disease among men. The cost-effectiveness was highest for "younger patients, for those with additional coronary risk factors (e.g., smoking or hypertension), and for those whose course of therapy is of less than lifelong duration. Conversely, it is lowest for older patients, for those with no additional coronary risk factors, and for those who are treated for a lifetime." Their results suggest that drug therapy "may not be cost-effective for all patients with elevated cholesterol levels, especially those over 65 years of age.

Failure to reduce plasma cholesterol by dietary modifications directs attention to the use of drugs. Several lipid-lowering drugs are available, five of which — nicotinic acid (niacin), cholestyramine, colestipol, probucol, and mevinolin — are approved in the United States and Canada for treatment of elevated LDL cholesterol. Clofibrate and several analogs are approved in some European countries.

Drug therapy in hyperlipoproteinemia is summarized in Table 5-7. None of the currently available hypolipidemic drugs are effective in type I hyperlipoproteinemia.

In familial type I hyperlipoproteinemia dietary fat intake of 25 gm/day or less markedly decreases triglyceride levels, resolves eruptive xanthomas, and relieves abdominal pain. Initially, a fat-free diet may be required, but at least 1% of the total calories should consist of linoleic acid. Fat-soluble vitamins should supplement the diet. Carbohydrates are substituted for fat.

A low cholesterol intake (less than 300 mg/day), a sharp restriction of saturated fat, and an increase in unsaturated fat intake (unsaturated:saturated ratio of approximately 2:1) are the dietary goals in type II hyperlipoproteinemia.

Elevated LDL levels in the familial type II disorder, due to a genetic deficiency of LDL receptors, requires dietary and drug therapy. For the heterozygous familial type II disorder (5% of all individuals suffering from heart attacks who are less than 60 years of age) one-half of LDL receptors are normal in number and can be stimulated to increase in activity when hepatic cholesterol levels are depleted (bile acid sequestrants, cholestyramine, and colestipol). If the response is less than desired, mevinolin or niacin is added. The homozygous familial type II hyperlipoproteinemia resists all drug therapy. Recently, success in lowering plasma LDL levels has been reported after liver transplant with restoration of LDL receptor activity.

Dietary restriction to achieve ideal body weight, followed by a low-cholesterol, low-saturated fat diet may be the only treatment required for type III hyperlipoproteinemia. If drugs are required, then clofibrate (or gemfibrozil) usually reduces lipids to normal and causes regression of xanthomas. Niacin may also be effective.

Type IV hyperlipoproteinemia requires: (1) weight reduction, (2) a low-carbohydrate, low-alcohol diet, (3) replacement of carbohydrates with unsaturated fats (especially omega-3 fatty acids), and (4) limitation of daily cholesterol intake to 500 mg. Drug therapy is rarely necessary.

For type V hyperlipoproteinemia, the first step is weight reduction with a high-protein, low-fat maintenance program. Alcohol restriction may be necessary to prevent abdominal pain. These measures are usually all that are necessary to reduce plasma lipid levels. Some cases require drugs to lower the lipids. The most effective drugs are clofibrate, gemfibrozil, or niacin. Norethindrone may be useful in women and oxandrolone in men to prevent abdominal pain when plasma lipid levels remain high.

Niacin: Mediated Reduction of Very Low Density Lipoproteins and Low Density Lipoproteins

USES AND/OR ACTIONS

Niacin (but not niacinamide) reduces the rate of VLDL synthesis and thereby the plasma LDL levels. As a consequence, VLDL- and LDL-cholesterol levels are reduced, and the drug is useful in types IIA, IIB, III, IV, and V hyperlipoproteinemias and may decrease the incidence rate of recurrent nonfatal MI. However, incidence rates of atrial fibrillation and other arrhythmias may be increased. Therefore, caution should be exercised if niacin is given to patients with established ischemic heart disease. In a 9–15-year follow-up of patients with ischemic heart disease, an approximately 10% decrease in the death rate from cardiac causes was reported [8].

PHARMACOKINETICS

Absorption

Niacin is rapidly absorbed, with peak concentrations occurring at about 45 minutes. Reportedly, approximately 88% of a 3-gm dose is recovered in the urine, suggesting that intestinal absorption is almost complete.

Metabolism

Niacin has a high hepatic extraction ratio; therefore, plasma clearance may be reduced in patients with hepatic impairment. Niacin is contraindicated in patients with cirrhosis.

Elimination

Renal clearance of niacin appears to depend on plasma concentration.

Table 5-7. Drug therapy in hyperlipoproteinemia

Type IIA	Type IIB	Type III	Type IV	Type V
Heterozygotes Cholestyramine resin: LDL should decrease 20–40%; VLDL variable increase in type IIB possible. Alternatively, colestipol hydrochloride plus niacin.	Cholestyramine resin: The sequestrant should decrease LDL 25–35%; niacin will have an effect on LDL (15–30%) and should decrease VLDL 35–50%	Niacin: VLDL should decrease 40–80% with diet alone. HDL should increase.	Niacin: LDL and VLDL should decrease > 30%; HDL should increase.	Niacin: LDL should decrease 30%, VLDL up to 70%.
Niacin*, particularly in type IIB: LDL should decrease 15–35%; VLDL should decrease 40%; HDL should increase.		Clofibrate: VLDL should decrease 40–80%; LDL is decreased.	Gemfibrozil: VLDL should decrease > 30%; HDL should increase.	Gemfibrozil: VLDL should decrease > 30%; HDL should increase.
Probucol: LDL should decrease 10–20%; HDL may decrease 10–40%.		Gemfibrozil (Lopid): VLDL should decrease > 30%; HDL should increase.		Norethindrone acetate: Use in women only — initial and maintenance: 5 mg/day (premenopausal women should receive drug 21 days/month to permit regular menses). VLDL should decrease 10–15%.
Mevinolin: LDL should decrease >30%; HDL may slightly increase with large doses.				

Dextrothyroxine sodium: initially, 1 mg/day; maintenance, 4–8 mg/day. LDL should decrease 15–30% with diet alone.

Homozygotes
Cholestyramine resin: 4–8 gm 4 times/day with meals; should be started in childhood.

Oxandrolone: For use in men, 2.5 mg 3 times/day (investigational use). VLDL and triglyceride should decrease 60%. Chylomicrons should decrease.

Key: LDL = low density lipoprotein; VLDL = very low density lipoprotein, HDL = high density lipoprotein.
*Less effective than cholestyramine resin or colestipol in patients w/familial type IIA
Source: Modified from American Medical Association, *Drug Evaluations* (6th ed.). Chicago: American Medical Association, 1986.

Distribution

Niacin rapidly disappears from the blood and is concentrated mainly in the liver, but some is also found in adipose tissue and the kidneys.

ADVERSE EFFECTS

Therapeutic doses of niacin may cause pruritus, flushing, headache, paresthesias, nausea, and other symptoms of gastrointestinal irritation. Flushing may persist in up to 10–15% of patients. Small initial doses with gradual increases reduces severity of pruritus, flushing, and symptoms of gastrointestinal irritation (nausea, flatulence, diarrhea) in most patients. Large doses may activate peptic ulcer, impair glucose tolerance, or produce liver damage and hyperuricemia. These reactions are usually reversible when therapy is discontinued. Rarely, anaphylaxis will be seen following intravenous administration.

TOXICITY

Toxic amblyopia is a rare complication.

PRECAUTIONS

Cardiovascular

Niacin potentiates the effects of ganglionic blocking agents. Therefore, concomitant use in hypertensive patients may lead to orthostatic hypotension. Liver function tests should be performed periodically in all patients.

DOSAGES

Adult: *Oral* — initially, 100 mg 3 times daily, increase to 2–6 gm daily in 3 divided doses with or after meals. Doses as high as 9–12 gm daily may be required.

DOSAGE FORMS AND STRENGTHS AVAILABLE

Nicotinic acid 50 mg* in containers of 100, 300, 500, and bulk.
Generic niacin 100 mg* in containers of 100, 300, 500, and bulk.
Generic niacin 500 mg in containers of 100 and bulk.
Nicolar (contains tartrazine) **500 mg** in containers of 100.

Niacin is particularly well suited when used in combination with bile acid sequestrants (see below), since niacin inhibits LDL production and bile acid sequestrants increase LDL breakdown.

If niacin fails to normalize LDL levels or if the patient cannot tolerate the drug, other drug therapy should be considered. Selection of an alternate drug should be guided by the concentrations of triglyceride-rich VLDL fraction. If the fasting triglyceride level exceeds 250 mg/dl, the fibric acid derivatives gemfibrozil, clofibrate, or probucol might be considered.

---

* Available without prescription

Clofibrate (Atromid-S): Mediated Reduction in Low Density Lipoproteins and Type III Hyperlipoproteinemia

USES AND/OR ACTIONS

Clofibrate is most often used for type III hyperlipoproteinemia. When used with appropriate dietary regulation, clofibrate is uniformly effective in decreasing LDL levels without shifting the levels of other lipoproteins in type III patients. Xanthomas may regress. Improvement in individuals with peripheral vascular disease associated with type III disorder has been reported. Because of the risks associated with its use, clofibrate is generally restricted to type III hyperlipoproteinemia. Clofibrate has no effect on the apoprotein E-III deficiency associated with this disorder. Clofibrate reduces VLDL levels in type IIB heterozygotes. However, homozygous and heterozygous type IIA patients usually do not respond. Clofibrate reduces VLDL levels in type IV and V abnormalities, although a reciprocal increase may be seen in these patients.

Diabetes Insipidus

Clofibrate has significant antidiuretic action in patients with mild to moderate central diabetes insipidus. When used for diabetes insipidus, clofibrate appears to increase the release of ADH from the neurohypophysis. There is no evidence that the peripheral action of ADH is enhanced.

Hepatic

Clofibrate may inhibit the hepatic release of lipoproteins, particularly VLDL.

Metabolic

Clofibrate may accelerate the catabolism of VLDL and LDL, increase the fecal excretion of neutral sterols, inhibit cholesterol synthesis, and alter the metabolism of some lipoprotein apoproteins. Clofibrate reportedly potentiates lipoprotein lipase activity and increases apo A-I levels and may increase HDL concentration.

The major effect of clofibrate in hyperlipoproteinemia is the reduction of VLDL, but the hypocholesterolemic effect is moderate in most patients. A rebound increase in cholesterol and triglyceride concentrations is often observed after clofibrate is discontinued. Clofibrate interferes with the binding of serum free fatty acids to albumin. Clofibrate has been reported to reduce serum fibrinogen levels and may diminish platelet adhesiveness.

PHARMACOKINETICS

Absorption

At doses up to 2 gm/day, absorption is complete.

Metabolism

Clofibrate undergoes rapid hydrolysis to an active metabolite, chlorophenoxyisobutyric acid (CPIB). Peak CPIB concentrations are usually attained in 3–6 hours. The mean half-life is 1.7 hours, but there are wide individual variations.

Elimination

The mean plasma elimination half-life of CPIB is 15.1 hours.

Distribution

Plasma binding decreases as the dose increases and is associated with increased plasma clearance. Approximately 40–70% is recovered in the urine as a glucuronide ester of CPIB.

Other

The therapeutic plasma concentration for hypolipidemic activity without side effects has not been determined.

ADVERSE EFFECTS

Cardiovascular

Potentially serious effects on cardiac muscle have rarely occurred; in these cases, serum creatine phosphokinase (CPK) levels were increased, sometimes accompanied by frank myositis with asthenia, myalgia, and malaise. Elevated levels may persist when other serum enzymes return to normal and the patient becomes asymptomatic. In patients with chest pain, increased serum transaminase (SGOT) and CPK levels may be caused by clofibrate rather than by MI.

Gastrointestinal

Nausea, vomiting, diarrhea, dyspepsia, and flatulence occur in about 10% of patients initially, but usually disappear with continued therapy. Cholelithiasis may occur.

Hepatic

Clofibrate causes hepatomegaly in animals, but similar changes have not been observed in humans. However, reversible elevations in SGOT and glutamic pyruvate transaminase (SGPT) levels have been noted.

Hematologic

Leukopenia can occur infrequently.

Musculoskeletal

Potentially serious effects on skeletal muscle have occurred rarely; in these cases, serum CPK levels were increased, sometimes accompanied by frank myositis with asthenia, myalgia, and malaise. Elevated levels may persist when other serum enzymes return to normal and the patient is asymptomatic.

Neurologic

Drowsiness may occur infrequently.

Skin

Rash and alopecia areata may appear infrequently.

PRECAUTIONS

Cardiovascular

The Coronary Drug Project Trial utilized clofibrate for the long-term management of men with established ischemic heart disease, and no definitive evidence was obtained supporting a reduced total mortality with this drug. Furthermore, the incidence of peripheral vascular disease, pulmonary embolism, thrombophlebitis, angina pectoris, increased heart size, arrhythmias, and intermittent claudication were all significantly increased. The incidence of cholelithiasis also increased twofold, and feminizing effects (decreased libido, breast tenderness) were occasionally noted. Therefore, clofibrate should not be given indiscriminately to patients who have had an MI.

The results of a large primary prevention trial of clofibrate conducted in Europe confirms the need for caution in the use of this drug. In this study, the incidence of nonfatal MI was reduced significantly, but the total number of deaths and gastrointestinal disorders, especially cholelithiasis, increased significantly.

Gastrointestinal

Cholelithiasis may occur.

Hepatic

Patients on long-term therapy must be closely supervised. In those with impaired renal or hepatic function, clofibrate must be used with caution and in reduced doses, as delayed detoxification and excretion make the duration of action unpredictable. Enhanced secretion of cholesterol into bile can increase saturation of gallbladder bile with cholesterol; consequently, the risk of cholesterol gallstones is increased approximately twofold.

Other

SGOT, SGPT, and CPK values should be determined periodically. Dietary regulation must continue during drug therapy, as the effects of diet and drugs are additive.

Pregnancy/Lactation

Clofibrate is CONTRAINDICATED during pregnancy and should not be given to nursing mothers, as it may be excreted in milk.

Pediatric

Clofibrate is not recommended for use in children, since data are insufficient to determine its safety in this age group.

DRUG INTERACTIONS

Coumadin Anticoagulants

Clofibrate potentiates the action of coumadin anticoagulants. The dosage of anticoagulants must be reduced by at least one half, and prothrombin times should be determined frequently, especially during initiation of therapy. Phenytoin action and tolbutamide action are both potentiated by clofibrate.

DOSAGES

Adult: *Oral* — 500 mg 3 or 4 times daily.

CLOFIBRATE DOSAGE FORMS AND STRENGTHS AVAILABLE

Atromid-S (Ayerst) 500 mg capsules in containers of 100.

Gemfibrozil (Lopid): Mediated Reduction of Hypertriglyceridemia-Hyperlipidemia

USES AND/OR ACTIONS

Gemfibrozil is structurally related to clofibrate and should be reserved for high-risk types III, IV, and V hyperlipoprotein phenotypes with severe hypertriglyceridemia (> 750 mg/dl) who respond inadequately to diet and other triglyceride-lowering drugs.

Gemfibrozil appears to reduce incorporation of long-chain fatty acids into newly formed triglycerides, thus reducing VLDL production in the liver. It inhibits synthesis of the VLDL carrier, apoprotein, which also decreases VLDL production. Gemfibrozil has effects similar to those of clofibrate in reducing cholesterol, triglycerides, and LDL cholesterol, but is more effective in elevating HDL cholesterol and the HDL cholesterol/total cholesterol ratio.

Intermediates of cholesterol synthesis did not accumulate in animal studies. Fibrinogen levels also were not affected.

PHARMACOKINETICS

Absorption

Peak plasma levels are attained in 1–2 hours.

Metabolism

Plasma levels are proportional to the dose. No evidence of accumulation has been demonstrated. The half-life is estimated to be 1.5 hours.

Elimination

Seventy percent of gemfibrozil is excreted unchanged, primarily in the urine.

ADVERSE EFFECTS

In general, adverse effects are similar to those encountered with clofibrate administration.

Gastrointestinal

Gastrointestinal disturbances can occur.

Hepatic

Hepatocellular enlargement, with no changes in liver function, was found in some animal species.

Metabolism

Transient elevations in serum transaminase levels have been reported.

Skin

Rash can occur.

PRECAUTIONS

Hepatic

Gemfibrozil is contraindicated in patients with severe hepatic disease, including biliary cirrhosis, and in patients with preexisting gallbladder disease.

Direct comparisons of cholesterol saturation indices after administration of clofibrate and gemfibrozil revealed similar data, suggesting that the risk of developing cholelithiasis is the same for both drugs.

Renal

Gemfibrozil is contraindicated in patients with severe renal dysfunction.

Endocrine

Blood glucose levels may be elevated in some patients, although doses of 800 mg/day do not impair the control of diabetes when an oral hypoglycemic agent or insulin is administered. Gemfibrozil should be used with caution in diabetics, and blood glucose levels should be monitored in all patients.

Metabolism

Dietary regulation must continue during drug therapy, as effects are additive.

Pregnancy/Lactation

Use of hypolipidemic drugs during pregnancy and lactation is not advocated because their safety has not yet been determined.

DRUG INTERACTIONS

Coumadin Anticoagulants

Gemfibrozil inhibited platelet aggregation in animal studies. It has less effect on unbound coumadin levels than an equivalent dose of clofibrate. However, frequent determination of prothrombin times is advised if gemfibrozil and coumadin are given concomitantly.

DOSAGES

Adult: *Oral:* 600 mg twice daily, one-half hour before breakfast and dinner.

DOSAGE FORMS AND STRENGTHS AVAILABLE

Lopid 300 mg capsules in amounts of 100.

Cholestyramine Resin (Questran): Modulation of Cholesterol Absorption and Low Density Lipoproteins

USES

Cholestyramine resin remains a first-line drug to treat type IIA hyperlipoproteinemia as an adjunct to dietary or other drug regimens.

Heterozygous Type II Disorder

Some success has been achieved with a combination of cholestyramine, niacin, and proper diet. More recently, cholestyramine and an inhibitor of the rate-limiting enzyme for cholesterol synthesis (see below) has been used with some success in the treatment of familial homozygous type II hyperlipoproteinemia; however, this disease is particularly resistant to therapy. Usual doses of cholestyramine resin decrease LDL in type IIB hyperlipoproteinemia but may increase VLDL (triglyceride) levels slightly. Cholestyramine does not reduce VLDL or triglyceride levels and may aggravate hyperprebetalipoproteinemia in types III, IV, and V hyperlipoproteinemias.

Hepatic

The major effect in hyperlipidemia is to increase the rate of LDL removal by increasing LDL receptor activity.

Hematologic

Cholestyramine resin should decrease LDL by 15–30% over diet alone in type IIA disorder. There may be a variable increase in VLDL in type IIB.

PHARMACOKINETICS

Cholestyramine resin is not absorbed from the gastrointestinal tract.

ADVERSE EFFECTS

Gastrointestinal

Bloating, epigastric distress, mild nausea, constipation, and occasional diarrhea can occur, but these symptoms usually subside with continued therapy. Steatorrhea, weight loss, and malabsorption syndrome have been rarely reported. With excessive doses, constipation often occurs. Many patients require a treatment such as high fluid intake and regular use of a mild laxative.

Skin

Rash and perianal irritation have been reported rarely.

TOXICITY

Since cholestyramine resin is not absorbed, no systemic toxicity has been observed.

PRECAUTIONS

Cholestyramine may rarely interfere with the absorption of fat; therefore, an associated deficiency of fat-soluble vitamins (A, D, and E) may also occur, requiring supplementation. Vitamin K deficiency may develop and result in a bleeding tendency due to hypoprothrombinemia.

Dietary regulation must continue during drug therapy, as diet and drug effects are additive. Some investigators suggest that folate deficiency occurs during long-term treatment in patients, especially children. Children may require 5 mg of folic acid daily.

Pregnancy/Lactation

Use of hypolipidemic drugs during pregnancy is not advocated, as their safety has not yet been determined.

INTERACTIONS

Anticoagulants

Mild lengthening of prothrombin time without bleeding has been reported. The dosages of concomitantly administered anticoagulants should be monitored closely.

The following may be absorbed when given concomitantly with cholestyramine resin and should be taken at least 1 hour before or 4 hours after cholestyramine: coumadin, antibiotics, barbiturates, digitalis, phenylbutazone, thiazide diuretics, iron compounds, and thyroid.

DOSAGES

Cholestyramine preparation should be suspended in 120–180 ml of water or, when necessary, in pulpy juices, mashed banana, applesauce, gelatin, or cooked cereal. The drug should never be swallowed dry because of the hazard of esophageal irritation or blockage.

Adult: initially 4 gm (1 packet or 1 rounded teaspoonful) 4 times daily with meals and at bedtime. Depending on the response, this may be increased to 6 gm 4 times daily. A dosage of 24 gm daily divided into 2 or 3 doses has been shown to be equally effective.

Children over 6 years: dosage has not been definitively established; 8 twice daily with meals, increased to a maximal total daily dose of 24 gm.

Children under 6 years: dose has not been established.

Colestipol Hydrochloride (Colestipol): Modulation of Low Density Lipoprotein-Receptor Activity

USES AND/OR ACTIONS

Colestipol hydrochloride may be considered an alternative to cholestyramine in patients with type IIA hyperlipoproteinemia, although there is less experience with its use. In the heterozygous type II disorder, it is more effective in combination with niacin than when used alone.

Colestipol binds bile acids in the small intestine to prevent their reabsorption. The reduced level of bile acids promotes apoprotein B catabolism and increases the rate of conversion of cholesterol to bile acids in the liver.

The major effect in hyperlipidemia is to increase the rate of LDL removal by increasing LDL receptor activity.

PHARMACOKINETICS

Since colestipol is not absorbed from the gastrointestinal tract, no systemic toxicity is reported.

ADVERSE EFFECTS

Gastrointestinal

Bloating, mild nausea, and constipation may occur but usually subside with continued therapy. Epigastric distress and diarrhea occur occasionally, and, rarely, vomiting and/or irritation of the tongue may occur.

With excessive doses, steatorrhea, weight loss, and malabsorption syndrome may occur. Constipation is a frequent problem, and many patients require treatment such as high fluid intake and regular use of a mild laxative.

Skin

Rash and perianal irritation are rare reactions.

PRECAUTIONS

Metabolic

Since colestipol may rarely interfere with the absorption of fat, an associated deficiency of fat-soluble vitamins (A, D, and E) may also occur and require supplementation. Vitamin K deficiency may develop and result in a bleeding tendency due to hypoprothrombinemia. Its level should be monitored.

Dietary regulation must continue during therapy, as the effects of diet and drugs are additive. Some investigators suggest that folate deficiency occurs during long-term treatment, and patients, especially children, should receive 5 mg of folic acid daily, if necessary.

Pregnancy/Lactation

Use of hypolipidemic drugs during pregnancy is not advocated, as their safety has not yet been determined.

Pediatric

Some investigators suggest that folate deficiency occurs during long-term treatment and patients, especially children, should receive 5 mg of folic acid daily, if necessary.

DRUG INTERACTIONS

Anticoagulants

Mild lengthening of prothrombin time without bleeding has been reported. The dosages of concomitantly administered anticoagulants should be monitored closely.

The following may be absorbed when given concomitantly with colestipol and should be taken at least 1 hour before or 4 hours after colestipol: antibiotics, barbiturates, digitalis, iron compounds, phenylbutazone, thiazide diuretics, coumadin, and thyroid.

DOSAGES

Adult: 15–30 gm daily (mixed with 120–180 ml of suitable liquid) in 2–4 divided doses with meals (should be given 1 hour before or 4 hours after other drugs).

Children: Safety and effectiveness has not been definitely established; 10–15 gm daily divided into 2 doses (mixed with fluids at the morning and evening meals) has been used in children with familial type II hyperlipidemia.

DOSAGE FORMS AND STRENGTHS AVAILABLE

Colestid water-insoluble beads (oral powder) in 500 gm bottles or 5 gm packets.

Probucol (Lorelco): Mediated Reduction in Low Density Lipoproteins and High Density Lipoproteins

USES AND/OR ACTIONS

Probucol reduces LDL levels in nonfamilial type IIA hyperlipoproteinemia. It is less effective than cholestyramine or colestipol in the familial variety. However, because probucol reduces HDL levels proportionately more than LDL levels, its usefulness is limited. Until further data are collected, probucol should be used only when more effective hypocholesterolemic drugs are inadequate or contraindicated. When hypercholesterolemia persists, probucol may be used with agents that decrease serum triglyceride levels in type IIB, III, and IV cases.

Probucol appears to increase the fractional rate of catabolism of LDL, which may be responsible for the increase in fecal bile acid excretion. Probucol is thought to block one of the early steps in cholesterol biosynthesis because the cholesterol precursors, desmosterol and 7-dehydrocholesterol, do not accumulate in patients.

PHARMACOKINETICS

Absorption and Distribution

The absorption is limited. High peak levels are attained if probucol is administered with meals. Probucol accumulates slowly in fatty tissues following prolonged administration.

Metabolism

Blood levels increase gradually for 3 or 4 months with continuous oral administration and remain relatively constant thereafter. There is no correlation between blood concentrations and hypocholesterolemic effect.

Elimination

The major pathway of excretion is through the biliary system; renal clearance is negligible.

ADVERSE EFFECTS

Cardiovascular

Cardiotoxic effects, especially dysrhythmias, have been produced in some rhesus monkeys fed high-cholesterol, high-fat diets. These effects, however, have not been reported in humans.

Gastrointestinal

The most common, and usually transient, side effects include nausea, abdominal pain, flatulence, and diarrhea.

Hepatic

Transient elevations are reported for plasma values of serum transaminases, alkaline phosphatase, bilirubin, uric acid, blood urea nitrogen, and blood glucose.

Hematologic

Eosinophilia can occur.

Neurologic

Angioedema, headache, dizziness, and paresthesias can occur.

Skin

Excessive or fetid perspiration can occur.

TOXICITY

Cardiotoxic effects, especially dysrhythmias, have occurred in rhesus monkeys fed high-cholesterol, high-fat diets but have not been observed in humans.

PRECAUTIONS

Cardiovascular

Because of cardiovascular effects, especially dysrhythmias, as produced in monkeys, probucol is not advocated for patients with arrhythmias.

Metabolic

Dietary regulation must continue during therapy, as the effects of diet and drugs are additive.

Pregnancy/Lactation

No adverse effects are clinically apparent, but probucol should not be given to pregnant or lactating women. Women of childbearing age should exercise strict birth control measures both during and for 6 months after therapy is discontinued. It is not known whether probucol is excreted in human milk, but mothers being treated with probucol should not breast-feed their infants.

DRUG INTERACTIONS

Bile Acid Binding Resins

Probucol may have an additive effect when given concomitantly.

DOSAGES

Adult: 500 mg with the morning and evening meal.
Children: the safety and efficacy of probucol has not been established. Some investigators have given 250 mg twice daily with meals to children weighing less than 27 kg and 500 mg twice daily with meals to children weighing more than 27 kg.

DOSAGE FORMS AND STRENGTHS AVAILABLE

Lorelco 250 mg tablets in containers of 120.

Mevinolin: A Drug That Inhibits Cholesterol Synthesis

All but a small percentage of the total body cholesterol is synthesized from two-carbon acetate groups (see above). An early rate-limiting enzyme in cholesterol biosynthesis, HMG–CoA reductase is regulated by receptor-mediated LDL catabolism (see Fig. 5-2). Consequently, increasing receptor-mediated LDL catabolism (as with cholestyramine) or suppressing cholesterol synthesis are two therapeutic strategies for treating type II hyperlipoproteinemia.

Insight into potential pharmacologic means of influencing HMC-CoA reductase was provided by observations that *Penicillium citrinum* produces a metabolite (compactin) that inhibits the enzyme [9]. Compactin in doses of 30–60 mg/day significantly decreased serum cholesterol in heterozygous patients with type IIA familial hypercholesterolemia. The drug significantly reduced plasma cholesterol and triglycerides in the lipoproteins IDL and LDL without altering the levels of VLDL or HDL.

Compactin was subsequently replaced by mevinolin (lovastatin) isolated from a strain of *Aspergillus terreus,* as a potent inhibitor of HMG-CoA reductase [1]. Mevinolin given to normal volunteers and in patients with type IIA familial hypercholesterolemia was generally well tolerated and caused substantial reductions in plasma levels of LDL-cholesterol. Results from a multicenter trial of mevinolin in patients with non-familial type II hyperlipoproteinemia have been published [1986], and the promise of significant lowering of total cholesterol and LDL-cholesterol by a well tolerated drug appears to be at hand.

Mevinolin exerts a dose-related reduction of plasma cholesterol by lowering LDL-cholesterol. Mevinolin slightly but significantly raises the plasma HDL-cholesterol level when given at a high dose. Mevinolin lowers the plasma triglyceride level.

PHARMACOKINETICS IN ANIMALS

Mevinolin is the inactive and precursor form of a potent HMG-CoA reductase inhibitor, a β-hydroxy acid. Mevinolin is not completely absorbed from the gastrointestinal tract. The absorbed drug undergoes extensive first-pass extraction in the liver (perhaps 80%). Within the liver, mevinolin is transformed into lactone and hydroxy acid forms.

Excretion of mevinolin in feces (83%) is largely from the metabolites in bile plus the unabsorbed drug. Considerable enterohepatic re-entry of active HMG-CoA reductase inhibitors appears to occur. In addition to excretion through the bile, mevinolin metabolites are eliminated in the urine (10%).

Both mevinolin and its beta-hydroxy acid metabolite are highly bound (> 95%) to plasma proteins. Both cross the blood-brain and placental barriers. Plasma concentrations of mevinolin and metabolites increase linearly in doses ranging from 60–120 mg, with peak concentrations at 2–4 hours. Steady state is achieved within 2–3 days, with little accumulation of inhibitors.

ADVERSE EFFECTS

Myalgia and Myositis

Approximately 0.5% of patients may develop elevated creatinine phosphokinase levels. The drug should be stopped with the appearance of myositis.

Gastrointestinal

Approximately 10% of patients treated with mevinolin complain of mild or transient gastrointestinal disturbances, such as flatulence and diarrhea.

Hepatic

A dose-related mild increase in serum transaminase levels can occur. Approximately 2% of patients receiving mevinolin for 1 year or longer will develop persistent increases in serum amino transferases requiring drug cessation.

Ophthalmologic

Lens opacification may develop (approximately 13% incidence) without loss of visual acuity.

As pointed out in consideration of the cost-effectiveness of cholestyramine, selection of patients in the top tenth percentile for cholesterol levels (see Table 5-5) who are refractory to diet and are having a poor response with other anti-lipid drugs and are less than 65 years of age are candidates for mevinolin. Mevinolin is currently marketed at a price that may amount to $2,000–3,000 per year. Bile acid sequestrants cost less than half the price of mevinolin.

For quick reference, a summary of therapeutic modulation of hyperlipoproteinemias is given in Table 5-8.

Table 5-8. Summary of therapeutic modulation of hyperlipoproteinemias

Hyperlipo-proteinemia	VLDL	LDL	HDL	Total cholesterol
Type IIA and IIB				
Fish oil	↓	↓	↓	↓
Olive oil	↓	↓	↑→	↓→
Vegetable oil	↓→	→	↓→	↓→
Drugs				
Niacin	↓	↓		↓
Probucol		↓	↓	↓
Cholestyramine	↑→	↓		↓
Colestipol		↓		↓
Mevinolin		↓	↑→	↓
Type III				
Niacin	↓	↓		↓
Clofibrate	↓	↓	↑→	↓
Gemfibrozil	↓	↓	↑	↓

Key: VLDL = very low density lipoprotein; LDL = low density lipoprotein; HDL = high density lipoprotein; ↓ = decrease; ↑ = increase; ↓→ = moderate decrease; ↑→ = moderate increase.

Hormonal Therapy in the Management of Hyperlipoproteinemia

Norethindrone Acetate (Aygestin, Norlutate)

USES AND/OR ACTIONS

Results of recent studies have shown that when norethindrone, a progestational agent, is used in conjunction with an appropriate diet, there are decreases in VLDL and chylomicrons and decreases in HDL and apoprotein A in some women with type V hyperlipoproteinemia. There is a concurrent increase in post-heparin lipolytic activity (PHLA), and abdominal pain and pancreatitis are ameliorated. Norethindrone has also been tried in women with types III, IV, or V hyperlipoproteinemia in whom estrogens or combination oral contraceptives caused undesirable effects (hypertriglyceridemia and decreased PHLA). However, recent studies have shown that progestins may elevate serum cholesterol levels. Therefore, until more experience has accumulated, norethindrone should be reserved for women with type V hyperlipoproteinemia who are refractory to established therapy. Its use in men is not advocated because of its estrogenic activity.

DOSAGES

Women: 5 mg daily. Premenopausal women should receive the drug 21 days per month to permit regular menses.

DOSAGE FORMS AND STRENGTHS AVAILABLE

Aygestin (Ayerst) 5 mg tablets.
Norlutate (Parke-Davis) 5 mg tablets.

Oxandrolone (Anavar)

USES AND/OR ACTIONS

Oxandrolone, an anabolic steroid with weak androgenic properties, is a synthetic derivative of testosterone. It reduces triglyceride levels (affecting both VLDL and chylomicrons) by increasing PHLA but has little effect on cholesterol and LDL, although LDL cholesterol increased slightly in a few patients. HDL cholesterol is decreased, apparently through stimulation of hepatic lipase and increased LDL catabolism.

The use of oxandrolone in hyperlipidemia is investigational and should be reserved for men with severe symptomatic hypertriglyceridemia who are refractory to more conventional agents.

ADVERSE EFFECTS AND PRECAUTIONS

Oxandrolone should not be used in women because of its virilizing effect or in children because it may cause premature epiphyseal closure and alter sexual development.

Since oxandrolone may induce edema, it should be used cautiously in men with cardiac, renal, or hepatic disease and should not be given with adrenal corticosteroids or corticotropin. The dosages of anticoagulants may have to be reduced in patients receiving oxandrolone.

DOSAGES

Men: 2.5 mg 3 times daily.

DOSAGE FORMS AND STRENGTHS AVAILABLE

Anavar (Searle) 2.5 mg tablets.

Ethinyl Estradiol

Estrogens were used to treat hyperlipidemia after it was found that women, compared to men, have lower serum beta lipoprotein (LDL), higher alpha lipoprotein (HDL, particularly HDL_2), and decreased susceptibility to atherosclerosis and ischemic heart disease until after the menopause. However, estrogens are unsuitable for men, because they have feminizing effects, elevate VLDL and triglyceride concentrations, and increase the levels of several blood clotting factors.

In a long-term trial in men with established ischemic heart disease, estrogens increased the incidence of thromboembolism and cardiovascular complications. They also have been reported to increase mortality from cancer. In women, estrogens may elevate VLDL levels and decrease PHLA. They also are reported to cause abdominal pain and pancreatitis in women with type V hyperlipoproteinemia.

Dextrothyroxine Sodium (Choloxin)

USES AND/OR ACTIONS

Of the thyroid analogues, dextrothyroxine has the highest ratio of hypolipidemic to calorigenic activity. The drug reduces LDL by increasing LDL receptor activity in both euthyroid and hypothyroid patients. It also may increase the rate of conversion of cholesterol to bile acid by limiting bile acid synthesis through stimulation of the enzyme 7 α-hydroxylase. The decrease in serum cholesterol may range from 15–30% and is greatest in patients with the highest baseline concentrations. Maximal effects appear in 1–2 months.

Dextrothyroxine is indicated only in type IIA hyperlipoproteinemia. It has no consistent effect on VLDL in the usual dosage range and thus is seldom useful in patients with types III, IV, or V patterns. Currently, dextrothyroxine should be used only in patients with severe type II hyperlipidemia who are at high risk and cannot tolerate more conventional therapy, because it increases mortality in patients with established ischemic heart disease.

ADVERSE EFFECTS

Untoward effects occur frequently, are usually caused by metabolic stimulation, and generally mimic the symptoms of hyperthyroidism. Weight loss appears to be the first sign of hypermetabolism. Related effects include nervousness, insomnia, tremors, hyperhidrosis, and menstrual irregularity. Some patients report altered taste sensations, vertigo, and diarrhea during the first 6 weeks of therapy, but these reactions subside spontaneously. Rash and pruritus may develop in patients who are hypersensitive to iodine.

PRECAUTIONS

Dextrothyroxine should be used judiciously, if at all, in pregnant women and nursing mothers, because effects on the fetal and neonatal thyroid gland are unknown. The drug also must be given cautiously to patients with hypertension, hepatic disease, or renal disease.

The use of dextrothyroxine in a long-term trial (Coronary Drug Project) in men with established ischemic heart disease was discontinued because of increased mortality in patients with arrhythmias, angina pectoris, or multiple infarctions. Therefore, dextrothyroxine should not be given to patients with preexisting ischemic heart disease or arrhythmias, especially those with ventricular premature contractions.

DRUG INTERACTIONS

In some diabetic patients, prolonged use of dextrothyroxine decreases glucose tolerance, which may necessitate increasing the dose of hypoglycemic agents. Since this drug augments the effect of oral anticoagulants (probably by increasing receptor affinity), the dose of the latter may require reduction by approximately one-third, and prothrombin times should be determined more frequently. Dextrothyroxine should be withdrawn 2 weeks before elective surgery if the use of anticoagulants is contemplated.

PHARMACOKINETICS

The pharmacokinetics of dextrothyroxine are essentially the same as those of levothyroxine.

DOSAGES

Euthyroid adults: initially, 1 mg daily for 1 month; the daily dose may be increased by increments of 1–2 mg at intervals of at least 1 month until a satisfactory reduction of serum cholesterol is achieved or a maximal daily dose of 8 mg is reached. In patients receiving digitalis, the maximal dose is 4 mg daily.

Children: initially, 0.05 mg/kg daily; this dose may be doubled after 1 month. The dose is increased by increments of 0.05 mg/kg at monthly intervals until a satisfactory reduction of serum cholesterol is observed or a maximal dose of 5 mg daily has been reached.

DOSAGE FORMS AND STRENGTHS AVAILABLE

Choloxin (Flint) 1, 2, 4, and 6 mg tablets.

References

1. Alberts, A. W., et al. Mevinolin: A highly potent competitive inhibitor of hydroxymethylglutaryl-coenzyme A reductase and a cholesterol-lowering agent. *Proc. Natl. Acad. Sci. USA* 77:39, 1980.

2. Arntzenius, A. C., et al. Diet, lipoproteins and the progression of coronary atherosclerosis: The Leiden Intervention Trial. *N. Engl. J. Med.* 312:805, 1985.
3. Aschoff, L. *Lectures in Pathology*. New York: Hoeber, 1924.
4. Blankenhorn, D. H., et al. Beneficial effects of combined colestipol-niacin therapy on coronary atherosclerosis and coronary venous bypass grafts. *J.A.M.A.* 257:3233, 1987.
5. Breslow, J. L. Genetic regulation of apolipoproteins. *Am. Heart J.* 113:422, 1987.
6. Brown, M. S., and Goldstein, J. L. A receptor-mediated pathway for cholesterol homeostasis. *Proc. Natl. Acad. Sci. USA* 76:3330, 1979.
7. Brown, M. S., and Goldstein, J. L. Lipoprotein metabolism in the macrophage: Implications for cholesterol deposition in atherosclerosis. *Annu. Rev. Biochem.* 52:223, 1983.
8. Canner, P. L. Mortality in coronary drug project patients during nine-year post-treatment period. *J. Am. Coll. Cardiol.* 8:1245, 1986.
9. Endo, A., et al. Inhibition of cholesterol synthesis in vitro and in vivo by ML-236A and ML-236B, competitive inhibitors of 3-hydroxy-3-methyl-glutaryl-coenzyme A reductase. *Eur. J. Biochem.* 77:31, 1977.
10. Frick, M. H., et al. Helsinki Heart Study: Primary-prevention trial with gemfibrozil in middle-aged men with dyslipidemia. *N. Engl. J. Med.* 317:1244, 1987.
11. Grande Covian, F. Second international colloquium on monounsaturated fats. Olivae, IVnd year-N°-17, June, 1987.
12. Harris, W., et al. The comparative reductions of the plasma lipid and lipoproteins of dietary polyunsaturated fats: Salmon oil versus vegetable oil. *Metabolism* 32:179, 1983.
13. Hashida, R., et al. Transcellular transport of lipoprotein through arterial endothelial cells in monolayer culture. *Cell Struct. Funct.* 11:31, 1986.
14. Hegele, R. A., et al. Apoprotein B-gene DNA polymorphism associated with myocardial infarction. *N. Engl. J. Med.* 315:1509, 1986.
15. Kemper, H. J., et al. Association of cholesterol concentrations in low density lipoprotein, high density lipoprotein, and high density lipoprotein subfractions, and of apolipoproteins A1 and A11, with coronary stenosis and left ventricular function. *J. Lab. Clin. Med.* 109:19, 1987.
16. Kornitzer, M., et al. Belgian heart disease prevention project. *Lancet* 1:1066, 1983.
17. Krause, D. M., et al. Intermediate density lipoproteins and progression of coronary artery disease in hypercholesterolemic men. *Lancet* 2(8550):62, 1987.
18. Kromhout, D., et al. The inverse relation between fish consumption and 20-year mortality from coronary heart disease. *N. Engl. J. Med.* 312;1205, 1985.
19. Lees, R. External imaging of human atherosclerosis. *J. Nucl. Med.* 24:154, 1983.
20. Lipid Research Clinics Coronary Primary Prevention Trial (LRC-CPPT). Consensus Conference. *J.A.M.A.* 253;2080, 1985.
21. Oster, G., and Epstein, A. M. Cost-effectiveness of antihyperlipemic therapy in the prevention of coronary heart disease. *J.A.M.A.* 258:2381, 1987.

22. Phillipson, B., et al. Reduction of plasma lipids, lipoproteins and apoproteins by dietary fish oils in patients with hyperglyceridemia. *N. Engl. J. Med.* 312:1210, 1985.
23. Roberts, A. B., et al. Selective accumulation of low density lipoproteins in damaged arterial wall. *J. Lipid Res.* 24:1160, 1983.
24. Samuel, P. Report to the American Heart Association meeting, 1986. *Cardiovasc. News* 6:27, 1987.
25. Stehbens, W. F. The role of hemodynamics in the pathogenesis of atherosclerosis. *Prog. Cardiovasc. Dis.* 18:89, 1975.
26. Vartiainen, E., et al. Effects of dietary fat modifications on serum lipids and blood pressure in children. *Acta Paediatr. Scand.* 75:396, 1986.
27. Weinberg, R. B. Lipoprotein metabolism: Hormonal regulation. *Hosp. Prac. [Off.]* 22:125, 1987.

Selected Reading

CHOLESTEROL

Brown, M. S., and Goldstein, J. L. A receptor-mediated pathway for cholesterol homeostasis. *Science* 232:34, 1986.

Grundy, S. M. Cholesterol and coronary heart disease. *J.A.M.A.* 256:2849, 1986

Martin, M. J., et al. Serum cholesterol, blood pressure, and mortality: Implications from a cohort of 361,662 men (MRFIT Program). *Lancet* 2(8513):933, 1986.

Vega, G. L., and Grundy, S. M. Mechanisms of primary hypercholesterolemia in humans. *Am. Heart J.* 113:493, 1987.

LOVASTATIN

Bilheimer, D. W., et al. Lovastatin and colestipol stimulate receptor-mediated clearance of low-density lipoproteins from plasma in familial hypercholesterolemia heterozygotes. *Proc. Natl. Acad. Sci. USA* 80:4124, 1983.

Tobert, J. A., et al. Cholesterol-lowering effect of lovastatin, an inhibitor of 3-hydroxy-3 methylglutaryl coenzyme A reductase in healthy volunteers. *J. Clin. Invest.* 69:913, 1982.

LIPOPROTEINS

Eisenberg, S., and Levy R. I. Lipoprotein metabolism. *Adv. Lipid Res.* 13:1, 1975.

Fredrickson, D. S., et al. Fat transport in lipoproteins — an integrated approach to mechanisms and disorders. *N. Engl. J. Med.* 276:32, 94, 148, 215, 273, 1967.

Havel, R. J. Classification of hyperlipidemias. *Annu. Rev. Med.* 28: 195, 1977.

Jackson, R. L., et al. Lipoprotein structure and metabolism. *Physiol. Rev.* 56:259, 1976.

Weinberg, R. B. Lipoprotein metabolism: Hormonal regulation. *Hosp. Pract. [Off.]* 22:125, 1987.

LOW DENSITY LIPOPROTEINS

Goldstein, J. L., and Brown, M. S. The low-density lipoprotein pathway and its relation to atherosclerosis. *Annu. Rev. Biochem.* 46:897, 1977.

Hashida, R., et al. Transcellular transport of lipoprotein through arterial endothelial cells in monolayer culture. *Cell Struct. Funct.* 11:31, 1986.

Roberts, A. B., et al. Selective accumulation of low-density lipoproteins in damaged arterial wall. *J. Lipid Res.* 24:1160, 1983.

HIGH DENSITY LIPOPROTEINS

Barr, D. P., et al. Protein-lipid relationship in human plasma in atherosclerosis and related conditions. *Am. J. Med.* 11:480, 1951.

Miller, G. J., and Miller, N. E. Plasma high-density lipoprotein concentration and development of ischaemic heart disease. *Lancet* 1:16, 1975.

Norum, R. A., et al. Familial deficiency of apolipoproteins A-1 and C-111 and precocious coronary artery disease. *N. Engl. J. Med.* 306:1513, 1982.

GENETIC CONSIDERATIONS OF LIPOPROTEINS AND ATHEROSCLEROSIS

Breslow, J. L. Genetic regulation of apolipoproteins. *Am. Heart J.* 113:422, 1987.

Hegele, R. A., et al. Apoprotein B-gene DNA polymorphism associated with myocardial infarction. *N. Engl. J. Med.* 315:1509, 1986.

Law, A., et al. Common DNA polymorphism within coding sequence of apolipoprotein B gene associated with altered lipid level. *Lancet* 1(8493):1301, 1986.

Maciejko, J. J., et al. Apolipoprotein A-1 as a marker of angiographically assessed coronary artery disease. *N. Engl. J. Med.* 309:385, 1983.

Sidd, J. J., et al. Coronary artery disease in identical twins: A family study. *N. Engl. J. Med.* 274:55, 1966.

MACROPHAGES AND ATHEROGENESIS

Aquel, N. M., et al. Monocytic origin of foam cells in human atherosclerotic plaques. *Atherosclerosis* 53:265, 1984.

Gerrity, R. G. The role of the monocyte in atherogenesis. 1. Transition of blood-borne monocytes into foam cells in fatty lesions. *Am. J. Pathol.* 103:181, 1981.

Kleirfeld, D. M. Identification of foam cells in human atherosclerotic lesions as macrophages using monoclonal antibodies. *Arch. Pathol. Lab. Med.* 109:445, 1985.

Mitchinson, M. J., and Ball, R. Y. Macrophages and atherogenesis. *Lancet* 1:146, 1987.

Intravascular Thrombogenesis and Thrombolysis

A major challenge in contemporary cardiology is the regulation of intravascular thrombogenesis and the dissolution of intravascular thrombi. The challenge is vexatious because a balanced intrinsic action and a reaction system maintains the normal fluidity of blood, yet the systems must respond promptly to locally perturbing imbalances. Thus, at sites of arterial or venous wall injury, thrombogenesis is induced by activation of blood coagulation stimulated by blood platelet aggregation, which, in turn, activates processes involved in the dissolution of an intravascular thrombus. With intense vascular wall injury, the reaction systems (thrombolysis) are often inadequate, and systemic drug intervention is required to avoid the consequences of serious and, at times, lethal thrombogenesis.

Intravascular Blood Coagulation: Thrombogenesis

Thrombogenesis in vivo is the result of a series of steps leading to the production of a fibrin clot (Fig. 6-1). It occurs at sites of endothelial cell destabilization that activate either the intrinsic or extrinsic pathway leading to the conversion of fibrinogen to fibrin. In the intrinsic pathway, the proenzyme factor XII, or the Hageman factor, is converted to the enzyme factor XIIa. In turn, factor XIIa converts factor XI to XIa. The subsequent coagulation reactions proceed on the surface of blood platelets. Factor XIa activates factor IX to IXa and, in the presence of factor VIII and platelet phospholipid and calcium (Ca^{2+}), activates factor X to Xa. Alternatively, factor X can be activated by products of the extrinsic pathway. With tissue injury, tissue thromboplastin (factor III) is released to form a complex with and activate factor VII, which, in the presence of Ca^{2+}, activates factor X. Activation of a tissue thromboplastin and of factor X with tissue injury requires a few seconds, while activation via the intrinsic pathway requires many minutes.

Activated factor X plus Ca^{2+}, factor V, and platelet phospholipid activate factor II (prothrombin), which is then cleaved to form thrombin. The thrombin is detached from the platelet surface and converts fibrinogen (factor I) to fibrin. In this latter conversion, two peptides are removed from each of the α (fibrinopeptides A) and β (fibrinopeptide B) chains, and spontaneous gelation of fibrin monomers then follows. After gelation, the fibrin polymer is stabilized by covalent bonds that confer relative resistance to proteolysis by plasmin.

This complicated series of reactions making up the intrinsic or extrinsic system amplifies and enhances activity severalfold at each stage. Such amplification is essential, since a gradual generation of thrombin with a slow conversion of fibrinogen to fibrin would prove ineffective, as platelet aggregates and fibrin threads are swept along by the rapidly moving bloodstream.

```
                    ┌─────────┐
                    │ Tissue  │
                    │ injury  │
                    └─────────┘
         Intrinsic pathway   Extrinsic pathway
                    ↓              ↓
                Factor XII    Release of tissue
Destabilized endothelium  (Hageman)   Thromboplastin (factor III)
     or                      ↓
Subendothelial collagen  Factor XIIa
                                     Factor VII ──→
         Factor XI ──→ Factor XIa    Ca²⁺ ──→

         Factor IX ──→ Factor IXa
         Factor VIII ──→
         Platelet phospholipid ──→
         Ca²⁺ ──→

                  Factor X ──→ Factor Xa
                  Factor V →
                  Platelet phospholipid →
                  Ca²⁺ →

                  Prothrombin ──→ Thrombin
                  (factor II)
                        Fibrinogen ──→ Fibrin
```

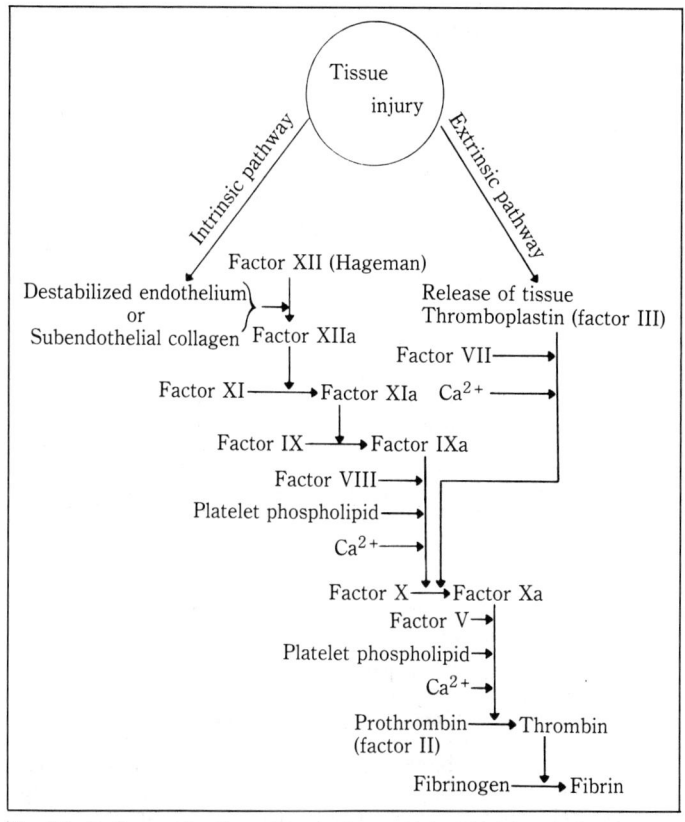

Fig. 6-1. Pathways for thrombogenesis: rapid (extrinsic) and slow (intrinsic). Factor X is activated from either the intrinsic or extrinsic pathway. Activated factor X in the presence of Ca^{2+}, factor V, and platelet phospholipid activates prothrombin to form thrombin. (From J. Hirsh. *Advances in Antithrombotic Therapy*. Monograph by Du Pont Pharmaceuticals, 1984.)

The body has a number of natural anticoagulants that serve to maintain the fluidity of blood. Key in the scheme of natural anticoagulants is the intact vascular endothelium. Thrombomodulin, a cell-surface thrombin-binding protein, converts thrombin into a protein C activator (Fig. 6-2). Protein C is a vitamin K-dependent glycoprotein that activates the fibrinolytic system by cleaving factors V and VIII and by releasing plasminogen activator from the endothelium. (Activated protein C functions as an anticoagulant by inactivating factors VIIIa and Va. A monoclonal-antibody assay to measure protein C levels [4.03 μg per ml] and levels from 55- to 65% of normal are consistent with heterozygous deficiency. However, detection of low protein C levels were not detectably associated with a risk of thrombosis [35]. The development of assays of protein C activation should

```
Intrinsic pathway
       |
Factor IX ──→ Factor IXa
Factor VIII ──→         ←──────┐
Platelet phospholipids ──→     │
Ca²⁺ ──→                       │
                               │
Factor X ──→ Factor Xa         │        ──→ Thrombomodulin
Factor V ──→       ←──┐        │   Protein C ↘ Activated
Platelet phospholipids ──→     │              protein C
Ca²⁺ ──→                       │   Endothelial cell
Prothrombin ──→ Thrombin
       Fibrinogen ──→ Fibrin
```

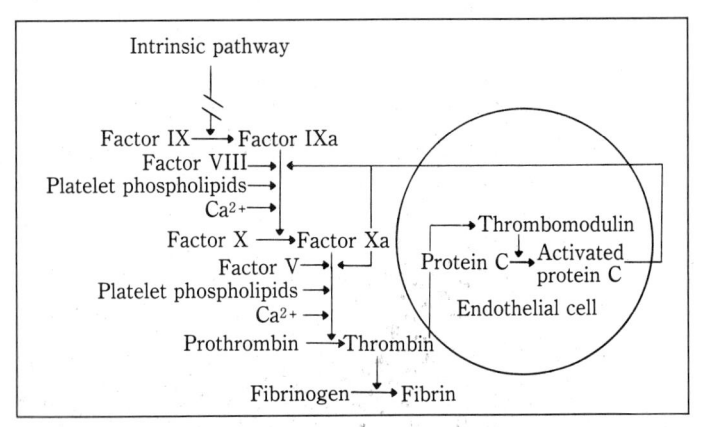

Fig. 6-2. Protein C, a natural anticoagulant, on the surface of endothelial cells through an endothelial cell receptor, thrombomodulin. Activated protein C counteracts factors VIII and V of the intrinsic coagulation pathway and thereby limits the generation of thrombin (From J. Hirsh. *Advances in Antithrombotic Therapy.* Monograph by Du Pont Pharmaceuticals, 1984.)

provide an important index of a predisposition to thrombosis formation in vivo.)

Another anticoagulant product of the intact endothelial cells is the surface heparin/heparan molecules. These molecules bind circulating antithrombin III. Antithrombin III, an α_2-proteinase inhibitor, is a glycoprotein that binds directly to the serine active site of thrombin, inhibits coagulation, and neutralizes thrombin and factor Xa. In many instances, thromboembolic disease is the clinical manifestation of anti-thrombin III deficiency.

α_2-macroglobulin, a tetrahedral glycoprotein, functions primarily as a protease inhibitor backup and acts via a steric entrapment of proteinases. A rapid clearing of proteinase α_2-macroglobulin complex by macrophages and the reticuloendothelial system then follows.

α_2-antiplasmin is a glycoprotein that functions as a primary inhibitor of plasmin (see section on intravascular thrombolysis below) and acts by blocking lysine-binding sites of fibrinogen crosslinked into clot.

Intravascular Thrombolysis

Resolution of a thrombus requires an enzymatically catalyzed reaction leading to a breakdown of the fibrin clot. The system consists of: (1) circulating plasminogen, a proenzyme; (2) enzymes in blood, endothelial cells, and tissues (i.e., tissue-type plasminogen activator [t-PA], which converts plasminogen to plasmin); and (3) natural inhibitors of plasmin or t-PA (Fig. 6-3).

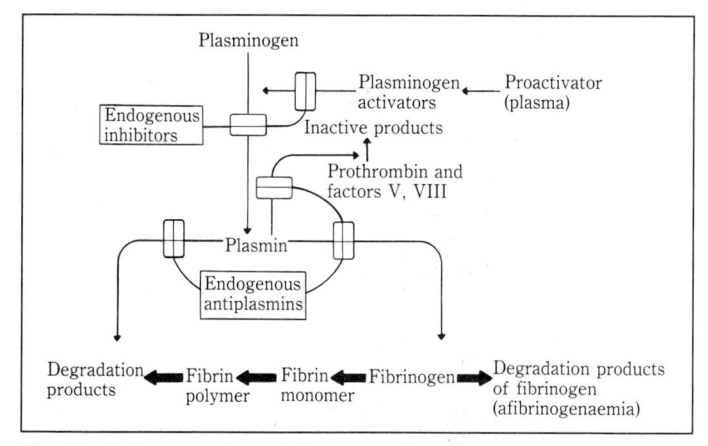

Fig. 6-3. Endogenous fibrinolytic system. Proactivator plasminogen is converted to plasminogen and then to plasmin, a proteolytic enzyme with selectivity for fibrinogen and degradation products of the fibrin polymer. The numerous sites for endogenous inhibition or antiplasmins are shown in the inset rectangles.

Activators of plasminogen, such as t-PA, are released by local trauma, thrombi, or other stimuli such as neurohumoral factors. Plasmin is a member of the serine protease class of proteolytic enzymes and digests fibrin as well as fibrinogen to fibrinogen degradation products (Fig. 6-3). Fibrinogen degradation products, in turn, inhibit the conversion of fibrinogen to fibrin. Plasmin also hydrolyzes prothrombin; factors V, VIII, and XII; the first component of complement; and prekallikrein. The natural plasmin inhibitors in blood, such as α_2-antiplasmin, limit the action of plasmin and reduce the amounts of the serine proteases so that plasma plasmin levels are immeasurable.

Most important for restricting plasmin action to fibrin is the avid binding of plasminogen to the t-PA fibrin complex through plasminogen-lysine binding sites. Thus, plasminogen is not readily converted to plasmin in the circulation but is converted to plasmin at the fibrin surface of the clot. Fibrin greatly enhances t-PA activation of plasminogen, since the forming plasmin is inhibited relatively slowly by α_2-antiplasmin as the lysine binding sites of plasmin are occupied by fibrin. By these processes, plasmin digests fibrin before enzyme inhibition occurs. With the breakdown of fibrin, the products, along with the activator and remaining plasmin, are released into the blood and bound by inhibitors, thus preventing fibrinolysis in the systemic circulation.

Convergence of Tissue Kinins, Complement Activation, Thrombogenesis, and Thrombolysis

A source of unceasing admiration is the convergence of powerful and self-catalyzing processes initiated by tissue injury — for

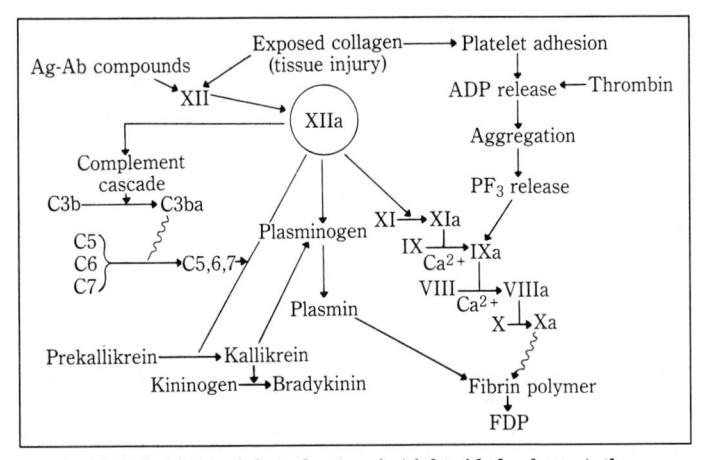

Fig. 6-4. Interrelation of thrombogenesis (right-sided columns), thrombolysis (center), complement activation, and kinin activation (left-sided columns): Plasma factor XII (three peptide chains joined by disulfide bonds) becomes activated by collagen, vascular membrane, and antigen-antibody (Ag-Ab) compounds and joins to the high molecular weight kininogen (prekallikrein) to become an enzyme with a specificity for factor XI.

example, cellular chemotaxis, thrombogenesis, and thrombolysis (see Fig. 6-4). Tissue injury activates local kinins and initiates the complement cascade to regulate blood flow and cell attraction (chemotaxis) to the site. Once the cells arrive, they release cytokines (i.e., interleukins) for cell-cell interactions. Consequently, antagonistic systems of thrombogenesis and thrombolysis are activated by factors common to the kinins and complement systems. The convergence of these complex processes is ample testimony of the incredible capability of vascular tissue to respond to injury and to initiate and modulate responses that maintain the integrity of and remodel arteries and veins as dynamic conduits for blood transportation.

Blood Platelets

Blood platelets are fascinating circulating complex organelles (1–5 microns in length) number 150–400,000/ml of blood and are derived from the bone megakaryocytes. Blood platelets remain in the circulation for approximately 10 days. In their day-to-day circulation, platelets do not adhere to each other, nor do they attach to the endothelial surface. Dramatic changes in platelet status, however, follow disruption or alteration of the endothelial surface of arteries and veins. Then platelets aggregate and adhere to the modified endothelial cells or to the underlying basement membrane collagen.

AGGREGATION AND/OR ADHESION

Platelet aggregation and/or adhesion initiates a secretory process during which subcellular granules are extruded, and mitogenic (platelet-derived growth factor) and permeability factors, proteolytic enzymes, adenosine diphosphate (ADP), serotonin, histamine, antiheparin, β-thromboglobulin, and epinephrine are released. Aggregation activates phospholipase A_2, which acts on the platelet membrane phospholipids to catalyze the release of arachidonic acid, the substrate for the cyclo-oxygenase product, cyclic endoperoxide prostaglandins (PGG_2 and PGH_2). PGG_2 is subsequently converted to thromboxane A_2 (TxA_2) by thromboxane synthetase and PGH_2 is converted to PGE_2. (See Chap. 4 for details on prostaglandin formation.)

Aggregate platelets participate in thrombogenesis by releasing platelet factor 3 (PF_3) (see Fig. 6-4) and by providing a lipid or lipoprotein surface that protects coagulation enzymes from inactivation by plasma proteinase inhibitors. Consequently, fibrin formation is localized within and around aggregated platelets. Additionally, coagulation proteins are present in the α-granules of platelets (fibrinogen, factors V and VIII, and platelet factor 3, in the cytosol (factor XIII), and in the membrane (factor XI). Finally, the platelet surface contributes to surface-mediated zymogen activation of plasma factors XII, XI, X, and prothrombin (factor II).

Although many drugs interfere with platelet function, the three most commonly used are aspirin, dipyridamole, and sulfinpyrazone.

ANTIPLATELET THERAPY

Antiplatelet agents, or antithrombotic drugs, suppress platelet function and are used primarily for arterial thrombotic disease.

Aspirin

Acetylsalicylic acid inhibits adenosine diphosphate (ADP) release and thereby decreases platelet aggregation and synthesis of TxA_2 and PGE_2 by irreversibly inhibiting cyclo-oxygenase for the life of the platelet. The net effect is to reduce the release and the subsequent aggregation of platelets. The results of several large multicenter transient ischemic attacks showed a substantial reduction in the number of attacks and a decrease in strokes and deaths in patients using 1–1.3 gm daily of aspirin [22]. The reduction of death was predominantly in men. However, the studies did not answer the question of the optimal dose or the value of low-dose aspirin. Aspirin is ineffective in the secondary prevention of stroke and has unproven benefit in the secondary prevention of myocardial infarction (MI).

Dipyridamole

The distinctive chemical compound, the pyrimidopyrimidine ring, was introduced as a general smooth muscle relaxant.

USES AND/OR ACTIONS

A summary of prospective comparisons of aspirin plus dipyridamole with aspirin alone was produced by Fitzgerald [15] and is reproduced as Table 6-1. No benefit was shown for combining aspirin with dipyridamole in treatment of transient ischemic attacks or in preventing strokes. The combination of aspirin and dipyridamole prevents early and late occlusion of saphenous vein aortocoronary bypass grafts (see below) and, when combined with a vitamin K antagonist anticoagulant (coumadin), may reduce the thromboembolism complications of prosthetic heart valves.

Dipyridamole usually does not significantly alter systemic blood pressure or blood flow in peripheral arteries. The drug increases coronary blood flow by selective dilatation of the coronary arteries. Dipyridamole purportedly stimulates the synthesis of prostacyclin (PGI_2) by vascular endothelium, inhibits cellular uptake and metabolism of adenosine, and increases the PGI_2 concentration at the platelet-vascular interface. Dipyridamole may augment the platelet-inhibiting action of aspirin. However, evidence in support of these latter actions of dipyridamole are contentious.

In rare clinical situations, dipyridamole decreases blood pressure and increases heart rate and cardiac output, largely as the result of dilatation of systemic resistance vessels.

Table 6-1. Prospective comparisons of aspirin and dipyridamole

Event	Dose/day Aspirin	Dipyridamole	Combination vs. aspirin alone	Comments
TIA, stroke	1 gm	225 mg	No difference	Both superior to placebo
TIA, stroke	325 mg	75 mg	No difference	No placebo group
Coronary-graft occlusion	975 mg	225 mg	No difference	
Peripheral vascular disease	330 mg	75 mg	Combination superior	Both superior to placebo More stenosing lesions in aspirin group before therapy

Key: TIA = transient ischemic attack.
Source: G. A. Fitzgerald. Drug therapy: Dipyridamole. Reprinted, with permission of *The New England Journal of Medicine* (316:1247, 1987).

PHARMACOKINETICS

Absorption and Distribution

Absorption is highly variable and may be low. Peak plasma concentrations using 50, 75, or 100 mg preparations showed a 7- to 15-fold variation.

Dipyridamole is highly bound to albumin and α_1-acid glycoprotein (91–99%). Uptake and binding to platelets is relatively slow.

Metabolism and Elimination

Dipyridamole is eliminated by biliary excretion as a glucaronide conjugate. Elimination is a triexponential function, with a terminal half-life of 10 hours. Dipyridamole is subject to enterohepatic recirculation. These elimination characteristics provide the rationale for a twice daily drug dosing.

Dipyridamole inhibits phosphodiesterase, the enzyme that degrades cyclic adenosine monophosphate (cAMP). The increase in cAMP levels stimulates PGI_2 synthesis and inhibits platelet aggregation and function.

ADVERSE EFFECTS

At the recommended doses of dipyridamole, reactions, in general, are minimal and transient.

Cardiovascular

Rarely, angina pectoris is aggravated with the initial doses of the drug.

Gastrointestinal

Approximately 10% of patients experience mild gastrointestinal distress.

Other

Approximately 10% of patients experience headaches, dizziness, nausea, flushing, or skin rashes.

PRECAUTIONS

Peripheral vasodilation leading to hypotension and syncope can occur.

DOSAGES

50 mg 3 times a day recommended for antiplatelet activity.

DOSAGE FORMS AND STRENGTHS AVAILABLE

Persantin (Boerhringer Ingelheim) **Tablets:** 25, 50, and 75 mg.
Generic tablets: 25, 50, and 75 mg.

Sulfinpyrazone

Sulfinpyrazone is a nonsteroidal anti-inflammatory drug related to phenylbutazone that was developed as a treatment for chronic gout. It is a powerful uricosuric agent.

USES AND/OR ACTIONS

Sulfinpyrazone, a potent inhibitor of renal tubular reabsorption of uric acid, prolongs platelet survival time, inhibits platelet release of ADP induced by collagen and epinephrine, and reduces platelet adherences to endothelial cells. The mode of action on platelets is uncertain; it may be a weak inhibitor of prostaglandin synthesis. Sulfinpyrazone reduces thrombotic complications of arteriovenous cannulae and early occlusion of saphenous vein aortocoronary grafts. Its reported benefit in the prevention of a second MI remains controversial.

PHARMACOKINETICS

Absorption and Distribution

The drug is well absorbed after oral administration and is bound to plasma proteins (98–99%). The uricosuric effect may persist for as long as 10 hours.

Elimination

Approximately half of the dose appears in the urine within 24 hours as the unchanged drug. Most of the drug (90%) appears in the urine in an unchanged form.

ADVERSE EFFECTS

Gastrointestinal

Sulfinpyrazone causes gastrointestinal irritation (10–15%) and should not be given to patients with peptic ulcer disease.

Hypersensitivity Reactions

Rash, fever, and, rarely, depressed hematopoiesis may occur. These symptoms disappear upon discontinuance of the drug.

DRUG INTERACTIONS

The drug should be used with great caution if administered with simultaneously administered sulfonamides, as the drugs potentiate each other.

DOSAGES

400 mg in divided daily doses.

DOSAGE FORMS AND STRENGTHS AVAILABLE

Anturane (CIBA) **Tablets:** 100 mg and **capsules,** 200 mg.

Thrombus

Thrombi can be divided into three types:

1. Those that occur in areas of slow and disturbed flow — for example, in the deep veins. Such thrombi are composed primarily of fibrin, red blood cells, and a minimal number of platelets and are referred to as *coagulation thrombi*.
2. Those forming in areas of moderate but disturbed flow — for example, atria with atrial fibrillation; tend to be a mixture of fibrin, platelets, and red cells.
3. Those forming in high-flow systems — for example, arteries; are mainly platelet aggregates that are referred to as *white or platelet thrombi*.

Thrombi within arteries develop on top of and are complications of a perturbed atherosclerotic plaque. The most common sites for intra-arterial thrombi are destabilized plaques in: (1) coronary arteries and (2) cerebral arteries. Less frequent sites are renal arteries and the abdominal aorta. Thrombi within coronary arteries resulting in greater than 50% reduction of the lumen diameter are usually located in the proximal third of the three major epicardial vessels: left anterior descending (LAD), right (RCA), and circumflex (CxA) vessels. The perturbed or destabilized atherosclerotic plaques result from intramural hemorrhage, plaque fissuring, or balloon angioplasty. From clinical evidence (including angiography, surgery, and thrombolytic drug response), perhaps 90% of patients develop an acute transmural MI as the consequence of a proximally located occlusive thrombus in the coronary artery. In addition, judging from angiographic evidence (thrombogenesis) and levels of thrombus-derived fibrinopeptide A (thrombolysis) in plasma, intracoronary thrombi must be in a dynamic state of formation and dissolution during the initial 24 hours of a transmural MI.

Atherosclerosis obstruction and thrombus formation in coronary arteries are end-stage morphologic events in the natural history of ischemic heart disease. The thrombotic-related component of ischemic heart disease was assessed in a prospective manner in 1511 Caucasion males 40–64 years of age [34]. Subsequently, 109 experienced their first major ischemic heart-disease event. High levels of factor VII and fibrinogen proved to be more closely associated with the subsequent appearance of ischemic heart disease than serum cholesterol (by one standard deviation). The risk of ischemic heart disease in individuals with high fibrinogen levels was greater in young than older men. Myocardial infarction and spontaneous intravascular thrombogenesis is reported with factor XII deficiency (factor XII is important in plasminogen-dependent fibrinolysis) (see Fig. 6-4).

Thrombi formed in high flow systems, such as arteries, are composed of platelet aggregates held together by strands of fibrin and are referred to as platelet or white thrombi. As the thrombus attracts more platelets because of its roughened surface, strands of fibrin tend to extend from the thrombus and attract red blood cells. Such "red tails" are readily detached and pass forward as emboli.

VASCULAR ENDOTHELIUM

Originally perceived as a passive surface, the endothelial cells are now known to influence and perhaps regulate arterial wall contraction and relaxation and structural wall remodeling. Endothelial cells actively inhibit blood clot formation. As referred to in the above discussion, two distinct anticoagulant mechanisms are triggered by contact with the endothelial cell surface: (1) surface heparin-heparan molecules, which bind circulating antithrombin III to accelerate the inactivation of coagulation proteases and (2) the production of a thrombin-binding protein, thrombomodulin, which alters the macromolecular specificity of thrombin and decreases its clot-forming catalysis.

Endothelial cells are the major source of the important prostaglandin prostacyclin (PGI_2). PGI_2 inhibits platelet aggregation and activation by raising platelet cyclic adenosine monophosphate. Ultimately, the relative rates of PGI_2 (endothelial cell) and TxA_2 (platelet) production may determine whether platelets aggregate onto endothelial cells.

SITES OF INTRAVASCULAR THROMBOGENESIS

Although thrombi may develop at various sites in the cardiovascular system, they present most commonly in the deep veins of the extremities, the endocardial surfaces (atria, ventricles, or valves), and in coronary and cerebral arteries.

A common site for thrombus formation is the deep veins of the extremities. Venous flow in the lower extremities depends on the contraction of surrounding skeletal muscles as they assist the antegrade passage of blood towards the heart. Venous disease or age-related changes that render venous valves incompetent, physical inactivity, prolonged sitting or bedrest (illness or surgery), and congestive heart failure, all reduce the venous blood flow and favor eddies, whirlpools, and stasis. Together, these factors increase the force and frequency of platelet collision, probably in the venous valve cusp pockets, and activate factors that are critical for platelets to become sticky. Aside from the local reaction to venous thrombosis, the major complication of deep vein thrombosis in the lower extremity is a life-threatening pulmonary emboli.

Since thrombus formation in the venous system results from reduced blood flow, the thrombi formed are coagulation thrombi. Coagulation thrombi consist of a loose fibrin matrix that traps large quantities of red blood cells and minimal numbers of leukocytes and platelets.

Thrombi may develop within the cardiac chambers in areas with regional reductions in atrial or ventricular contractility. Thrombi may also develop on the surfaces of diseased (rheumatic, myxoid degeneration) or artificial valves. The greatest risk of intracardiac thrombi is in shedding pulmonary, systemic, or cerebral emboli. In the atria or ventricles, where disturbance of blood flow is moderate, thrombi are a mixture of fibrin, red blood cells, and platelets.

Coronary artery thrombi or platelet (white) thrombi will be dealt with in greater detail in following pages.

Anticoagulants

Two major classes of anticoagulants, heparin and vitamin K antagonists, retard liver synthesis of clotting factors or accelerate their inactivation. By inhibiting thrombin generation, anticoagulants prevent or limit thrombogenesis.

MONITORING THE COAGULATION STATE

Anticoagulant therapy must be constantly monitored by appropriate coagulation tests. The five common coagulation tests are:

I. Bleeding time (modified Ivy method)
   A. Place a sphygmomanometer around the patient's upper arm and inflate to 300 mm Hg.
   B. With a disposable lancet, make three puncture wounds on the extensor surface of the forearm and start a stopwatch.
   C. Gently blot the bleeding points every 15 seconds with filter paper until bleeding has stopped from all three points.
   Normal: 7 minutes or less
II. Venous clotting time (Lee-White method)
   A. Perform venipuncture and start stopwatch as blood enters the syringe.
   B. Deliver 1 ml of blood to each of three 12 × 75 mm glass test tubes and incubate in a water bath at 37°C.
   C. After 5 minutes, incline the first tube gently to 90° and continue to do this every 1–2 minutes until clotting occurs. Handle the second and third tubes in the same manner. The venous clotting time is reported as the average clotting time of the second and third tubes.
   Normal: 6–15 minutes
III. Prothrombin time (One-step, quick)
   A. Blood is withdrawn into a solution containing oxalate, which precipitates Ca^{2+}.
   B. Incubate 0.1 ml plasma for 30–60 seconds.
   C. Add 0.2 ml Ortho brain thromboplastin (containing Ca^{2+}) and start stopwatch.
   Normal: 11–12 seconds
IV. Activated partial thromboplastin time (APTT) The partial thromboplastin time test is used to assess heparin effect; APT extracted from brain. Ca^{2+} and APT are added to the patients' plasma to determine clotting time. APT mimics factor XI and, thus, provides a sensitive test of stage 1 of the coagulation scheme.
   A. Take 0.1 ml cephalin (Ortho thrombofax reagent).
   B. Add 0.1 ml plasma and incubate 30–60 seconds.

C. Add 0.1 ml celite and wait exactly 60 seconds.
D. Add 0.1 ml CaCl$_2$ and start stopwatch.
Normal: 16–20 seconds

Heparin

USES AND/OR ACTIONS

Heparin, a negatively charged and highly sulfated mucopolysaccharide, is synthesized and stored in mast cell granules and extracted from bovine lung or porcine mucosal tissue. Commercial heparin is a straight chain anionic polysaccharide of variable molecular weight and, depending on the animal tissue source, may have differing physiologic and antigenic properties.

Heparin binds irreversibly to the lysine residue of a naturally occurring plasma protease inhibitor that is identical to activated factor X (Xa) and heparin cofactor antithrombin III (AT-III) (see above), producing a complex with a higher affinity for serine proteases than AT-III. Small amounts of heparin interact with AT-III to inactivate factor Xa and thereby prevent the conversion of prothrombin to thrombin; this is the basis for "low-dose therapy." Larger amounts of heparin interact with and inactivate the clotting factors XIIa, XIa, IXa, and kallikrein and prevent the conversion of fibrinogen to fibrin.

Heparin also reduces postprandial lipemia by activating lipoprotein lipase.

PHARMACOKINETICS

Metabolism

Heparin is metabolized mainly in the liver by heparinase and is excreted by the kidneys. Approximately 50% may be eliminated unchanged, particularly with large doses. The duration of action is dose-dependent; IV doses of 100, 200, and 400 units/kg have half-lives of 56, 96, and 152 minutes, respectively.

ADVERSE EFFECTS

Bleeding

The most important side effect of heparin administration is bleeding, and it occurs in approximately 5% of patients with therapeutic doses.

Drug-induced immune thrombocytopenia (2–5% of patients), a mild reduction in plasma platelet counts, is often associated with the induction of anticoagulation with heparin. The mild thrombocytopenia is probably due to a rapidly reversible platelet aggregation or sequestration. In some patients, the thrombocytopenia is profound and is promptly reversed upon the cessation of heparin therapy. Monitoring of plasma platelet counts is indicated in patients with hypersensitivity reactions or who seem to be likely to experience heparin refractoriness. The thrombocytopenia may appear after 3–4 days or may be delayed for a few weeks. It may be associated with increased immunoglobulins, that is, IgG and complement C3 levels, suggesting a heparin-mediated and complement-related platelet injury. Unlike the simple hypersensitivity reaction, the immune thrombocytopenia occurs more commonly with bovine-derived than porcine-derived heparin.

Hypersensitivity Reactions

Reactions consist of facial flush, urticaria, substernal distress, and asthmaticlike episodes. Because these individuals appear to have tolerance for epinephrine, an initial dose of 0.25 ml of 1:1000 dilution may need to be repeated for relief of symptoms.

Other

Other rare reactions include osteoporosis and spontaneous fractures when heparin is continued for at least 6 months, alopecia, and arterial thrombosis secondary to heparin-induced thrombocytopenia.

PRECAUTIONS

Pregnancy/Lactation

Since heparin cannot penetrate cell membranes, it does not cross the placenta or enter breast milk. The use of heparin during pregnancy is, however, associated with increased incidence of maternal hemorrhage, stillbirth, and prematurity.

DOSAGE REQUIREMENTS

Full-dose heparin is usually administered by intermittent, subcutaneous, or IV routes (intermittent injections, continuous drip, or constant infusion pump). Heparin is inactive when used orally. The IV route is preferred, although continuous infusion and intermittent injections appear to be equally effective in preventing thromboembolism.

In a prospective study of more than 200 patients, 140 receiving intermittent IV and 69 receiving a continuous infusion of heparin, major bleeding was 7 times more frequent in the intermittent groups than in the continuous infusion group. In addition, one-fourth less heparin was required in the continuous than in the intermittent groups. [18].

The onset of the anticoagulant effect is immediate following IV bolus injection of full therapeutic doses and occurs 20–30 minutes after subcutaneous injection. With continuous infusion, a 2– to 3–hour delay in the onset of the anticoagulant effect is avoided by injecting an initial bolus of 5000 units.

Heparin is oftentimes given for 7 or 10 days, and an oral anticoagulant is added during the last 3 or 4 days (see below).

MONITORING HEPARIN THERAPY

Present evidence indicates that repeated blood sampling with subcutaneous heparin for monitoring purposes (see below) is not required. However, since the response to heparin varies from patient to patient, one or two tests should be performed initially. Constant monitoring is required for IV heparin. Tests used to monitor heparin therapy are the whole blood clotting time (Lee-White), partial thromboplastin time (PTT), or activated partial thromboplastin time (APTT). The APTT is the most widely accepted.

Experimentally-induced thrombosis is prevented at values of APTT that are 1½–2 times normal (normal value of 40 seconds increase to 60–80 seconds).

DOSAGES

The dosage should be prescribed in units rather than in milligrams because the U.S.P. standard for potency is 120 units/mg of dry lung material and 140 units/mg dry weight of other sources. Most commercial preparations range from 140–190 units/mg. Consequently, doses expressed in milligrams have no therapeutic meaning. Additionally, the USP unit is approximately 10% greater than the international unit (IU), and this difference must be taken into account when dosing a patient.

Small doses usually are given to prevent thromboembolism; large doses are required to prevent propagation of a thrombus. Maximum large doses are required to block the thrombin-platelet interaction in acute pulmonary embolism.

IV infusion: *Adults:* initially, 5000 units into the tubing after starting the infusion; then 20,000–30,000 units daily at an initial rate of 0.5 unit/kg/min in 5% dextrose or isotonic sodium chloride. The rate is subsequently adjusted according to the results of clotting time tests.
Children: initially, 50 units/kg followed by 100 units/kg every four hours.
Intermittent IV: *Adult:* initially, 5000 units and 5000–10,000 units every 4–6 hours.
Subcutaneous: *Adult* (low-dose prophylaxis): 5000 units 2 hours before surgery and every 12 hours thereafter until patient is discharged or fully ambulatory. For full dose effects, adults require 10,000–20,000 units every 12 hours. At different sites (around iliac crest or over lower abdomen), a small needle (-27) and the smallest volume limits the complicating hematoma.
Intramuscular: Should not be used, as it causes tissue irritation, local bleeding, or hematoma, and the absorption is unpredictable.

Low-dose or mini-dose heparin as a prophylaxis during the postoperative period should take into consideration:

Hemostatic competence of the patient as revealed by the hematocrit, platelet count, prothrombin time, and partial thromboplastin time (see below).
Risk of bleeding, even with the low-dose heparin, particularly if

patients are receiving oral anticoagulants or platelet antiaggregating agents.

Low-dose heparin is inadequate during an active thrombotic process.

Indications for use of low-dose heparin to prevent deep vein thrombosis are:

Following abdominal, thoracic, or gynecologic surgery
Myocardial infarction with congestive heart failure
Non-hemorrhagic strokes
Acute respiratory failure

Individual Antithrombotic Drugs

Heparin Calcium

DOSAGE FORMS AND STRENGTHS AVAILABLE

Calciparine (American Critical Care) **sterile solutions:** 5000, 12,500, and 20,000 from porcine intestinal mucosa.

Heparin Sodium

DOSAGE FORMS AND STRENGTHS AVAILABLE

Generic solutions: 1000, 2500, 5000, 7500, 10,000, 15,000, 20,000, and 40,000 units/ml.
Liquaemin Sodium (Organon) 1000, 5000, 10,000, 20,000, and 40,000 units/ml.

Treatment of Heparin-Mediated Response or Toxicity

Protamine Sulfate

USES AND/OR ACTIONS

Protamine sulfate, with its strong electropositive charge, binds to and inactivates the negatively charged heparin to form a stable complex. Protamine has an anticoagulant action and prolongs clotting time.

Protamine sulfate is used to counteract heparin doses that cause hemorrhage or increase the risk of hemorrhage. Each milligram of protamine neutralizes 90–100 USP units of heparin activity. The reaction is almost instantaneous, and the effect persists for approximately 2 hours. Since the heparin effect may last longer than 2 hours, the need for blocking may reappear and a second protamine injection is necessary.

ADVERSE EFFECTS

Protamine is usually well tolerated and as much as 200 mg has been given in 2 hours with no untoward side effects. To prevent thrombotic complications, no more than 50 mg should be administered as a single bolus. Standard doses of protamine used to reverse the heparin effect (post-angiography or post-cardiopulmonary bypass) may reduce platelet number and function, and these platelet effects correlate positively with a prolongation of the bleeding time [56].

PRECAUTIONS

Diabetic patients treated with protamine zinc insulin are particularly sensitive to protamine. Hypersensitivity reactions may occur in patients allergic to fish, since protamine is obtained from salmon.

TOXICITY

Toxic manifestations include acute hypotension, dyspnea, and bradycardia.

DOSAGES

IV: *Adult:* total dose is based on the amount of heparin given over the previous 3–4 hours (mg protamine sulfate, dry material); neutralizes not less than 80 USP heparin units (lung tissue) and not less than 100 USP heparin units (intestinal mucosa). A solution of 10 mg/ml is injected slowly over 1–3 minutes, not to exceed 50 mg/ml in any 10-minute period.
Generic powder: Solution 10 mg/ml in 5- and 25-ml containers.

Vitamin K Antagonists

USES AND/OR ACTIONS

Coumarin derivatives (dicumarol), warfarin sodium (coumadin, panwarfin), warfarin potassium (athrombin-K), indandione derivative, and anisindone (Miradon) resemble vitamin K in their chemistry and antagonize vitamin K in vivo. Since vitamin K is essential for liver production of coagulation factors, vitamin K antagonists are useful clinically as anticoagulants. Of these compounds, warfarin sodium is the most commonly used because of its predictable clinical effects, including bioavailability, onset of action, and duration of effect.

The coumarin and inandione compounds block a unique vitamin K-dependent posttranslational modification of factors II, VII, IX, and X. A vitamin K-dependent mechanism converts several glutamate residues in the above factors to gamma carboxyglutamic acid (GLa) residue. Vitamin K undergoes a cycle of oxidation and reduction (liver), and coumarin prevents the reduction reaction; oxidized vitamin K is ineffective in the gamma carboxylation reaction. The carboxylated residues are necessary for binding calcium (Ca^{2+}) and in facilitating the orientation of clotting factors on a phospholipid surface of platelets in the process of generating thrombin formation. With prolonged warfarin administration, carboxylation of vitamin K-dependent factors is impeded, Ca^{2+} binding is depressed, coagulation is retarded, and thrombin formation is reduced.

PHARMACOKINETICS

Absorption

The coumarin derivatives and indandione are administered orally but are incompletely and erratically absorbed from the gastrointestinal tract. The drugs have a dose-dependent plasma half-life. Coumadin is more readily and completely absorbed than dicumarol; however, there is considerable variation in absorption from one individual to another with each compound.

Metabolism

Within the circulation, the drugs are bound to albumin (99%) and are therefore distributed only in the blood compartment. The drugs have a slow rate of degradation. The drugs accumulate in the liver, spleen, and kidney. About 15–50% of a therapeutic dose is metabolized daily. There is a considerable delay (up to 48 hours) between the time of peak plasma levels and the therapeutic response, as measured by the prothrombin time. The delayed therapeutic response is due to variations in the half-life degradation of factors II, VII, IX, and X ranging from 6–60 hours.

Elimination

The coumadin class of drugs are metabolized via side chain reduction, ring oxidation, and glucuronidization by enzymes of the hepatic endoplasmic reticulum. The metabolites appear in the urine.

ADVERSE EFFECTS

Hemorrhage

Hemorrhagic complications are the major concerns with the vitamin K antagonists. Once bleeding develops, it may be necessary to discontinue the vitamin K antagonist and administer vitamin K: For mild bleeding, a single dose of 1–5 mg of phytonadione (vitamin K) IV or 10–20 mg PO, for severe bleeding, 20–40 mg IV with additional doses at 4-hour intervals, as necessary (see below). The peak effect of oral vitamin K is 4–8 hours. IV doses of vitamin K greater than 2–5 mg result in rebound hypercoagulability and resistance to oral vitamin K antagonists.

Skin

Infrequently, other reactions occur, including dermatitis and necrosis of the breast, buttocks, thighs, abdomen, calves, and skin. Skin lesions may have sharply demarcated necrotic centers surrounded by erythematous, diascopy-positive rims and may appear weeks or months after initiating the vitamin K antagonist. Purple toe syndrome, alopecia, gastrointestinal irritation, and elevated transaminase levels may develop.

Recurrent skin necrosis has been associated with protein C deficiency and is most commonly seen in obese females who are given a large loading dose.

PRECAUTIONS

Anticoagulants should be used cautiously in the presence of mild liver or kidney disease, alcoholism, infective endocarditis, and drainage tubes in any orifice and/or with a history of gastrointestinal ulcers.

Pregnancy/Lactation

If anticoagulants are required during pregnancy or lactation, then subcutaneous heparin is the agent of choice (dose limited to 10,000 units twice daily). Vitamin K antagonist anticoagulants cross the placental barrier and are associated with a high incidence rate of birth defects, particularly those involving the central nervous system. About one-third of fetuses are stillborn or, if born alive, are abnormal. Vitamin K antagonist (anticoagulants) appear in the milk of lactating women but are not hazardous to the nursing infant.

Pregnant women with cardiac valve prostheses present a unique anticoagulation problem. In one series of 72 pregnancies, three with a tilting-disk mitral valve prosthesis had thrombosis in and around the valve (two were fatal) during heparin treatment. Abortion rates were similar whether or not heparin was substituted for the vitamin K antagonist (sixth to twelfth week of gestation, group I; after the seventh week of gestation, group II; or vitamin K antagonist given throughout gestation, group III). Vitamin K-related embryopathy occurred in 25 and 30% of group II and III pregnancies. The findings suggested that vitamin K antagonists are contraindicated from the sixth to the twelfth weeks of gestation [24].

INTERACTIONS

A number of drugs significantly prolong or decrease the activities of oral vitamin K antagonists. These interactions are summarized in Table 6-2.

DOSAGE REQUIREMENTS

A large loading dose followed by a gradual reduction to a maintenance dose is **no longer recommended.** The loading dose primarily depresses factor VII, which has a half-life of 4–6 hours. Factors IX and X decrease more slowly, but at the same rate, with

Table 6-2. Drugs that affect anticoagulant activity

Drugs that increase anticoagulant activity by:

Displacement of warfarin from plasma proteins	Increasing warfarin receptor-site activity
Aspirin (> 3 gm/day) Phenylbutazone Mefenamic acid Oryphenbutazone Sulfinpyrazone Ethacrynic acid Clofibrate	Dextrothyroxine Enzyme inhibition Disulfiram

Drugs that decrease anticoagulant activity by:

Reducing liver eyzyme activity	Reducing gastrointestinal absorption	Increasing clotting factor
Barbiturates Glutethimide Phenytoin Griseofulvin	Cholestyramine Colestipol	Rifampin

smaller doses administered daily. Benefits of the vitamin K antagonists are related largely to depression of factors IX and X.

A most common practice of overlapping heparin with an oral vitamin K antagonist for 4 or 5 days to provide optimum protection against recurrence of intravascular thrombogenesis is strongly supported by recent observations. The vitamin K antagonist inhibits hepatic synthesis of coagulation factors II, VII, IX, and X, as well as protein C. Protein C is a proenzyme that is activated by thrombin on the endothelial surface via an endothelial cell receptor, thrombomodulin. In turn, activated protein C inhibits the activated forms of factors V and VIII (see Fig. 6-2). Consequently, depletion of protein C before reducing the formation of factors IX, X, and II actually renders the patient hypercoagulable. By inactivating the activated forms of factors VIII and V, protein C affects an anticoagulant activity and facilitates thrombin, thus serving as part of a negative feedback mechanism that limits its own generation.

Benefits of vitamin K antagonists are largely due to the depression of factors IX and X. Modest to small doses of the antagonist, monitored by changes in the daily prothrombin times, avoids hyper-response and precipitous decreases in factor VII that could lead to major bleeding and skin necrosis, a manifestation of protein C depletion. Avoiding a loading dose minimizes the danger of hemorrhage in unusually sensitive patients (e.g., after major surgery; elderly, malnourished, or debilitated patients; and patients with infections, liver disease, or congestive heart failure).

MONITORING VITAMIN K ANTAGONISTS

The one-stage (Quick) prothrombin time test is used to regulate the dose of these drugs. The test estimates the combined activities of the complex of prothrombin, factors V, VII, X, and, to a minor extent, fibrinogen. Factor VII is the most responsive factor to vitamin K antagonists and therefore acts as the determinant of a routine prothrombin time during the first few days of therapy. With prolonged therapy, factor X shows the lowest activity. Therapeutic ranges of oral anticoagulants should raise the one-stage prothrombin time to values 1½–2 times greater than the control when expressed in seconds.

While adjusting the dose of oral anticoagulants, prothrombin time should be determined 3 times during the first week, twice the second week, and then weekly until the maintenance dose is established. Thereafter, the maintenance dose should be evaluated monthly.

Caution is necessary in interpreting the one-stage prothrombin time test in patients receiving full-dose heparin plus an oral anticoagulant. Heparin may prolong the one-stage prothrombin time, and determining APTT and thrombin time may be necessary to monitor the effect of the two anticoagulants.

CONTRAINDICATIONS OF VITAMIN K ANTAGONIST

Blood dyscrasia
Ulcerative lesions of the gastrointestinal tract
Severe renal or hepatic disease
Severe hypertension with current or postencephalopathy
Bacterial endocarditis, acute or subacute

Dicumarol (Abbott)

DOSAGES

Adult: 200–300 mg on day 1, followed by 25–200 mg daily using the prothrombin time (Quick) determination as a guide. Frequent dose adjustments may be necessary during the first 7–14 days as per the results of daily prothrombin times. The maintenance dose varies from 25 to 150 mg daily.

DOSAGE FORMS AND STRENGTHS AVAILABLE

Generic tablets: 25 and 50 mg.

Warfarin Sodium

Warfarin sodium is the drug of choice for oral anticoagulation.

DOSAGES

Adult: first day, 15 mg; second day, 10 mg; and third day, 10 mg, with daily prothrombin tests (Quick and APTT). Maintenance —2.5–10 mg, per prothrombin tests.

DOSAGE FORMS AND STRENGTHS AVAILABLE

Coumadin (Du Pont) **tablets:** 2, 2.5, 5, 7.5, and 10 mg.
Panwarfin (Abbott) **tablets:** 2, 2.5, 5, 7.5, and 10 mg.

Therapy of Overdose of Vitamin K Antagonists (Phytonadione, K_1)

Major unrelenting bleeding after discontinuation of the anticoagulant requires vitamin K and phytonadione (vitamin K_1) (Aqua-MEPHYTON, Mephyton, and Konakion).

Vitamin K is concentrated in the chloroplasts of plant leaves and in many vegetable oils. Isolation and elucidation of the chemical structure indicates at least two substances, vitamin K_1 and K_2. Vitamin K_1, or phylloquinone, is found in plants and is the natural vitamin K available for therapeutic use.

USES AND/OR ACTIONS

Vitamin K is an essential cofactor for the hepatic microsomal enzyme system that converts multiple glutamic acid residues to gamma-carboxyglutamic acid residues in factors II, VII, IX, and X and protein C.

Phytonadione, the natural fat-soluble vitamin K, is the preferred preparation to reverse hypoprothrombinemia secondary to oral anticoagulants. It has a more prompt, potent, and prolonged effect than the vitamin K analogues. Phytonadione reverses moderately excessive actions of the oral anticoagulants. Doses of 0.5–10 mg partially correct the prothrombin time in approximately 4–6 hours, and full correction is in 24 hours. When further oral anticoagulants are not required, then up to 10 mg of phytonadione may be used (large doses increase the resistance to oral anticoagulants for several days). If further therapy with warfarin sodium is contemplated, doses of phytonadione should be limited to 0.5–1 mg. The oral and subcutaneous routes are preferred, since administration of the vitamin in this fashion is less likely to cause adverse reactions. The phytonadione doses should be as low as possible, and prothrombin times should be determined frequently, since rapid restoration of coagulability presents the same hazards of intravascular clotting that stimulated the initiation of anticoagulant therapy.

When immediate correction of hypoprothrombinemia is necessary, transfusion of plasma or plasma concentrates rich in stable vitamin K-dependent clotting factors is indicated. Fresh frozen plasma or blood components (factors Va, VIII, and IX) may be required to limit transfusing large volumes of plasma.

ADVERSE EFFECTS

IV injections of phytonadione may cause flushing, hyperhidrosis, substernal tightness, cyanosis, acute peripheral vascular failure, shock and hypersensitivity reactions. Injections may be fatal.

Subcutaneous or intramuscular injections may result in local nodule formation, pain, or hematoma.

DOSAGES

Adults and children: 2.5–25 mg in divided doses daily for adults as well as children

DOSAGE FORMS AND STRENGTHS AVAILABLE

Mephyton (Merck, Sharp and Dohme): **Tablets:** 5 mg.
Menadion (K_3) (Lilly): **Tablets:** 5 mg.
Menadiol Sodium Diphosphate (K_4) (Synkayvite) (Roche): **Tablets:** 5 mg.

INTRAVENOUS, INTRAMUSCULAR, AND SUBCUTANEOUS INJECTION

The preparation may be diluted with 5% dextrose, 0.9% sodium chloride, or 5% dextrose and sodium chloride. For IV use, injection should not exceed 1 mg/min and should be used when the severity of hemorrhage warrants rapid reversal of the anticoagulation. For mild overdose of anticoagulant, 0.5–5 mg should be used; for moderate overdose, up to 10 mg is used; and for severe hemorrhage, 25 mg. Slow IV administration, monitored by frequent prothrombin time determinations, is recommended.

DOSAGE FORMS AND STRENGTHS AVAILABLE

IV, IM, and SQ

AquaMEPHYTON (K_1) (Lily): 2 mg/ml in 0.5 ml (1 mg/0.5ml) containers and 10 mg/ml in 1, 2.5, and 5 ml containers.

IM

Konakion (K_1) (Roche): 2 mg/ml in 0.5 ml containers and 10 mg/ml in 1 ml containers (**intramuscular use only**).

Menadiol Sodium Diphosphate, Vitamin K_4

DOSAGES

PO, SQ, IM, and IV: *Adult:* 5–15 mg once or twice daily; *children:* 5–10 mg once or twice daily.

DOSAGE FORMS AND STRENGTHS AVAILABLE

Synkavite (Roche) **tablets:** 5 mg.
Synkavite (Roche) **solution ampules:** 1 ml (5 mg/ml), 1 ml (10 mg/ml), and 2 ml (75 mg/2 ml).

Clinical Use of Antithrombotic Drugs

VENOUS THROMBOSIS AND PULMONARY EMBOLISM — HEPARIN PLUS WARFARIN SODIUM REGIMEN

Uses and/or Actions

The primary and best established use of anticoagulants is in the prevention of pulmonary emboli as part of the treatment of deep vein thrombosis. Since deep vein thrombosis consists primarily of a large fibrin component and red cells, the drugs of choice in preventing the formation or extension of the thrombi are anticoagulants.

Patients with deep vein thrombosis are usually treated with heparin for 7–10 days and then with oral anticoagulants for a period of weeks to months to prevent pulmonary emboli. A sequence of heparin and warfarin sodium was first developed in animal models because of the delayed anticoagulation effect of the vitamin K antagonists when compared to heparin. Now, with the recognition of differences in the metabolic turnover of the coagulation factors, including protein C, the need for combined and sequential heparin and warfarin therapy is recognized and proceeds according to the following scheme:

Initial 7 days: IV heparin.
From 7 to 10 days: IV heparin plus oral warfarin.
From 10 days to 3 months: oral warfarin.
Patients with recurrent venous thrombosis require long-term anticoagulation with oral warfarin.

Diagnosis of Deep Vein Thrombosis

Deep vein thrombosis of the lower extremity produces two phenomena of diagnostic importance: (1) inflammation of the venous wall and (2) venous obstruction. Inflammation of the venous wall is recognized by local tenderness in the upper mid-thigh, without evidence of inguinal lymphadenopathy and with a systemic temperature of less than 101°F. Deep saphenous vein obstruction is recognized by a prominence of the lower leg veins, increase in leg girth, and pretibial edema.

Laboratory evidence in support of a thrombus in the deep veins of the lower extremity is provided by the radiofibrinogen technique or by impedance phlebographic and Doppler ultrasound methods. The radiofibrinogen technique relies on the incorporation of fibrinogen into the thrombus and its detection by surface counting. The technique requires an active thrombus and sufficient time and an appropriate target to achieve the desired target-to-background ratio. The procedure is particularly useful in the early detection and follow-up of venous thrombi. The technique fails with prior heparin use and does not detect thrombi in the upper deep veins of the thigh or in the pelvis.

The impedance phlebographic and Doppler ultrasound methods involve cuff obstruction to venous outflow, thereby inducing a pool of blood in the leg veins. Following the release of the cuff, the speed of blood exiting the leg is measured. The impedance method monitors the behavior of calf resistance, while the Doppler method measures frequency shifts in the ultrasound signal return from the femoral vein or other veins. Both techniques have a low specificity in identifying superficial vein thrombi, but both have a high sensitivity and specificity in identifying deep venous thrombotic obstruction in the lower extremity.

A third objective evidence of venous thrombi comes from contrast phlebography and is the only means for directly demonstrating a thrombus; the limitations are its invasive nature and the local irritation produced by the contrast media.

RISKS FOR DEEP SAPHENOUS VEIN THROMBOSIS

Risks for venous thrombus in a lower extremity are:

I. Post-surgery
  A. Hip and knee surgery
  B. Extensive pelvic surgery
  C. Major amputation of a lower extremity
II. Prolonged immobility
  A. Congestive heart failure
  B. Advanced age
III. Chronic lung disease

Diagnosis of Pulmonary Embolism

While the sequences of IV heparin and coumadin are the accepted therapeutic strategy for preventing pulmonary emboli secondary to deep vein thrombosis of the lower extremity, identifying patients with pulmonary emboli continues to be a major clinical challenge. Clues to diagnosis of pulmonary embolism include: (1) history of previous deep vein thrombosis, (2) development of dyspnea or pleuritic chest pain, and (3) appearance of tachypnea. If these clues are accompanied by hypotension and signs of acute cor pulmonale, IV heparin should be initiated before diagnostic procedures are completed (chest x ray, arterial blood gases, electrocardiogram, impedance plethysmograms of the lower extremity, perfusion, and ventilation lung scans). If pulmonary embolism is suspected without hypotension and the scans are normal, the heparin may be discontinued and other causes sought for the acute cor pulmonale. If scans are consistent with pulmonary embolism and impedance plethysmograms and blood gases are abnormal, heparin should be continued and the diagnosis of pulmonary emboli accepted. If the lung scans are equivocal (or positive) but blood gases and impedance plethysmogram are normal, a pulmonary arteriogram should be performed. If the arteriogram shows filling defects or cutoffs in the pulmonary arteries, the IV heparin-warfarin sequence should be followed for 3 months.

Adjusted doses of SQ heparin (initial dose of 15,000 U adjusted thereafter to prolong the APTT to 50–70 seconds) is an effective and safe alternative to continuous IV heparin [11].

Low-dose heparin is effective in preventing venous thrombosis and reducing the risk of pulmonary embolism in patients undergoing elective surgical procedures (bone fracture reduction and pinning, hip surgery, open urologic procedures, and gynecologic malignancy).

Antiplatelet agents do not prevent, nor are they useful in, the treatment of venous thrombosis.

Coronary Artery Disease — Myocardial Infarction

The goals of antithrombotic therapy during and early after acute myocardial infarction are: (1) to increase the rate of stable coronary artery recanalization. Continuous electrocardiographic monitoring of ST-segment changes and serial coronary arteriography in 45 consecutive patients in the early stages of acute MI identified the effects of and the presence of intermittent coronary occlusion. The occlusions were reversed by intracoronary streptokinase and/or isosorbide dinitrate [20]; (2) prevention of venous thromboembolism; (3) prevention of arterial thromboembolism; (4) reduction of early recurrence or extension of MI (reinfarction) (particularly following thrombolytic therapy and/or coronary artery angioplasty), and (5) retardation of the progression of occlusive coronary artery disease by limiting the likelihood of intravascular thrombogenesis [7].

PREVENTION OF VENOUS THROMBOEMBOLISM

The incidence of lower extremity deep vein thrombosis following MI is given as 17–38%. Deep vein thromboses form early (3–5 days), and the incidence rate is increased by immobilization, heart failure, or shock. Anticoagulants decrease the incidence rate to less than 6%.

Prevention of deep vein thromboses and subsequent pulmonary emboli is the basis for the following regimen:

Early ambulation (within 1–3 days)
Immediate subcutaneous low dose heparin (5000 USP units every 8–12 hours) for patients over 70 years or those with anterior-septal MI, previous MI, heart failure or shock, prolonged immobilization, previous deep vein thrombosis or pulmonary emboli, obesity, or severe varicosities of the lower extremities.

PREVENTION OF ARTERIAL EMBOLIZATION

This complication is most severe with a mural thrombus that follows an acute transmural anterior-apical MI. The thrombus is detected by two-dimensional echocardiography (sensitivity 77–92% and specificity 88–94%) and begins its development within 2–7 days (50–75% within the first 48 hours). The incidence rates of cerebral emboli in acute MI are approximately 3–5%, of peripheral arterial emboli approximately 4%, and of emboli to the kidneys and lower extremities approximately 1%. The incidence rates are lowered by anticoagulants. Anticoagulation should be initiated after a large acute transmural antero-septal MI (peak creatine kinase level > 700 IU/liter or peak lactate dehydrogenase > 500 IU/liter or both).

RECOMMENDATIONS

Immediate IV bolus heparin is given, followed by IV infusion and a concomitant vitamin K antagonist, as outlined in the sections on venous thrombosis and pulmonary emboli. A vitamin K antagonist should be continued for 3 months.

EARLY RECURRENCE OF MYOCARDIAL INFARCTION

The incidence of recurrence during hospitalization is high in patients with subendocardial or non-Q wave MI, particularly within 10–18 days. The sequence is seen in obese females who have recurring chest pain during hospitalization. The incidence rate of reinfarction may be reduced by large doses of diltiazem (360 mg/day).

POST-MYOCARDIAL INFARCTION AND REINFARCTION

In post-myocardial infarction and reinfarction, the thrombus is predominantly a platelet-rich clot, since the coronary artery is a high-flow system and the initiating step in thrombus formation is platelet adhesion and aggregation.

DRUGS USED TO TREAT MYOCARDIAL INFARCTION

Anticoagulants

Anticoagulants given in the hospital reduce the incidence rate of venous thromboembolism and systemic emboli but have questionable value in reducing the mortality rates. Anticoagulants, heparin, and warfarin reduce the mortality of the post-MI period in patients with anterior and antero-septal infarcts and echocardiographic evidence of a mural thrombus. The low-dose heparin regimen appears to be as effective as the continuous IV heparin regimen.

Benefits of long-term therapy in survivors of acute MI are controversial. The Sixty Plus Reinfarction Study from the Netherlands [50] reported that anticoagulants given over a period of 2½ years following MI significantly reduced the rates of reinfarction from 15.9–5.7% and that the risk of bleeding did not negate the beneficial effects in preventing recurrent MI.

In an alternate consecutive case and randomized multicenter protocol, 728 patients (50–75 years of age) with Q-wave myocardial infarction 6–18 months previously showed a significant reduction in reinfarction rate with SQ heparin (12,500 IU) daily. The heparin reduced the cumulative general mortality rates but not the cardiovascular mortality rates. In addition to reduced myocardial reinfarction rate, fatal events secondary to strokes or pulmonary emboli were significantly reduced [38].

Antiplatelet Agents

The long-term use of aspirin may reduce the incidence rates of recurrent MI, presumably due to coronary artery thrombi.

Sulfinpyrazone has shown inconsistent benefits in reducing the incidence rates of myocardial reinfarction or sudden death when used on a long-term basis following MI. Dipyridamole, when used chronically following MI, is no more effective than aspirin.

Coronary Artery Disease — Unstable Angina Pectoris

In using thromboxane TxA_2 and PGI_2 synthesis as indices of platelet activation, 84% of patients with unstable angina were found to have phasic increases in the production of both prostaglandins associated with episodes of unstable angina. The data indicate a platelet activation during myocardial ischemia secondary to unstable angina [14]. As evidenced by high transcoronary TxA_2 levels, the myocardial circulation has an extraordinary capacity to synthesize TxA_2 in patients with unstable angina [37]. Patients with chronic stable angina had no increase in the formation of thromboxane A_2.

Increasingly, coronary angiographic profiles of intracoronary thrombi [64], coronary artery angioscopy [45], layered thrombi in patients who had fatal MI [13], and elevated serum levels of fibrinopeptide A [17] correlate intracoronary thrombogenesis with the syndrome of unstable angina pectoris. Since thrombogenesis in the high-flow rate coronary arteries is predominantly platelet-derived, one would expect abnormal production of thromboxane A_2, β-thromboglobin and platelet factor 4 (platelet specific proteins stored in platelets and granules and secreted during platelet activation) in patients with unstable angina pectoris.

DRUGS USED TO TREAT UNSTABLE ANGINA PECTORIS

Antiplatelet Drugs

In a multicenter, double-blind, placebo-controlled and randomized trial on 1266 men with unstable angina pectoris, the incidence rates of fatal as well as nonfatal MI were reduced by 51% in the 625 individuals using 324 mg of aspirin daily. "And the protective effect of the aspirin (51% reduction in mortality) was maintained for a 12-month follow-up period" [30]. This striking benefit was corroborated by an independent Canadian study [4]. In the latter study, the effects of 325 mg of aspirin 4 times/day were compared with those of sulfinpyrazone (800 mg daily), both drugs, or neither. The patients were entered into the trial within 8 days post-MI and were treated and followed up for 2 years. The aspirin group showed a 55% reduction in the risk of MI or cardiac death compared with the other three groups.

Anticoagulant Drugs

Heparin (subcutaneous and intermittent daily) was first used in more than 300 patients with unstable angina pectoris in 1959

[39]. More recently, full dose heparin regimens (7500–10,000 unit bolus followed by IV infusion to reach therapeutic anticoagulant levels) were given for 2 to 7 days, and repeat coronary angiograms revealed a reduction or disappearance of the thrombi [63]; however, no final conclusions have yet been made on the use of heparin therapy for unstable angina pectoris.

Aortocoronary Bypass Surgery

Grafting of saphenous veins or the internal mammary artery as bypass conduits from the aorta to a region distal to a critical narrowing of the coronary artery initiates an injury process in the artery wall and an acceleration of platelet aggregation and adhesion at the site of the vascular anastomosis. Saphenous vein graft occlusion rate may be 10–12% within 2 weeks after surgery and as high as 25% at 1 year. By 7 years, the majority of the vein grafts are markedly narrowed or completely obstructed. Most vein grafts display a significant reduction in caliber within 1 year. Graft failure rate is considerably lower with the internal mammary artery than with the saphenous vein.

Antiplatelet Drugs

In a prospective, randomized, double-blind trial in 407 patients in which dipyridamole was administered 2 days before surgery and aspirin administration was begun 7 hours following surgery, a significantly reduced frequency of early and late (11–18 months) vein graft failure was demonstrated (100 mg dipyridamole 4 times/day prior to surgery, 100 mg on the day of surgery and 1 hour after surgery) [6]. Dipyridamole (75 mg) and aspirin (325 mg) were continued 3 times/day thereafter. Another prospective study on a smaller number of patients who were started on low-dose aspirin (100 mg daily) immediately following surgery showed a lower incidence rate of ventricular arrhythmia and graft occlusion at 4 months after surgery than in the placebo-treated controls [31]. Aspirin or dipyridamole individually prevent lipid accumulation in primate vein bypass grafts [1]. Since aspirin, aspirin plus dipyridamole, and dipyridamole have not been tested in an alternate case study, the value of dipyridamole is presently uncertain (see above) [15].

An interesting experimental study identified a superiority of cod liver oil over aspirin-dipyridamole in preventing intimal hyperplasia in autologous vein grafts in dogs [28] and in modulating endothelium-dependent responses in porcine coronary arteries [47]. In the latter study, Yorkshire pigs maintained on a low (0.6 ml/kg/day) or a high (1.0 ml/kg/day) dose of cod liver oil for four weeks displayed augmented relaxations of proximal left anterior descending coronary artery rings (in vitro) to bradykinin, serotonin, adenosine diphosphate, and thrombin when compared to the response of tissue rings from control animals. Further platelet-induced contractions were significantly reduced in tissue rings with endothelium taken from the treated pigs and were comparable to tissue in rings without endothelium from control animals.

Valvular Heart Disease and Atrial Fibrillation

Intracardiac thrombi are mixed fibrin/red blood cell/platelet thrombi forming within the heart chamber. Platelet-rich thrombi form on the surface of valves. Patients with mitral valve disease and intermittent atrial fibrillation are particularly susceptible to intracardiac thrombi and embolic strokes or peripheral embolization. Anticoagulant therapy is indicated for fresh onset atrial fibrillation prior to cardioversion efforts and is usually discontinued within 2 weeks after the patient regains sinus rhythm.

ANTICOAGULATION WITH RECENT ONSET ATRIAL FIBRILLATION

The recommendations are to commence with full-dose IV heparin for 48 hours and add on warfarin. Warfarin is continued at therapeutic doses (as per prothrombin times) for a 2-week period. With chronic atrial fibrillation and a systemic or cerebral emboli, warfarin is administered permanently at therapeutic doses.

PROSTHETIC HEART VALVES

In a long-term follow-up of Starr-Edwards model 6000 prosthesis in the mitral position inserted between the years 1960–1966, aside from perioperative mortality, the greatest number of deaths were caused by cerebral embolism [32]. Other leading causes of death were congestive heart failure, MI, and sudden death. Porcine valves in the mitral position reduced the systemic arterial embolization rate, but early calcification and valve failure required reoperation at some point within the subsequent 5–10 years [43].

Platelet function is altered in patients with valvular heart disease, particularly those with aortic stenosis, and in many with prosthetic valves. Plasma β-thromboglobulin levels are increased; the increase is positively related to the incidence rate of systemic embolization. Platelet survival time is shortened and corrected by sulfinpyrazone and aspirin plus dipyridamole.

A randomized comparison of long-term anticoagulation with a placebo in preventing systemic embolization in patients with prosthetic valves is unlikely to be conducted, since the incidence rates of systemic embolization is sharply reduced or eliminated with warfarin plus dipyridamole.

Relative rates of thromboembolism with various prosthetic valves positioned in the mitral and the aortic valve regions are summarized in Table 6-3.

Cerebrovascular Disease

Anticoagulant therapy in cerebrovascular disease remains controversial, despite studies in patients with transient ischemic

Table 6-3. Relative rates of thrombembolism in prosthetic valves

Valve	Incidence rate ($+ \rightarrow + + + +$)
Mitral valve	
Starr-Edwards (bare struts)	+ + + +
Smeloff-Cutter	+ + + +
Beall	+ + → + + +
Bjork-Shiley	+ +
Lillehei-Kaster	+ + + +
Hancock xenograft (no anticoagulant)	+ → + +
Aortic valve	
Starr-Edwards	+ + → + + +
Smeloff-Cutter	+ → + +
Bjork-Shiley	+ → + +
Lillehei-Kaster	0 → + + +
Hancock xenograft (no anticoagulant)	+ +

Key: Incidence rates: lowest = +, highest = + + + +.

attacks, progressive or incomplete strokes, and presumed cerebral embolisms. One large randomized study suggested anticoagulants are more effective than aspirin in preventing stroke after transient ischemic attacks or minor strokes [41]; however, IV heparin has no demonstrable effect in preventing stroke progression in acute, partially stable strokes, and anticoagulants do not improve the outcome of patients with completed strokes. The main causes of unexpected bleeding in patients on long-term anticoagulant therapy are summarized in Tale 6-4.

Thrombolytics

Formation of fibrin as a consequence of the coagulation system is counteracted by a fibrinolytic system. The existence of a fibrinolytic system was recognized by Morgagni and John Hunter about 200 years ago when they noted that after sudden death blood remains uncoagulated. The term *fibrinolysis* was first recorded in the literature nearly 100 years ago.

The fibrinolytic system, outlined in Fig. 6-3, can be summarized as follows: Proenzyme (plasminogen) + activators in the presence of endothelial cells (t-PA), and tissue kinases (including urokinase) produces plasmin (a fibrinolytic fibrin-dissolving enzyme). Plasminogen activators appear in plasma following acute anoxemic episodes, surgery, electroshock, pyrogen administration, exercise, ischemia, and epinephrine administration.

The primary mechanism of thrombolysis is the direct result of diffusion and absorption of plasminogen activator into a thrombus. The intrinsic plasminogen of the fibrin clot is converted to plasmin by activators. Clot lysis by exogenous plasmin action appears to be limited. Since plasmin, a relatively nonspecific

Table 6-4. Main causes of unexpected bleeding in patients on long-term anticoagulant therapy

Occult lesion	Coagulation defect	Drug-drug interaction
Gastrointestinal	Hemophilia	Acetylsalicylic acid
Diaphragmatic hernia		Antibiotics
Duodenal ulcer	Von Willebrand's disease	Thyroid drugs
Stomach tumor		Quinidine
Colon tumor		Diuretics
Arteriovenous fistula	Malingering	Cimetidine
		Prolonged narcotics
Urinary	Psychoneurosis	Alcohol
Nephrolithiasis	Suicidal tendency	
Prostatic carcinoma		
Tumor		

serine protease, causes degradation of fibrinogen, coagulation factors, and plasminogen, the proteolytic effects give rise to fibrinogen degradation products (potent anticoagulants) and a systemic lytic state. These undesirable side effects of thrombolytic agents cannot be dissociated from the therapeutic effect. As a consequence, the thrombolytic agents, streptokinase or urokinase, regardless of the portal of injection, entail unavoidable risks.

When practical, before thrombolytics are used, a thrombus should be demonstrated by angiographic means. When time is critical, such as in the setting of MI, thrombolytics may be started prior to obtaining the angiographic evidence of an intravascular thrombus. For lower extremity deep vein thrombosis or pulmonary emboli, venography or pulmonary angiography is required.

The fibrinolytic system may be activated exogenously. Currently there are five activators being used intravenously to lyse coronary artery thrombi. These are streptokinase, anisoylated plasminogen-streptokinase activator complex (APSAC), urokinase, recombinant tissue plasminogen activator (t-PA), and recombinant pro-urokinase. Each of these agents has advantages and disadvantages [45].

ACUTE MYOCARDIAL INFARCTION

Patients experiencing MI at an early age, prior to 45 years, develop low tissue specific-plasminogen activator (t-PA) owing to high plasma levels of the t-PA inhibitor [23]. The level of the t-PA inhibitor appears to be positively related to serum triglyceride levels. Additional evidence of impaired plasminogen conversion as an independent risk factor for myocardial reinfarction comes from the results of a prospective cohort study of 109 unselected men with an initial MI before the age of 45. Sixteen patients had at least one reinfarction within 3 years. High plasma concentrations of fast-acting plasminogen activator inhibitor (PAI), high triglyceride levels and dyslipoproteinemia involving VLDL and HDL, poor left ventricular performance, and multi-vessel coronary artery disease were all independently related to reinfarction [21].

An overlap in values for PAI in patients with myocardial reinfarction and those in the non-reinfarction group limits the usefulness of this particular assay in singling out patients at risk for reinfarction. Distinguishing levels of extrinsic tissue plasminogen activator (t-PA) in plasma euglobulins, at the mere detection limit, more clearly identified patients at high risk for reinfarction when compared to those with high t-PA levels [25]. These findings suggest that young male patients with MIs may be predisposed to intracoronary thrombogenesis because of rapid inhibition of endogenous t-PA.

INTRACORONARY FIBRINOLYTICS

Efforts to lyse a coronary thrombus with intracoronary streptokinase began more than 25 years ago [2] raised a number of fundamental questions. These include:

1. **Frequency of thrombotic coronary artery occlusion in the pathogenesis of acute MI** — Early evidence suggesting a low incidence rate of thrombosis from postmortem examinations conflicted with contemporary angiographic and surgical recognition of thrombus in the proximal segments, usually in the left anterior descending coronary artery during the first 4 hours following MI [9]. Presently, consensus opinion in clinical cardiology circles holds that thrombus formation is the rule (perhaps > 80% incidence rate in the setting of acute transmural MI).

2. **The critical time for reversing ischemic injury and cell death** — Compelling evidence indicates irreversibility of myocardial injury within 60 minutes of ischemia. However, the 60-minute figure may not be absolute, since the possibility has been raised that injury and death of myocardial cells progresses in a wavelike manner from the subendocardial to the subepicardial region as the MI becomes transmural and may require 2–4 hours to be completed. Using the recovery of left ventricular function as a measurable endpoint of therapy in acute transmural MI due to a total occlusion of the left anterior descending coronary artery, it was learned that reperfusion by an adequate reconstitution of blood flow should be accomplished within 2–6 hours after the onset of symptoms. However, the ischemic myocardium may require days to months (see Fig. 4-2) before the optimal structure and function relationship of the left ventricle are regained. Therefore, follow-up estimates of left ventricular function after an acute transmural MI should be made around the tenth to fourteenth day, at 6 and 12 weeks after myocardial infarction.

The left ventricular function may be followed by serial measurements of the global ejection fraction by radionuclide techniques (LVEF) or by serially following regional wall motion using nuclear ventriculography or two-dimensional echocardiography. For nuclear ventriculography, the centerline method is used in which a line is drawn between end-diastolic and end-systolic silhouettes and 100 equally spaced cords are constructed perpendicular to the centerline. The length of the cords provide a means of quantifying regional motion. The extent of abnormality is defined by the number of contiguous cords within the infarct zone that are abnormal [10].

3. **Identification of acute MI candidates for fibrinolytic therapy** — patients experiencing chest pain for at least ½ and less than 4 hours who exhibit ST-T segment elevation in the electrocardiogram for at least one minute (0.1 mV) in the anterior chest leads ($V_1 \rightarrow V_6$) or in leads reflecting the inferior surface of the heart (standard II, III, and the augmented unipolar extremity lead, AVF) and are unresponsive to organic nitrates. Patients with high ST-T segment elevations in the anterior chest leads in the absence of Q waves are prime candidates. Those with elevations of the ST-T segments in the inferior leads benefit less remarkably from fibrinolytic therapy.

4. **Risks and benefits of intracoronary fibrinolytic therapy in patients with acute MI** — The consensus opinion of leading cardiologists is that the benefits of thrombolytic therapy far outweigh the risks. Intracoronary infusion of streptokinase recanalizes 75% of completely obstructed infarct-related arteries. Urokinase infused into coronary arteries causes recanalization in 62–94% of arteries and is associated with a less marked reduction in fibrinogen concentration and fewer complications than in patients infused with streptokinase. Combining intracoronary fibrinolysis with percutaneous transluminal coronary angioplasty, particularly in patients under 70 years of age with a thrombus in the proximal left anterior descending artery of less than 4 hours duration, appears to be the setting for maximal benefit.

   Immediate benefits include a significant reduction in 30-day mortality, particularly in patients with anterior wall MI when comparing randomized control (noninfused) with streptokinase-infused patients. Intracoronary streptokinase reduces 1-year mortality in only those patients in whom coronary artery reperfusion was documented. **Patients older than 70 years of age, however, show little improvement in 1-year mortality benefit and no significant improvement in left ventricular function.**

5. **What is the "natural" incidence rate of spontaneous fibrinolysis in the setting of acute MI?** Spontaneous fibrinolysis is part of the hemostatic mechanism(s) for maintaining the fluidity of the blood and has long been regarded as a "stress-related" phenomenon. Alimentary lipidemia inhibits fibriholysis, and plasma lipoproteins, VLDL and perhaps LDL, accelerate prothrombin activation.

   Fibrinolytic activity over the endothelial surface of arteries is higher in human atherosclerotic arteries than in the nonatherosclerotic region because of localized plasminogen activator on the surface of the atheromatous plaque. However, perturbation of the endothelial cells, as seen in a destabilization of an atherosclerotic lesion secondary to fissure or in intramural hemorrhage and after angioplasty, would be expected to abruptly reduce the fibrinolytic activity of the atheromatous plaque area, leading to platelet deposition and intravascular thrombogenesis. Apparently, a scenario of this nature under lies coronary artery thrombosis (particularly in the proximal left anterior descending artery) in perhaps 80% of patients with acute anterior and anteroseptal MI. Perhaps 15–20% of the time, spontaneous fibrinolysis may develop during the initial 12 hours [9].

INTRAVENOUS FIBRINOLYTICS

Intracoronary fibrinolytic therapy is a difficult and complex procedure, requiring the availability of special facilities for coronary artery visualization and arterial perfusion, and backup cardiovascular surgery within the first few hours after the onset of chest pain. An alternate approach was described in 1979 [57]. Thereafter, the results of a large number of clinical trials of high-dose brief-duration regimen support the conclusion that reduced mortality rates are seen in patients receiving streptokinase IV (1,500,000 units over one hour) in the setting of acute MI.

The European Cooperative Study Group for Streptokinase Treatment in Acute Myocardial Infarction (1979) administered the fibrinolytic agent within 5–12 hours after the onset of symptoms and reported a significant reduction in overall mortality rate during a 6-month observation period [57]. IV streptokinase (250,000 IU) was administered over the first 20 minutes, followed by 100,000 IU/hour for the next 24 hours. Subsequently, at least four studies reported favorable results from IV therapy: the Italian Group for the Study of Streptokinase in Myocardial Infarction (GISSI) (11,806 patients) [52]; the Netherlands Interuniversity Cardiology Institute Trial (533 patients) [48]; Western Washington Intravenous Streptokinase Trial (WWIST) (368 patients) [27]; and the Intravenous Streptokinase in Acute Myocardial Infarction (ISAM) Trial from the Federal Republic of Germany (1741 patients) [53]. The results are as follows:

1. Early treatment (within 1 hour after onset of pain) reduced in-hospital mortality by 47% (GISSI).
2. Treatment within 3 hours of pain onset was associated with a 23% mortality reduction (GISSI) (supported by results of the WWIST trial).
3. Treatment started between 3 and 6 hours reduced mortality by 17% (GISSI).
4. One-year survival curves remained significantly higher in the IV streptokinase group (GISSI) than in the untreated patients.
5. A relationship exists between patency achieved, limitation of infarct size, improved left ventricular ejection fraction, and mortality (Netherland study). In a double blind trial of 219 consecutive patients randomly assigned to streptokinase or to no streptokinase, within four hours after the onset of chest pain, left ventricular ejection fraction was significantly greater

in the group that was taking streptokinase when compared to the non-streptokinase group. The differences were seen in either anterior or inferior infarctions. Short-term survival was significantly higher in the streptokinase than in the non-streptokinase group [60].
6. Considering only anterior wall infarcts, mortality rate at 14 days was greater in untreated than in treated groups. Strikingly different results were found in patients suffering an inferior wall infarction (WWIST).
7. Special attention must be directed to the postinfarction period to prevent reocclusion and reduction in the incidence rate of late stenosis.

Details of special postinfarction, post-thrombolysis management are considered below.

While time of therapy institution following the onset of chest pain is the most important clinical factor influencing the potential benefit from either intracoronary or IV fibrinolytic therapy, other clues of a favorable outcome include:

I. Patient's age — mortality rate due to higher incidence rate of major hemorrhagic complications in patients older than 75 years of age: Hemorrhagic complications are more frequent in women than men and in patients with diabetes mellitus or systemic hypertension.
II. Electrocardiographic changes provide extremely useful information regarding the potential for (potentially) successful application of fibrinolytic therapy.
   A. Appearance of new Q waves, a high QRS score, and high ST-T segment elevation or depression (> 1 mm), particularly in leads reflecting an anterior wall infarction, should predict a greater effectiveness in limiting myocardial infarct size than with inferior wall infarction.
   B. Patients with high ST-T segment elevation or marked contralateral ST-T segment depression experience the optimum limitation of infarct size.
   C. No significant limitation of infarct size can be expected with low ST-T segment changes in the absence of Q waves when compared to high ST-T segment changes in the absence of Q waves.

CONTRAINDICATIONS FOR THE USE OF FIBRINOLYTIC AGENTS

1. Risk of intracranial hemorrhage with acute hypertension ($>$ 180 mm Hg systolic; > 110 mm Hg diastolic), poorly controlled chronic hypertension, any cerebrovascular pathology.
2. Risk of hemorrhage and potential for hemorrhagic disease (organ biopsy or aspiration within six weeks, traumatic cardiopulmonary resuscitation, severe liver or kidney disease or malignancy), > 75 years of age.
3. High titer of streptokinase antibodies and recent streptococcal infection, previous streptokinase 5 days to 6 months earlier.

FIBRINOLYTICS AND ANTICOAGULATION [29]

1. Pretreat with heparin (40 IU/kg) — IV bolus.
2. Streptokinase (400–500 IU/kg/min) — 1.5 million units (dilute 1.5 million units in 50-ml normal saline and infuse in ml/hr equal to patient's body weight [kg]).
3. Post-streptokinase, uninterrupted IV heparin (10–15 IU/kg/hr).
4. Maintain PTT at about 80 seconds (heparin requirements increase in the initial 24–48 hours).
5. Continue heparin prior to coronary angiography, angioplasty, or bypass surgery.
6. Switch to warfarin if there is no angioplasty or bypass surgery and continue for 2–3 months.

ANISOYLATED PLASMINOGEN-STREPTOKINASE ACTIVATOR COMPLEX

In the anisoylated plasminogen-streptokinase activator complex (APSAC), the plasminogen (lysyl groups that bind to fibrin) has been acylated at its enzyme center. The acylation is reversible with time, thereby regenerating fibrinolytic activity and producing sustained release pharmacokinetics (half-life of biological activity of 105 minutes), better binding to fibrin and accumulation within the thrombus, fewer side effects, and the possibility of administering a bolus rather than a prolonged infusion. While APSAC is an improvement over streptokinase, it retains many of the undesirable features of streptokinase, and it is more expensive than streptokinase.

Urokinase

Urokinase was originally prepared from urine but is now derived from growing human fetal kidney cells in tissue culture and has a half-life of 16 minutes in vivo. Urokinase is non-antigenic, and it is more clot selective than streptokinase [51]. Two million units as a bolus is reported to be effective as a thrombolytic when given within 3 hours after the onset of symptoms. Post-infusion coronary angiograms from patients given IV or intracoronary urokinase showed reperfusion rates similar to streptokinase [33]. One million IU of urokinase, when given by intracoronary injection, appears to be the dose required for optimal reperfusion rates [40].

Tissue-Type Plasminogen Activator: t-PA

A natural enzyme of endothelial cell (as well as other human tissue cells), t-PA and Pro-urokinase (Pro-UK) were first isolated from human myeloma cells [8] and now by recombinant DNA technology [55]. Both t-PA and Pro UK have a high affinity for fibrin and fibrin-bound plasminogen and a relatively low affinity for circulating plasminogen. Because of these differences in affinity, they are more clot selective and produce little or no depletion of fibrinogen.

By 1983, it was anticipated that t-PA was a clot-specific thrombolytic agent that might benefit patients with acute MI. Comparisons of IV t-PA and streptokinase in a single-blind, randomized trial established the superiority of t-PA in reestablishing coronary patency (70% vs. 55%) and in limiting the bleeding complications [59]. Subsequent trials indicate a 70% success rate for IV t-PA in effecting a rapid recanalization of coronary arteries [62]. In a prospective study, the Thrombolysis in Myocardial Trial (TIMI) (677 patients) [54], preinterventional and postinterventional coronary angiography revealed a two-fold greater success with t-PA than with IV streptokinase in lysing intracoronary thrombi. The rate of clot lysis is dose-related, and the therapeutic-to-toxic ratio is extremely high. Few drugs have such a wide safety margin. In experimental laboratory pretreatment, heparin significantly enhances the thrombolytic effect of t-PA, probably by preventing new fibrin formation and its incorporation into the thrombus during lysis (dog) [5].

Two forms of t-PA are under investigation: double- and single-stranded. The original recombinant DNA material, double-stranded (DS), is being replaced by a possibly more clot-selective single-stranded (SS) molecule. The half-life for the DS molecule is short (5–3 minutes) and even shorter for the SS form. Because of the extremely short half-life for each molecular form, heparin must be simultaneously given.

Comparison of fibrin specificity is given in Table 6-5 for the two t-PA forms. Infusions of 80 and 100 mg SS is accompanied by a lesser effect than the DS form on plasminogen, fibrinogen, and fibrinogen degradation products.

Platelet-mediated hemostatic defects are induced by t-PA, since plasminogen is also bound to platelet surface. As platelets aggregate, a platelet-specific protein, thrombospondin, is released from the alpha granules. Thrombospondin binds fibrinogen, fibrin, heparin, histidine-rich glycoprotein (GP), and plasminogen [49]. Thrombospondin-plasminogen-GP as a tri-molecular protein is activated by t-PA and the resultant plasmin disaggregate platelets and destabilizes the hemostatic plug. The effectiveness of t-PA in disaggregating platelets is greater than that of streptokinase or urokinase [12].

Table 6-5. Double- and single-stranded t-PA and plasma, plasminogen, and fibrinogen degradation products (3-hour IV infusion)

	DS—80 mg (n = 108)	SS—80 mg (n = 38)	SS—100 mg (n = 44)
Plasminogen (percent decrease)	56 ± 16	28 ± 11	30 ± 43
Fibrinogen (percent decrease)	33 ± 23	3 ± 23	10 ± 41
Fibrinogen degradation products (μg/ml)	94 ± 106	27 ± 75	47 ± 74

Key: DS = double-stranded; SS = single-stranded; patients = number in parenthesis. Results are mean ± standard deviation for samples drawn 2 hours post-infusion.
Source: Adapted from H. S. Mueller. Different fibrinolytic potencies of two forms of recombinant tissue-type plasminogen activator. NHLBI thrombolysis in myocardial infarction trial [abstract]. *Clin. Res.* 34:631A, 1986; and A. K. Rao. Differential effects in-vivo of predominantly single-chain and double-chain recombinant tissue plasminogen activator on plasma fibrinogen and fibrinolyte system [abstract]. *Clin. Res.* 34:337A, 1986.

T-PA-mediated activation of platelet-bound plasminogen leads to the degradation of platelet surface glycoproteins along with Von Willebrand factor, surface factors responsible for platelet adhesion and aggregation [46].

Thus, t-PA affects all aspects of platelet-mediated hemostasis by (1) inhibiting adherence and aggregation; (2) disaggregating platelet masses; (3) lysing stabilized platelet plugs; and (4) affecting the coagulation mechanisms.

PREVENTING REOCCLUSION AFTER SUCCESSFUL THROMBOLYSIS

After successful clot lyses, approximately 30% of patients experience coronary artery reocclusion. Most reocclusions are due to thrombus reformation on the destabilized atherosclerotic plaque (see Chaps. 4 and 5). Rethrombosis occurs with similar frequencies in patients receiving streptokinase, urokinase, or double- or single-stranded t-PA.

Therapy directed at the prevention of coronary artery reocclusion includes:

Reduction of lumen-narrowing directly (angioplasty) or indirectly (coronary bypass grafting), possibly in the early hours after the MI (within 24–48 hours)

Heparin immediately upon admission to the hospital (5000 U/IV bolus) followed by IV infusion (1000 U/hour) to maintain APTT between 1.5 and 2.5 times the control value for at least 5 days (APTT should be assessed less than 8–12 hrs after initiating thrombolytic therapy to determine the lower limit of therapeutic control). After 5 days, subcutaneous heparin (10,000 U every 12 hrs) should be continued for an additional 5 days.

Platelet-inhibitor therapy (80 mg aspirin/day) started within 24 hrs and continued for 5 days and then increased to 325 mg/day. Long-term platelet inhibitor therapy is then instituted.

A randomized trial of IV t-PA (n = 72 and placebo n = 66) within 4 hours after the onset of an acute myocardial infarction with subsequent randomization to elective coronary angioplasty on the third hospital day (n = 42) and without angioplasty (n = 43) showed a patency rate of 66% for the t-PA group and 24% for the placebo group. Left ventricular ejection fraction (LVEF) was greater in the t-PA than in the placebo group. Angioplasty improved LVEF after exercise (but not at rest) and reduced the incidence of post-infection angina [19]. Also documented was a reduced incidence of clinical congestive heart failure in the treated group (14%) compared with the placebo group (33%).

STATUS OF FIBRINOLYTICS CIRCA 1988

The 5 thrombolytics in use or under investigation are compared in Table 6-6.

Table 6-6. Comparative pharmacologic and clinical features of thrombolytic preparations for acute myocardial infarction

Feature	SK	APSAC	UK	t-PA	Pro-UK
Clot binding	+++	+++	+	+++	++++
Plasminogen activation	++++	++++	+++	++	++
Clot specificity (fibrinolysis versus fibrinogenolysis)	+	++	++	+++	+++
Antigenicity	++++	+++	0	?	?
% Reperfusion (treatment < 3 hours)	31.55	44.64	66	62.80	67
Simultaneous heparin	0	0	0	+++	+++
Allergic side-effects	+	+	0	?	?
Expense	+	++	+++	++++	++++

Key: SK = streptokinase; APSAC = anisoylated plasminogen-streptokinase activator complex; UK = urokinase; t-PA = recombinant tissue plasminogen activator; pro-UK = pro-urokinase; ? = unknown; 0 = none; + = weakly positive; ++ = positive; +++ = strongly positive; ++++ = very strongly positive.
Source: Modified from S. Sherry. Appraisal of various thrombolytic agents in the treatment of acute myocardial infarction. *Am. J. Med.* 83 (Suppl. 2A):31, 1987.

MANAGEMENT OF HEMORRHAGIC COMPLICATIONS [29]

For minor bleeding, pressure dressings should be applied. Anticoagulation should be discontinued if bleeding cannot be controlled. For moderate bleeding, the anticoagulant should be reversed with protamine sulfate for heparin, fresh frozen plasma for warfarin. For severe bleeding: (1) If fibrinogen < 100 mg%, administer 5–10 IU cryoprecipitate; (2) transfuse blood as needed; (3) consider epsilon amino caproic acid; and (4) consider surgical control of bleeding site.

OTHER INDICATIONS FOR FIBRINOLYTICS

Pulmonary Embolism

Streptokinase and urokinase are considered to be agents of choice in selected patients with acute, massive, and life-threatening pulmonary emboli (emboli large enough to occlude two-thirds or more of the main branches of the pulmonary artery or equivalent vessels, that cause acute right-side heart failure with or without shock, dyspnea, and progressive deterioration). In patients with preexisting lung or heart disease with pulmonary hypertension, the embolism must be confirmed by pulmonary angiography. Thrombolytics are useful only within 5–7 days after the embolism.

Deep Venous Thrombosis

Thrombolytics are useful in deep vein thrombosis that is less than 72 hours in duration. Expected success rate in lysing the thrombus may be greater than 60%. The major benefit is the preservation of vein valvular function.

Occluded Arteriovenous Cannulae

Installation of the thrombolytic into the occluded cannulae in chronic renal dialysis patients may salvage the shunt and avoid surgery.

Peripheral Artery Thrombosis

Thrombolytic therapy may be effective if the thrombus is less than 72-hours old. For emboli, embolectomy using a Fogarty balloon catheter is the usual approach.

Baseline Laboratory Data

Prior to therapy, the following data should be collected: thrombin time (TT), activated partial thromboplastin time (APTT), prothrombin time (PT), hematocrit, fibrinogen concentration, and platelet count. The TT and APTT values should be less than twice the normal control times if therapy is to be continued.

ADVERSE EFFECTS

Bleeding

(See Management of Hemorrhagic Complications, above.)

Allergic Reaction

Streptokinase is a foreign protein and may cause allergic reactions such as chills, bronchospasm, rash, malaise, or anaphylactoid reactions. If these reactions are severe, then the thrombolytics must be discontinued and 40–80 mg of hydrocortisone should be given IV. Hypersensitive subjects may be premedicated with corticosteroids, such as prednisolone (25 mg), and an antihistamine IV. In general, urokinase causes fewer allergic reactions.

PRECAUTIONS

Thrombolytic therapy should be undertaken with care in patients who have had recent cardiopulmonary resuscitation, as well as those with subacute bacterial endocarditis, mitral disease with atrial fibrillation, hepatic or renal disease, diabetic retinopathy, septic thrombophlebitis, and infected AV cannula. It should be undertaken with care also in pregnant women (first 18 weeks) and in patients of advanced age (> 75 years).

Drug Evaluations

Streptokinase

PHARMACOKINETICS

The half-life of streptokinase is biphasic: fast, 11–13 minutes, and slow, 83 minutes. Activity ceases upon discontinuance of the enzyme.

DOSAGES

The powder is reconstituted with isotonic sodium chloride or 5% dextrose for injection to a volume of approximately 45 ml and stored at 2–4°C. The enzyme should be used within 24 hours. Shaking should be avoided.

IV: *Adult:* in acute MI, 750,000 IU during the first 10–15 minutes and the remaining 250–750,000 IU over 60 minutes (total dose = 1–1.5 million IU).
Other indications: Initial loading dose of 250,000 IU over 30 minutes followed by 100,000 IU/hour (24 hours for pulmonary embolism, 24–72 hours for arterial thrombosis or embolism, and 72 hours for deep vein thrombosis).
After treatment is discontinued and the thrombin time decreased to less than 2 times normal values (usually 2–4 hours), heparin is infused in a dose that prolongs the APTT by 20–30 seconds.

Intra-arterial-occluded AV cannulae: 250,000 IU diluted in 2 ml into each limb of the cannula over a 30-minute period, followed by clamping of the cannula for 2 hours.

Intracoronary: Prior to angiography, 5,000–10,000 units of heparin are given interarterially. After the obstructed artery is identified, streptokinase is started by ostial infusion through the angiographic catheter. For delivery through catheters in the coronary artery, the enzyme is infused at the clot site, 20,000 IU initially, then 2000 units/min, with spot angiograms every 15 minutes to monitor clot lysis. Infusion is continued until reperfusion occurs (usually a total of 150,000–250,000 IU) and for 30–60 minutes thereafter. Following intracoronary infusion, heparin IV is maintained for a clotting time 2–3 times normal. Warfarin sodium and dipyridamole or aspirin plus dipyridamole is continued for 3 months.

INTRAVENOUS ADMINISTRATION DURING ACUTE MYOCARDIAL INFARCTION

Details are given above.

DOSAGE FORMS AND STRENGTHS AVAILABLE

Kabikinase (Pharmacia) **powder** (lyophilized): 250,000, 600,000, and 750,000 IU.

Streptase (Hoecht-Roussel) **powder** (lyophilized): 250,000 and 750,000 IU.

Urokinase

Urokinase is nonantigenic and causes less severe allergic reactions than streptokinase. It may be used if streptokinase resistance is high. The powder, reconstituted with sterile water only, must be used immediately.

DOSAGES

IV: *Adult:* 4400 IU/kg infused over 10 minutes followed by continuous infusion of 4400 IU/kg/hour for 12–24 hours; thereafter, heparin followed by oral anticoagulants, as with streptokinase

Intracoronary: three reconstituted vials are added to 500 ml of 5% dextrose in water (1500 IU/ml). After a bolus dose of 2,500–10,000 units of heparin and the angiogram, 6000 IU/min (4 ml/min of solution) are given for up to 2 hours. Usually requires 500,000 IU to achieve thrombolysis. Progress is monitored by angiography every 15 minutes.

DOSAGE FORMS AND STRENGTHS AVAILABLE

Abbokinase (Abbott) **powder** (lyophilized): 250,000 IU with 25 mg mannitol and 45 mg sodium chloride.

Abbokinase open catheter (lyophilized): 5000 IU with 15 mg mannitol and 1.7 mg sodium chloride.

Abbokinase occluded catheter: 5000 IU/ml **gently** instilled by tuberculin syringe in amounts equal to volume of catheter. Aspiration of clot and urokinase solution is attempted after 5–10 minutes.

t-PA

USES AND/OR ACTIONS

Clot lysis is induced by intracoronary injection of t-PA in 70–90% of patients with a total thrombotic occlusion of a coronary artery. Results of early trials indicate a success rate of 75% recanalization of thrombotic coronary occlusion with IV t-PA (TIMI Study Group) [54].

t-PA has a low affinity for circulating plasminogen activator but has a high affinity for fibrin. Because both the activator and plasminogen bind in close proximity to fibrin, plasminogen is activated on the fibrin surface. Its effect on the clot is sustained. The recommended dose is a 10 mg bolus followed by 50 mg in 1 hour and 20 mg each at 2 and 3 hours for a total dose of 100 mg. The observed incidence of intracranial bleeding in over 3,000 patients treated with Alteplase was 0.4%.

PHARMACOKINETICS

Metabolism and Elimination

The half-life of t-PA is only 5–8 minutes in the circulation. Consequently, the systemic effects of t-PA are promptly reversed by discontinuance of the enzyme, while the local clot-lysing effects continue. Therefore, invasive procedures (coronary arteriograms and/or angioplasty) can be safely carried out in the presence of thrombolysis. Additionally, thrombolysis is more rapid with t-PA than with streptokinase or urokinase.

Current Status of t-PA

The Food and Drug Administration has approved the genetically engineered product t-PA for use in the management of acute myocardial infarction. In all, t-PA (Alteplase, Activase, Genentech, Inc.) has been tested in more than 4000 patients in the United States.

Therapy Directed Towards Limiting Myocardial Reperfusion Injury and Thrombogeneity

As reviewed in Chap. 4, reperfusion of an ischemic myocardium is accompanied by tissue injury mediated by:

I. Generation of O_2 free radicals, O_2^-, OH· by endothelial cells causing:
   A. Peroxidation of lipid components of cellular and mitochondrial membrane.
   B. Increased vascular thrombogeneity and endothelial cell permeability.
   C. Chemostatic-mediated leukocyte migration, accumulation, and activation with the generation of additional free radicals. Neutrophils possess an NADPH oxidase on the cell surface (see Fig. 4-3), which is responsible for the production of superoxide anion. The neutrophils also possess a myeloperoxidase that generates CLO^- via hydrogen peroxide.

   The ischemic myocardium releases proteases that activate the complement system (see Fig. 6-4). The initial stimulus for neutrophil binding to endothelial cells is probably C5a. As a result of this binding, the permeability of macromolecules into the vessel wall is increased. The combined effect of C5a, neutrophils and prostaglandins, produces the greatest permeability of the endothelial cells. The net effect is a marked production and release of free radicals.
II. Peroxidation of membranes activates phospholipases and releases arachidonic acid, the precursor of prostaglandins. Conversions of prostaglandins lead to additional free radicals, and the formation of a particular prostaglandin, thromboxane A_2 (TxA_2) appears to mediate infarct extension.
III. Increase in coronary resistance due to the release of powerful vasoconstrictors (from endothelial cells).

IV. Immediate burst of norepinephrine release during the initial minute of reperfusion.

Presently, therapy during the period of immediate reperfusion is limited to anticoagulant therapy (heparin and antiplatelets). Application of therapy directed toward the reduction of free-radical generation, limiting endothelial cell injury and complement activation, and buffering the effect of the norepinephrine surge, has appeared in surgical journals and should be a promising direction for myocardial reperfusion injury following drug-induced thrombolysis or percutaneous coronary angioplasty.

The most direct means of limiting the production of oxygen metabolites are by:

1. Xanthine oxidase inhibitor — may be particularly beneficial in preventing endothelial cell damage, vascular injury, and thrombogeneity (see Fig. 4-4).
2. Free radical scavengers and antioxidants — recombinant human superoxide dismutase administered after 90-minute coronary artery occlusion limits reperfusion injury and reduces infarct size along the vascular distribution in the canine model [26]. Other free radical scavengers reported to be effective in preserving left ventricular function after myocardial reperfusion include catalase and hydroxyl radical scavenger and mannitol. Mannitol also decreases capillary endothelial and myocardial cell swelling [61].
3. Agents that limit lipid peroxidation — peroxidase (decreases OH generation and inactivates lipid peroxides and hydroxides), the antioxidant, Q_{10} and reduced glutathione (GSH) (oxidizes and inactivates free radicals and lipid peroxides), GSH plus the antioxidant vitamin E (alpha tocopherol) (blocks lipid peroxidation and limits neutrophil-mediated endothelial cell injury by enhancing prostacyclin production) [58].
4. Inhibitors of platelet aggregation — both heparin and t-PA have an anti-aggregation effect on platelets (see above under t-PA). Drugs such as aspirin decrease the production of thromboxane A_2 (TxA_2) by inhibiting thromboxane synthetase. Other drugs may block TxA_2 receptors. Nonsteroidal anti-inflammatory agents must be used with extreme caution (or not at all) in the setting of MI and reperfusion because of an associated attenuation of myocardial repair and post-infarction scar thinning.
5. Antineutrophilic agents — neutrophil attraction to the injured myocardium may be limited by reducing platelet aggregation and the subsequent appearance of free radicals and lipid peroxidation. Antineutrophilic antibodies, directed toward neutrophil depletion in the injured myocardium, are promising experimental approaches; however, no clinically useful approaches are currently available.

THERAPY DIRECTED TOWARD LIMITING RESTENOSIS FOLLOWING PERCUTANEOUS TRANSLUMINAL CORONARY ANGIOPLASTY

Percutaneous transluminal coronary angioplasty (PTCA) destabilizes the atherosclerotic lesion and, like other destabilizers (fissures, intramural hemorrhage, and plaque rupture), powerful and self-catalyzing processes of cellular chemotaxis, thrombogenesis, and thrombolysis (see Fig. 6-4). Collectively, the processes are in sufficient balance so that the repair process does not lead to restenosis. Approximately one-fourth to one-third of all patients receiving PTCA develop restenosis within 6 months after the procedure. Key in the restenosis process is endothelial cell dysfunction and platelet deposition and the subsequent organization of thrombus.

Like all tissue repair processes, modulation of the tissue injury (PTCA) response is seminal to effectively limiting restenosis. Tissue injury and repair are influenced by numerous locally generated hormones referred to as autocoids. Such autocoids or chemical messengers include structurally small (endothelial-derived relaxation factor, $.O_2^-$, $\cdot OH^-$, H_2O_2, serotonin, catecholamines, histamine), intermediate (prostaglandins, interleukins), kinins (bradykinin, endothelial-derived growth factors, platelet-derived growth factors), and large macromolecules (negatively charged heparin-like aggregates of glycosaminoglycans and perhaps collagen and elastin fragments [3]. Systemic hormones in large amounts (corticoids) may transiently limit the repair of tissue injury. But in the order of natural events, the highest priority is given to the autocoids as modulators of tissue injury and repair.

That is not to say that efforts to limit the injury-repair process underlying restenosis following PTCA are being neglected. Drugs such as the calcium channel blockers were tested and found to be worthless. Dipyridamole, as an antiplatelet drug, when used alone was also ineffective. At the end of 1987, the following may have anti-restenosis potential:

1. Long balloon inflation time (90 seconds).
2. Aspirin, although the dose is unsettled. One regimen empirically uses 975 mg in 3 divided doses, beginning a day before PTCA until one hour before the procedure and thereafter 80–325 mg/day for at least 6 months [16].
3. Anticoagulants. IV heparin is routinely given prior to and during PTCA (10,000 U) and continued (800–1000 U/hour) overnight, but the effectiveness of a short-term (2–5 hours) or long-term (24 hours) heparin treatment as an anti-stenosis regimen remains uncertain. In some centers, continuous (24 hours) IV heparin is reserved for patients with thrombus or intimal dissection following PTCA.
4. Diet. Fish oils (cod liver oil and omega-3 unsaturated fatty acids) may possess unique properties for limiting the generation of chemical messengers of exuberant fibrosis following PTCA. Early results with eicosapentaenoic acid (EPA, a 20-carbon omega-3 fatty acid) suggest a reduced post-PTCA restenosis rate, but other studies fail to support this finding. The final word on fish oil or on vegetable oils such as olive oil remains to be written.
5. Life-style change. Controlling diabetes mellitus, reducing serum cholesterol, and discontinuing cigarette smoking, the identified risk factors for post-PTCA reocclusion [44], may reduce the frequency rate of restenosis.

References

1. Boreboom, L. E., et al. Aspirin or dipyridamole individually prevent lipid accumulation in primate vein bypass grafts. *Am. J. Cardiol.* 55(5):556, 1985.
2. Boucek, R. J., and Murphy, W. P., Jr. Segmental perfusion of the coronary arteries with fibrinolysin in man following a myocardial infarction. *Am. J. Cardiol.* 6:525, 1960.
3. Boucek, R. J. Factors affecting wound healing. *Otolaryngol. Clin. North Am.* 17(2):243, 1984.
4. Cairns, J. A., et al. Aspirin, sulfinpyrazone or both in unstable angina. *N. Engl. J. Med.* 313:1396, 1985.
5. Cercek, B., et al. Enhancement of thrombolysis with tissue-type plasminogen activator by pretreatment with heparin. *Circulation* 74(3):583, 1986.
6. Chesebro, J. H., et al. Effect of dipyridamole and aspirin on late vein-graft patency after coronary bypass operations. *N. Engl. J. Med.* 310:209, 1984.
7. Chesebro, J. H., and Fuster, V. Antithrombotic therapy for acute myocardial infarction: Mechanisms and prevention of deep venous, left ventricular, and coronary artery thromboembolism. *Circulation* 74 (5 pt 2):[I]1, 1986.
8. Collen, D., et al. Purification of human tissue-type plasminogen activator in centigram quantities from human melanoma cell culture fluid and its conditioning for use in-vivo. *Thromb. Haemost.* 48:294, 1982.
9. De Wood, M. A., et al. Prevalence of total coronary occlusion during the early hours of transmural myocardial infarction. *N. Engl. J. Med.* 303:897, 1980.
10. Dodge, H. T. Advantages and applications of the centerline method for characterizing regional ventricular function. *Circulation* 74(2):293, 1986.
11. Doyle, D. J., et al. Adjusted subcutaneous heparin or continuous intravenous heparin in patients with acute deep vein thrombosis. *Ann. Int. Med.* 107:441, 1987.
12. Erlemeir, H. H., et al. Risk of intracoronary versus intravenous thrombolysis in acute myocardial infarct [abstract]. *Circulation* 74 (Suppl. II):11, 1986.
13. Falk, E. Unstable angina with fatal outcome: Dynamic coronary thrombosis leading to infarction and/or sudden death. Autopsy evidence of recurrent mural thrombosis with peripheral embolization culminating in total vascular occlusion. *Circulation* 71:699, 1985.
14. Fitzgerald, D. J., et al. Platelet activation in unstable coronary disease. *N. Engl. J. Med.* 315:983, 1986.
15. Fitzgerald, G. A. Drug therapy: Dipyridamole. *N. Engl. J. Med.* 316:1247, 1987.
16. Fuster, V., et al. Review article. Platelet-inhibitor drugs' role in coronary artery disease. *Prog. Cardiovasc. Dis.* 29:325, 1987.
17. Gallione, A., et al. Fibrin formation and platelet aggregation in patients with severe coronary artery disease: Relationship with the degree of myocardial ischemia. *Circulation* 72:27, 1985.
18. Glazier, R. L., and Crowell, E. B. Randomized prospective trial of continuous vs. intermittent heparin therapy. *J.A.M.A.* 236:1365, 1976.

19. Guerci, A. D., et al. A randomized trial of intravenous tissue plasminogen activator for acute myocardial infarction with subsequent randomization to elective coronary angioplasty. *N. Engl. J. Med.* 317:1613, 1987.
20. Hackett, D., et al. Intermittent coronary occlusions in acute myocardial infarction. *N. Engl. J. Med.* 317:1055, 1987.
21. Hamsten, A., et al. Plasminogen activator inhibitor in plasma: Risk factor for recurrent myocardial infarction. *Lancet* 2(8549):3, 1987.
22. Hamsten, A., et al. Increased plasma levels of a rapid inhibitor of tissue plasminogen activator in young survivors of myocardial infarction. *N. Engl. J. Med.* 313:1557, 1985.
23. Harker, L. A. Review article. Clinical trials evaluating platelet-modifying drugs in patients with atherosclerotic cardiovascular disease and thrombosis. *Circulation* 73:206, 1986.
24. Iturbe-Alessio, I., et al. Risks of anticoagulant therapy in pregnant women with artificial heart valves. *N. Engl. J. Med.* 315:1390, 1986.
25. Jespersen, J., and Gram, J. Fibrinolysis and recurrence of myocardial infarction [letter to editor]. *Lancet* 2(8556):461, 1987.
26. Jolly, S. R., et al. Canine myocardial reperfusion injury. Its reduction by the combined administration of superoxide dismutase and catalase. *Circ. Res.* 54:277, 1984.
27. Kennedy, J. W. Streptokinase for the treatment of acute myocardial infarction: A brief review of randomized trials. *J. Am. Coll. Cardiol.* 10 (5 Suppl. B):28B, 1987.
28. Landymore, R. W., et al. Comparison of cod-liver oil and aspirin-dipyridamole for the prevention of intimal hyperplasia in autologous vein grafts. *Ann. Thorac. Surg.* 41:54, 1986.
29. Lew, A. S. I.V. Streptokinase in acute myocardial infarction: Practical considerations. *Cardio* October 1986, p. 29.
30. Lewis, H. D., et al. Protective effects of aspirin against acute myocardial infarction and death in men with unstable angina. *N. Engl. J. Med.* 309:396, 1983.
31. Lorenz, R. L., et al. Improved aortocoronary bypass patency by low-dose aspirin: Effects on platelet aggregation and thromboxane formation. *Lancet* 1(8389):1261, 1984.
32. Macmanus, Q., et al. The Starr-Edwards model 6000 valve. A 15-year follow-up of the first successful mitral prosthesis. *Circulation* 56:623, 1977.
33. Mathey, D. G., et al. Intravenous urokinase in acute myocardial infarction. *Am. J. Cardiol.* 55:878, 1985.
34. Meade, T. W., et al. 1,511 Caucasian males, 40–64 — prospective study. *Lancet* 2(8506):533, 1986.
35. Miletich, J., Sherman, L., and Broze, G., Jr. Absence of thrombosis in subjects with heterozygous protein C deficiency. *N. Engl. J. Med.* 317:991, 1987.
36. Mueller, H. S. Different fibrinolytic potencies of two forms of recombinant tissue-type plasminogen activator. NHLBI thrombolysis in myocardial infarction trial [abstract]. *Clin. Res.* 34:631A, 1986.
37. Neri Serneri, G. G., et al. Abnormal cardiocoronary thromboxane A_2 production in patients with unstable angina. *Am. Heart J.* 109:732, 1985.
38. Neri Serneri, G. G., et al. Effectiveness of low-dose heparin in prevention of myocardial reinfarction. *Lancet* 1(8539):937, 1987.

39. Nichol, E. S., et al. Virtue of prompt anticoagulant therapy in impending myocardial infarction: Experiences with 318 patients during a 10-year period. *Ann. Int. Med.* 50:1158, 1959.
40. Ohyagi, A., et al. Dose of urokinase for intracoronary thrombolysis in patients with acute myocardial infarction. *Clin. Cardiol.* 10:453, 1987.
41. Olsson, J.-E., et al. Antiocoagulant vs. antiplatelet therapy as prophylactic against cerebral infarction in transient ischemic attacks. *Stroke* 11:4, 1980.
42. Rao, A. K. Differential effects in-vivo of predominantly single-chain and double-chain recombinant tissue plasminogen activator on plasma fibrinogen and fibrinolyte system [abstract]. *Clin. Res.* 34:337A, 1986.
43. Schoen, F. J., et al. Long-term failure rate and morphological correlations in porcine bioprosthetic heart valves. *Am. J. Cardiol.* 51:957, 1983.
44. Shaw, R. E., et al. Clinical and morphologic factors in prediction of restenosis after multiple vessel angioplasty [abstract]. *J. Am. Coll. Cardiol.* 7:63A, 1987.
45. Sherman, C. T., et al. Coronary angiography in patients with unstable angina pectoris. *N. Engl. J. Med.* 315:913, 1986.
46. Sherry, S. Appraisal of various thrombolytic agents in the treatment of acute myocardial infarction. *Am. J. Med.* 83 (Suppl 2A):31, 1987.
47. Shimokawa, H., et al. Effects of dietary supplementation with cod liver oil on endothelium-dependent responses in porcine coronary arteries. *Circulation* 76:898, 1987.
48. Simoons, M. L., et al. Early thrombolysis in acute myocardial infarction: Limitation of infarct size and improved survival. *J. Am. Coll. Cardiol.* 7:717, 1986.
49. Silverstein, R. L., et al. Platelet thrombospondin forms a trimolecular complex with plasminogen and histidine-rich glycoprotein. *J. Clin. Invest.* 75:2065, 1985.
50. Sixty Plus Reinfarction Study Research Group. A double-blind trial to assess long-term anticoagulant therapy in elderly patients after myocardial infarction. *Lancet* 2(8202):989, 1980.
51. Tennant, S. N., et al. Intracoronary thrombolysis in patients with acute myocardial infarction: Comparison of the efficacy of urokinase with streptokinase. *Circulation* 69:756, 1984.
52. The GISSI Study Group. Effectiveness of intravenous thrombolytic treatment in acute myocardial infarction. *Lancet* 1(8478):397, 1986.
53. The ISAM Study Group. A prospective intravenous streptokinase in acute myocardial infarction study. Mortality, morbidity and infarct size at 21 days. *New Engl. J. Med.* 314:1465, 1986.
54. The TIMI Study Group. The thrombolysis in myocardial infarction (TIMI) trial: Phase 1 findings. *N. Engl. J. Med.* 312:932, 1985.
55. Van de Werf, F., et al. Coronary thrombolysis with intravenously administered human tissue-type plasminogen activator produced by recombinant DNA technology. *Circulation* 69:605, 1984.
56. Velders, A. J., and Wildeveur, C. R. Platelet damage by protamine and the protective effect of prostacyclin. An experimental study in dogs. *Am. Thorac. Surg.* 42:168, 1986.
57. Verstraete, M., et al. Streptokinase in acute myocardial infarction. *N. Engl. J. Med.* 301:797, 1979.

58. Verstraete, M. Prevention of thrombosis in arteries: Novel approaches. *J. Cardiovasc. Pharmacol.* 7:5191, 1985.
59. Verstraete, M., et al. Randomized trial of intravenous recombinant tissue type plasminogen activator versus intravenous streptokinase in acute myocardial infarction. *Lancet* 1(8433): 842, 1985.
60. White, H. D., et al. Effect of intravenous streptokinase on left ventricular function and early survival after acute myocardial infarction. *N. Engl. J. Med.* 317:850, 1987.
61. Willerson, J. T., et al. Influence of hypertonic mannitol on ventricular performance and coronary blood flow in patients. *Circulation* 51:1095, 1975.
62. Williams, D. O., et al. Intravenous recombinant tissue-type plasminogen activator in patients with acute myocardial infarction: A report from the NHLBI thrombolysis in myocardial infarction trial. *Circulation* 73:338, 1986.
63. Wolf, N. Heparin and unstable Angina. *Cardiovascular News* May 1986, p. 11.
64. Zack, P. M., et al. The occurrence of angiographically detected intracoronary thrombus in patients with unstable angina pectoris. *Am. Heart J.* 108:1408, 1984.

Selected Reading

BLOOD PLATELETS

Geastow, E., et al. Platelet-inhibiting drugs in the prevention of clinical thrombotic disease. *N. Engl. J. Med.* 293:1296, 1975.

Walsh, P. N. Platelets and coagulation proteins. *Fed. Proc.* 40:2086, 1981.

Weiss, H. J. Platelet physiology and abnormalities of platelet function. *N. Engl. J. Med.* 293:531

ENDOTHELIAL CELLS

Campbell, J. H., and Campbell, G. R. Endothelial cell influences on vascular smooth muscle phenotype. *Am. Rev. Physiol.* 48:295, 1986.

Goldberg, I. D. The Endothelium: Injury and Repair of the Vascular Wall. In S. Kalsner (ed.), *The Coronary Artery*. New York: Oxford University Press, 1982.

Simionescu, M., and Simionescu, N. Functions of the endothelial cell surface. *Am. Rev. Physiol.* 48:279, 1986.

Smith, W. L. Prostaglandin biosynthesis and its compartmentation in vascular smooth muscle and endothelial cells. *Ann. Rev. Physiol.* 48:251, 1986.

Vanhoutte, P. M., et al. Modulation of vascular smooth muscle contraction by the endothelium. *Ann. Rev. Physiol.* 48:307, 1986.

CORONARY THROMBOSIS

Friedman, M., and Van den Bovenkamp, G. J. The pathogenesis of coronary thrombus. *Am. J. Pathol.* 48:19, 1966.

Davies, M. J., and Thomas, A. C. Plaque fissuring — the cause of acute myocardial infarction, sudden ischaemic death, and crescendo angina. *Br. Heart J.* 53:363, 1985.

McGovern, V. J. Reactions to injury of vascular endothelium with special reference to the problem of thrombosis. *J. Path. Bacteriol.* LXIX:283, 1955.

Uchida, Y., et al. Fiberoptic observation of thrombosis and thrombolysis in isolated human coronary arteries. *Am. Heart J.* 112:691, 1986.

THROMBOLYSIS

Sherry, S. Setting thrombolysis in action. *Drug Ther.* 7:23, 1977.

Sullivan, J. M. Streptokinase and myocardial infarction. *N. Engl. J. Med.* 301:836, 1979.

Verstraete, M. Biochemical and clinical aspects of thrombolysis. *Semin. Hematol.* 15:35, 1978.

ANTICOAGULANT DRUGS

Breckenridge, A. Oral anticoagulant drugs: Pharmacokinetic aspects. *Semin. Hematol.* 15:19, 1978.

Brozovic, M. Oral anticoagulants in clinical practice. *Semin. Hematol.* 15:27, 1978.

Deykin, D. Current status of anticoagulant therapy. *Am. J. Med.* 72:659, 1982.

ANTIPLATELET DRUGS

Fuster, V., and Chesebro, J. H. Antithrombotic therapy: Role of platelet-inhibitor drugs. *Mayo Clin. Proc.* 56:102, 185, 285, 1981.

VITAMIN K

Dam, H., and Doisy, E. A. In *Nobel Lectures: Physiology or Medicine, 1942–1962*. New York: Elsevier, 1964.

Gallop, P. M., Lian, J. B., and Hauschka, D. J. Carboxylated calcium-binding proteins and vitamin K. Basic science for clinicians. *N. Engl. J. Med.* 302:1460, 1980.

Index

The abbreviations *f* and *t* stand for figure and table, respectively.

Abbokinase. *See* Urokinase
ACAT, 267
ACE inhibitors. *See* Angiotensin-converting enzyme inhibitors
Acebutolol (Sectral)
  dosages of, 178, 244
  ISA in, 175
  pharmacokinetics of, 178
Acetazolamide (Diamox), 29
Acetylcholine release, 15
N-Acetylcysteine, 231
  conjugates of, 165
  tolerance of, 232
Acetylsalicylic acid, 309
Action potential(s), 6, 62–65
  amiodarone effects on, 119
  atrial, 73–74
  autonomic control of heart rate and, 67–69
  decreased, 101
  early and delayed afterdepolarizations following, 69, 70*f*
  effects of class agents on, 78*t*, 78–84
  maximum, 98
  mechanisms of, 63–65
  phase 0 of, 65–67
    slowing of, 213
  phase 3 of, 66*f*
  phase 4 of, 76, 77*f*
  prolonged, 83
  rate of, 63
  reduced amplitude of, 77
  refractory period of, 65
  ventricular, digitalis effects on, 73–74
Activase. *See* t-PA
Adalat. *See* Nifedipine
Adenosine, 76
  antiarrhythmic properties of, 84–85
  efficacy of, 85
  mechanism of action of, 85
  side effects of, 85
Adenosine diphosphate (ADP) inhibition, 309
Adenosine monophosphate, 228
Adenosine triphosphate, 76, 226, 228
  antiarrhythmic properties and efficacy of, 84–85
  side effects of, 85
Adrenergic blockade, 193
Adrenergic neuron blockade, 191, 197
Adrenergic neurotransmission, impaired, 188, 191

Adrenocorticosteroids
  plus loop diuretics, 170
  plus thiazides, 169
Adrenoreceptors, 23. *See also* Alpha adrenoreceptors; β adrenoreceptors
  activities of, 1–2
β-Adrenoreceptors, 2, 239
  agonists, 23. *See also specific agents*
  desensitization and decrease of, 48
  down-regulation of, 2
  reduced, 48–49
Afterdepolarizations
  delayed, 72
  early, 69–72
Afterload, 1
  modulation of, 6–7, 28–29
  reduced, 14, 30
Agranulocytosis, 106
  with captopril, 210
  with procainamide, 92
Albuterol sulfate, 48
Aldactone. *See* Spironolactone
Aldoclor. *See* Methyldopa-chlorothiazide tablets
Aldomet. *See* α-Methyldopa
Aldoril. *See* Methyldopa-hydrochlorothiazide tablets
Aldosterone
  blockage of, 3
  increased levels of, 32
  receptors for, 167
  stimulation of release of, 208–209
Allopurinol, 158
Alpha adrenergic activity, 176
Alpha adrenoreceptors, 144, 200
Alpha-agonists, 203
Alteplase. *See* t-PA
Amblyopia, toxic, 282
Amenorrhea, 167
American Heart Association dietary recommendations, 275–276
Amiloride (Miradol), 29, 166
  dosages of, 168
  drug interactions of, 171
  with hydrochlorothiazide, 169
  with digitalis, 46
  mechanism of action of, 167
Aminophylline
  effects of, 85
  interactions of with beta blockers, 182–184
Amiodarone, 46, 83
  adverse effects of, 121–122
  interaction of with digitalis, 47
  patient monitoring with, 122
  pharmacokinetics of, 120–121
  pharmacology of, 119–120

Amiodarone—*Continued*
  preparations and dosages of, 122
  therapeutic use of, 120
Amphotericin B, 169
  interaction of with digitalis, 43
Amrinone lactate, 49–50
ANA. *See* Antinuclear antibody (ANA) determination
Anasarca, 29
Anavar. *See* Oxandrolone
Angina (pectoris), 218
  beta blockers and, 114–117, 239
  calcium channel blockers for, 246–247, 250
  with dipyridamole, 311
  drugs used to treat, 230–255, 331–332
  silent, 247–248
  stable, 246
  unstable, 248
    calcium channel blockers for, 246
    treatment for, 331–332
  variant, 246–247
Angioplasty, 229, 342
  calcium channel blockers for, 249–250
  percutaneous transluminal coronary, 225, 229, 230
    limiting restenosis following, 348–349
Angiotensin, 4, 142, 205
Angiotensin I, 208
Angiotensin II, 208
  blockage of, 32
  circulating levels of, 4, 29, 32
  reduced activity of, 209
Angiotensin-converting enzyme inhibitors, 32–33, 148, 153, 208
  drug reactions with, 212
  hemodynamics of, 209
  for left ventricular diastolic dysfunction, 51
  mechanism of action of, 208–209
  precautions for, 33
  for primary hypertension, 150–152
  side effects of, 209
  specific agents, 210–212
  therapeutic use of, 209
Anhydron. *See* Chlothiazide
Anisidone (Miradon), 320
Anisoylated plasminogen-streptokinase activator complex (APSAC), 335, 340–342
ANP. *See* Atrial natriuretic peptide
Antiarrhythmic drugs. *See also* Arrhythmias, agents for; *specific agents*
  classes I through IV, summary tables, 60–61
Anticoagulants
  for angina, 331–332
  in anti-restenosis therapy, 349
  with cerebrovascular disease, 333–334
  with cholestyramine resin, 289–290
  colestipol with, 291
  coumadin, 286, 288
  dextrothyroxine with, 299
  monitoring coagulation state and, 315–316
  for myocardial infarction, 330
  specific agents, 316–319
  vitamin K antagonists, 320–322
Anticoagulation
  with atrial fibrillation, 333
  drugs affecting, 323*t*
  fibrinolytics and, 340
  monitoring of, 315–316
Antihypertensive drugs
  categories of, 148–149
  combination drug therapy guidelines for, 149
  identifying, 147–148
  mono-drug therapy guidelines for, 149
  stepped care approach with, 149–150
Antineutrophilic agents, 348
Antinuclear antibody (ANA) determination, 89, 93
Antioxidant defense mechanisms, 227–228
Antioxidants, 348
Antiplasmin, 306
Antiplatelet drugs, 331–332
Antiplatelet therapy, 308–313
Antithrombin III, 306
Antithrombotic drugs, 319
  clinical use of, 327
Anturane. *See* Sulfinpyrazone
Aortocoronary bypass surgery for angina, 332
AP. *See* Action potential
APD. *See* Atrial action potential duration
Apoproteins, 261
  A, 296
  B and E receptors for, 266
  composition and charge differences in, 262
  function of, 264
  genes coding for, 268
Apresoline. *See* Hydralazine
APTT. *See* Thromboplastin time, activated partial
AquaMEPHYTON. *See* Phytonadione
Aquatag. *See* Benzthiazide
Aquatensen. *See* Methylclothiazide
Arachidonic acid, 277, 347
Arginine vasopressin, 3
Arrhythmias
  agents for
    actions of, 62, 76–77
    association and dissociation with sodium channel of, 79–82

Class I, 78–82, 106–112
Class Ia, 86–98
Class Ib, 98–106
Class II, 82–83, 112–119
Class III, 83–84, 119–124
Class IV, 83–84, 124–127
classification of, 60t, 61t, 75–76
effects of, 76–84
interactions of, 128–138t
specific agents, 84–127
use dependence of, 79
clinical guides to therapy for, 54–62
digitalis and, 41, 73–75, 100–101
drugs that induce, 58
with flecainide, 109
mechanisms of, 59–62, 69–72
with myocardial ischemia, 230
probucol and, 293
reentrant
reversal of, 77
termination of, 105
treatment of, 120
refractory, 110, 120
supraventricular, 107
ventricular, 96, 99, 103, 105, 113–114
worsening of, 108
Arterial blood flow, in atherosclerosis, 259–260
Arterial changes with hypertension, 144–145
Arterial embolism, prevention of, 329–330
Arterial hypertension. *See* Hypertension, arterial
Arterial smooth muscle
relaxation of, 206
factors affecting, 220t
spasm, 247
Aspirin, 309
plus captopril, 212
Asthma, drug-induced, 113, 115, 116, 117
Atenolol (Tenormin), 114, 179, 244
plus chlorthalidone (Tenoretic), 182–183
preparations and dosages of, 115
Atherosclerosis. *See also* Coronary heart disease, risk factors
cholesterol levels and risk of, 258
decreased susceptibility of, 297
diet and, 271, 272–277
drug management of, 277–296
genetic basis for, 268
hormonal therapy in prevention of, 296–299
hypercholesterolemia and, 260
hypertension with, 144
identifying high risk factors for, 268–271
lipoproteins and, 265–268
phenotypes of, 270t

pathogenesis theories of, 258–260
precocious, 264, 268
protection from, 248
thrombi and, 313
Atherosclerotic plaques, 246, 266, 313
ATP. *See* Adenosine triphosphate
Atrial action potentials, 16, 73–74
Atrial fibrillation
cardiac autonomic nerve plexus pathology and, 68
treatment of, 120, 125, 333
Atrial flutter, 125
Atrial natriuretic peptide, 2–3
Atrial tachyarrhythmias, 82
Atrioventricular (AV) block, 14, 87
with amiodarone, 121
with calcium channel antagonists, 213, 215
with procainamide, 92
third-degree, 126–127
with verapamil, 127, 252
Atrioventricular conduction system, 57f
disturbances of, 116
Atrioventricular nodal rhythms, 69
Atrioventricular pathways, 56, 57f
Atromid-S. *See* Clofibrate
Atropine, 42
Autocoids, 349
Autoimmune hemolytic anemia, 194
Automaticity
abnormalities of, 69–73
increased, 73, 75
reversal of, 76
Autonomic effects input, damping of, 173
Autonomic nervous system
amiodarone effects on, 120
in coronary artery blood flow, 220–221
AV junctional tachycardia, 38, 42
AVP. *See* Arginine vasopressin
Aygestin. *See* Norethindrone

Baroreceptors, 205
reflexes, 141
reset of, 172
response of, 209
Bendroflumethiazide (Naturetin), 160
Benzthiazide (Aquatag, Exna, Proaqua), 160
Beta adrenoceptors. *See* β-Adrenoceptors
Beta Blocker Heart Attack Trial (BHAT), 12, 241–242
Beta blockers, 12, 75, 171–172, 186
with ACE inhibitors, 209
adverse effects of, 174, 177
for angina pectoris, 239
antiarrhythmic effects of, 112
basis for, 82–83

Beta blockers—*Continued*
  antihypertensive uses of, 150–152, 176–177
    in elderly, 151
    mechanism of, 172–173
    organ systems in, 173–174
  beneficial effects of, 175, 240
    mechanism of, 242–243
  beta and alpha adrenergic activity, 176
  cardioselective, 112–114, 172, 174–175, 177
  definition of, 112
  with diuretics, 182–183
  drug interactions of, 183–186
  hemodynamic effects of, 173
  lipid profile effects of, 175–176
  membrane stabilization by, 176
  with myocardial infarction, 240–242
  for myocardial ischemia, 229
  plus nifedipine, 250
  nonmetabolized, 178
  patient age and, 239
  pharmacokinetics of, 178
  pharmacologic properties of, 172*t*, 174–176
  for prolonged repolarization, 55
  risk factors and, 147
  serum lipids and, 265
  side effects of, 112–113
  specific agents, 114–119, 178–182, 243–246
  in stepped care approach, 150
  sympathomimetic activity of, 172, 173, 175
  plus theophylline, 184
  therapeutic uses of, 113–114
  verapamil and, 251
  water and lipid solubility of, 176
Beta-adrenergic receptors, 112
  antagonists. *See* Beta blockers
  blocking activity of, 176
  subtypes of, 174
BHAT, 12, 241–242
Bile acid binding resins, 293
Bipyridine derivatives, 49–50
Blocardren. *See* Timolol
Blood clotting factors. *See* Coagulation factors
Blood flow. *See* Coronary artery blood flow
Blood pressure
  blood flow and, 259–260
  control of, 199
  drugs that lower, 186, 209
  elevated, 141. *See also* Hypertension
  lowered, 152–153, 173, 192–193. *See also* Antihypertensive drugs
    by vasodilation, 205
  precipitous fall in, 210, 211

Blood vessels, calcium channel antagonists effects on, 213–214
Bone marrow depression, 106
Bradyarrhythmias, 41, 58
Bradycardia
  with beta blockers, 177
  with calcium channel antagonists, 215
  with diltiazem, 126
  with nitrates, 232
  with propranolol, 116
  treatment of, 120
  with verapamil, 127
Bradycardia-tachycardia syndrome, 57
Bretylium, 83
Bretylium tosylate, 75, 91
  adverse effects of, 124
  patient monitoring with, 124
  pharmacology of, 122–123
  pharmacokinetics of, 123
  preparations and dosages of, 124
  therapeutic use of, 123
Bronchospasm
  with beta blockers, 174–175, 177
  drug-induced, 113
  reduced, 114
Bumetanide (Bumex), 165–166
Bumex. *See* Bumetanide
Butopanine, 48

Calan. *See* Verapamil
Calciparine. *See* Heparin calcium
Calcium
  accumulation of following myocardial injury, 249
  and hypertension, 143, 148
  intracellular concentrations of, 14, 156
    increased, 21
  intracellular-extracellular concentration of, 14–15
  release from intracellular storage pools of, 213
Calcium channels, 22*f*, 84
  activation of, 64
  antagonists, 149, 213
    adverse effects of, 215
    effects of, 213–214
    pharmacokinetics of, 214–215
    specific agents, 215–216
    therapeutic use of, 214
  blockers, 84, 349
    action of, 124–125
    for hypertension, 151–152
    for ischemic heart disease, 246–250
    pharmacokinetics of, 254*t*
    pharmacology of, 125
    specific agents, 126–127, 250–253
    therapeutic use of, 125
Calcium chloride, parenteral, 43
Capoten. *See* Captopril

Index

Captopril (Capoten), 31, 148
  adverse effects of, 210
  plus aspirin, 212
  plus chlorpromazine, 212
  in chronic congestive heart failure treatment, 32–33
  dosages of, 29, 211
  plus loop diuretics, 212
  pharmacokinetics of, 210–211
  precautions for, 33
Cardiac action potential. *See* Action potential(s)
Cardiac arrhythmias. *See* Arrhythmias
Cardiac asystole, 47
Cardiac cell membrane
  ion flux regulation in, 13
  neurotransmitter receptors and calcium channel in, 22*f*
Cardiac contractility, 213, 215
Cardiac dilatation, 4
Cardiac electrical activation, 62–63
Cardiac hypertrophy, 143–144
Cardiac output, 1
  with beta blocker therapy, 173
  increased, 8, 31
  reduced, 8, 30
Cardilate. *See* Erythrityl tetranitrate
Cardiomyopathy, hypertrophic, 234
Cardiotonic glycosides. *See also* Digitalis glycosides
  dosages of, 18–19, 33
  factors guiding selection of, 20
  pharmacokinetic properties of, 17–18
  source and chemical characteristics of, 16–17
Cardiotoxicity, 292–293
Cardiovascular disease, hypertensive, 147–148
Cardiovascular dysfunction, 99
  with disopyramide, 97
  with mexiletine, 104
  quinidine-induced, 88
Cardioversion. *See* Electrical cardioversion
Cardizem. *See* Diltiazem
Catapres. *See* Clonidine
Catecholamines
  release of, 123
  cardiac stimulation by, 242
  circulating, 113, 173
    high levels of, 1–2, 32, 49, 192, 228–229
  excessive, 113
  hypersensitivity to, 124
  inotropic action of, 22
Central nervous system
  adverse drug effects on, 99–100, 110, 115–117, 122, 177
  in beta blocker antihypertensive effects, 174
  neurotransmitter depletion in, 188

Cerebral ischemia, 232
Cerebrovascular disease, 333–334
Chest pain, control of, 240. *See also* Angina
Children
  causes of acute heart failure in, 6*t*
  clofibrate for, 285
  colestipol for, 291, 292
  deslanoside dosages for, 35–36
  dextrothyroxine in, 299
  digitalization of, 20
  digoxin for, 34–35, 47
  diuretic dosages for, 28
  nonglycosidic drugs for, 23
  probucol in, 293
  vasodilators for, 8
Chlorophenoxyisobutyric acid (CPIB), 284
Chlorothiazide (Diuril, SK-Chlorothiazide), 159
  plus reserpine, 189
Chlorpromazine
  plus beta blockers, 184
  plus captopril, 212
  plus guanethidine/guanadrel, 202
Chlorthalidone (Hygroton), 162
  plus atenolol (Tenoretic), 182–183
Chlothiazide (Anhydron), 160–161
Cholecystitis, 159
Cholelithiasis, 284–285, 287
Cholesterol. *See also* Hypercholesterolemia; Hyperlipidemia; Lipoproteins
  atherosclerosis and, 258, 265
  biosynthesis of, 294
  conversion of acetate to, 261*f*
  dietary, 261, 272
  fish oil-derived fatty acids and, 276–277
  intracellular homeostasis of, 265–267
  modulation of absorption of, 288–290
  precursors of, 292
  reduced, 113
  removal from cells, 267
  serum levels of, 260
    elevated, 271, 272*f*
    requiring treatment, 270*t*
  with thiazide therapy, 158–159
  thrombi and, 313
  transport of, 263
  unesterified, 261
Cholesterol ester hydrolase, 267
Cholestyramine, 278
  cost-effectiveness of, 295
  interaction of with digitalis, 42–43
Cholestyramine resin (Questran), 288–290
Choloxin. *See* Dextrothyroxine sodium
Chylomicrons, 263, 296
Cimetidine, plus beta blockers, 185
Cinchonism, 88

Circus-movement tachycardia, 58t
Cisplatin, plus ethacrynic acid, 170–171
Clofibrate (Atromid-S), 278–279
  adverse effects of, 284–285
  dosages of, 286
  drug interactions with, 286
  pharmacokinetics of, 283–284
  precautions with, 285
  uses and actions of, 283
Clonidine (Catapres), 151, 153, 196
  adverse effects of, 196
  plus beta blockers, 184
  dosages of, 196–197
  plus propranolol, 202
  risk of rebound hypertension with, 195–196
  therapeutic use of, 195
Clonidine hydrochloride-chlorthalidone tablets (Combipres), 201
Coagulation, intravascular, 304–306
Coagulation factors, 297, 304
  heparin and, 316
  inhibition of synthesis of, 323
  modification of, 320
  vitamin K antagonists and, 323–324
  XII deficiency, 313
Colchicine, 158
Cold extremities, beta blockers and, 175, 177
Colestid. See Colestipol
Colestipol, 278, 290–291
  adverse effects of, 290–291
  and digitalis toxicity, 42, 47
  dosages of, 291–292
  drug interactions with, 291
Collagen deposition, 224
Combipres. See Clonidine hydrochloride-chlorthalidone tablets
Compactin, 294
Complement activation, 307–308
Conduction
  abnormalities of, 69–73, 177
  block of, 99
    one-way, 77, 83
  velocity of, 65–67, 71, 77, 81–83
Congestive heart disease, 41
Congestive heart failure
  acute
    causes of, 4–5, 6t, 7t
    diuretics for, 7–8
    modulation of preload and afterload in, 6
    therapeutic end points for, 5
    vasodilator therapy for, 8–26
  beta blockers for, 12, 177
  causes of in adults, 7t
  causes of in children, 6t
  chronic
    causes of, 26–27, 50–51
    modulation of myocardial contractility in, 33–50
    modulation of preload and afterload in, 28–29
    therapeutic end points for, 27–28
    vasodilators for, 29–33
  compensatory responses to, 1–4
  with disopyramide, 97
  end-stage, 2
  with flecainide, 109
  manifestations of, 1
  mortality and Killip classification of, 7t
  sites for therapeutic intervention in, 2f
  with ventricle dilation, 144
  with verapamil, 127
Corgard. See Nadolol
Corneal lipofuscin deposits, 121
Coronary arteries
  blood flow in
    anatomic considerations of, 218–219
    autonomic nervous system in, 220–222
    physiologic considerations of, 219–220
  bypass surgery for, 249–250
  "clean," with angina-like distress, 248
  disease of, 144, 224
    diet and, 271
    modifying risk factors for, 270–271
    treatment for, 329–332
  intramural, 248
  lesions in. See Angina
  obstructions in, 246
  reocclusion of, 342
  spasm of, 247
  stenosing lesions in, 222–223
  stenosis-subendocardial region vulnerability, adaptation to, 222–223
  thrombotic occlusion of, 336
    myocardial ischemia with, 228–229
Coronary Drug Project Trial, 285
Coronary heart disease, risk factors, 268–271
Corticosteroids, 121
  inflammatory reaction and, 224
  with oxandrolone, 297
Corticotropin, 169
Corzide. See Nadolol-bendroflumethiazide tablets
Coumadin. See also Warfarin sodium
  anticoagulants, 170, 286, 288
  derivatives of
    adverse effects of, 321–322
    pharmacokinetics of, 321
    uses of, 320–321
  plus heparin, 328

Cyclic adenosine monophosphate (cAMP), 22–23
  increased intracellular concentration of, 49
Cyclic guanosine monophosphate (cGMP), 49, 219
Cyclic nucleotide phosphodiesterases, 22
Cyclic nucleotides, 49
Cyclo-oxygenase, 224
  inhibitors, 31
Cyclo-Prostin. *See* Epoprostenol sodium
Cysteine conjugates, 165
Cysteine disulfide, 210

Death, sudden
  with beta blocker withdrawal, 114-116, 118
  with left ventricular hypertrophy, 144
Deep vein thrombosis, 327–328
  fibrinolytics for, 343–344
  prevention of, 329
  risks for, 328
Demi-regroton, 190
Depolarization
  diastolic, 69, 98
  mechanisms of, 62–63
  phase 4 of, 75–76
  premature ventricular, 94, 103
  rate of, 62
    increased, 100
    maximum, 75
Depolarization wave, 59–62
  in reentry, 71
  vagal impulses and, 67
Dermatitis, allergic contact, 232
N-Desethylamiodarone, 121
Desipramine, plus guanethidine/guanadrel, 202
Deslanoside
  in adults, 35
  chemical characteristics of, 17
  dosages of, 35–36
  factors guiding selection of, 20
  onset of action of, 19
  pharmacokinetic properties of, 17–18
  source of, 16
  switching from intravenous to oral administration of, 21
Dextroamphetamine, 202–203
Dextrothyroxine sodium (Choloxin), 298–299
Diabetes
  clofibrate and, 283
  control of, 349
  dextrothyroxine with, 299
  gemfibrozil and, 287
  insulin-dependent, 113
  poorly controlled, 264, 268
Diamox. *See* Acetazolamide

Diazoxide, 153
Dicumarol, 324
Diet
  in anti-restenosis treatment, 349
  cholesterol in, 272
  lipid-lowering, 272–277
  monounsaturated and polyunsaturated oils in, 276
  saturated fat in, 273–276
Digitalis
  arrhythmias induced by, 100–101
  arrhythmogenic properties of, 73–74
  for chronic congestive heart failure, 27
  concentrations of, 12–13
  with diuretics, 27
  effects of, 27, 73–74
    on electrocardiogram, 73–74, 75t
    on sympathetic nervous system, 14–15
    vagal, 15–16
  goal of therapy with, 27–28
  inotropic action of, 14
  interactions of with other drugs, 42–47
  limitations of with acute congestive heart failure, 12
  mediation of myocardial inotropy by, 13–14
  myocardial sensitivity to, 37
  plus thiazides, 170
  toxicity of, 16, 20, 36–37
    electrocardiogram in diagnosis of, 37–38
    extracardiac symptoms of, 38–39
    factors influencing myocardial tolerance and, 39–41
    treatment of, 39, 41–42
Digitalis glycosides, 12–13, 76. *See also specific agents*
  benefits of vagal stimulation induced by, 16
  in children and adolescents, 20
  dosages of, 18–19, 33–36
  factors guiding selection of, 20
  in geriatric patients, 20–21
  interactions with other drugs, 42–47
  mechanism of action of, 13–14
  nonspecific tissue binding of, 32
  pharmacokinetic properties of, 17–18
  pharmacologic properties of, 16
  plasma assays of, 36
  source and chemical characteristics of, 16–17
  sympathetic nervous system and, 14–15
  toxicity of, 19, 36–42
  vagal effects of, 15–16
Digitalis lanata, 16
Digitalis purpurea, 16

Digitoxin
  dosages of, 19, 35
  factors guiding selection of, 20
  glomerular filtration and blood levels of, 41
  pharmacokinetic properties of, 17
  plasma assays of, 36
  toxicity of, 42
Digoxin, 44–45
  bioavailability of, 18, 34
  concentrations of, 12–13
  dosages of, 19, 21, 34–35
  fab fragments of antibody to, 42
  factors guiding selection of, 20
  glomerular filtration and blood levels of, 41
  increased serum levels of, 32, 46
  pediatric considerations for, 47
  pharmacokinetic properties of, 17–18
  plasma assays of, 36
  plateau blood levels of, 19
  source and chemical characteristics of, 16–17
  plus spironolactone, 171
  toxicity of, 47
Dihydropyridine calcium antagonists, 84
Dilatrate-SR. *See* Isosorbide dinitrate
Diltiazem (Cardizem), 213
  adverse effects of, 126, 215, 253
  before angioplasty, 250
  plus beta blockers, 184
  dosages of, 126, 215, 253
  effects of, 83
  interaction of with digitalis, 47
  for left ventricular diastolic dysfunction, 51
  for myocardial ischemia, 252–253
  pharmacokinetics of, 125–126, 214
  uses and actions of, 125, 253
Dipyridamole (Persantin), 309
  adverse effects of, 253, 311
  for angina, 332
  antiplatelet effect of, 349
  aspirin and, 310*t*
  dosages of, 255, 311
  effects of, 85
  following myocardial infarction, 331
  pharmacokinetics of, 311
  precautions for, 311
  uses and actions of, 310
Disopyramide, 46
Disopyramide phosphate, 95–97
  dosages of, 97–98
Diulo. *See* Metolazone
Diupres dosage, 189
Diurcardin. *See* Hydroflumethiazide
Diuretics. *See also specific agents*
  with ACE inhibitors, 209
  in adults, 28–29
  beta blockers and, 182–183
  in children and adolescents, 28
  classes of, 154
  with clonidine, 196
  with digitalis, 27
  digitalis toxicity and, 39–41
  effects of, 7–8
  interactions of, 169–171
  intravenous, 6, 7–8
  loop, 153, 163–166, 170
    plus captopril, 212
  in monotherapy or combined, 154
  potassium-depleting, 43–44
  potassium-sparing, 41, 166–168
    with thiazides, 158, 168–169
  reserpine with, 188–190
  side effects and treatment of, 29
  in stepped care approach, 150
  with sympathetic depressants, 201–202
  thiazide, 151, 155–159
    risk factors and, 147
    specific drugs, 159–162
  thiazidelike, 162–163
  types of, 148
Diuril. *See* Chlorothiazide
Diutensin-R, 189
Divalent cations, 143
Dobutamine, 23–25
  contraindications for, 24
  dosages of, 25
  hypersensitivity to, 124
Dopamine, 23, 25
  dosages of, 25–26
  hypersensitivity to, 124
Dopexamine, 48
Doppler ultrasound, 327–328
Dyrenium. *See* Triamterene
Dyspnea, 1, 5
Dysrhythmias, 37, 38*t*. *See also* Arrhythmias

ECG. *See* Electrocardiography
Ectopic pacemakers, 82
Edecrin. *See* Ethacrynic acid
Edema, 28–30, 196, 198
EDRF. *See* Endothelial cell-derived relaxation factor
Effective refractory period, 65, 81
  prolonged, 77, 82–84
  reduced, 15, 16, 82
Eicosopentaenoic acid, 277
Elderly
  digitalization of, 20–21
  digitalis toxicity in, 38–39
  diuretic therapy for, 29
Electrical cardioversion, 54, 91, 123, 233
Electrocardiogram
  amiodarone effects on, 119–120
  digitalis effects on, 37–38, 73–74, 75*t*
  disopyramide effects on, 96
  encainide effects on, 107
  flecainide effects on, 109

NAPA effects on, 95
procainamide hydrochloride and, 90–91
QT interval of, 54–55
quinidine effects on, 86
Electrophysiologic testing, indications for, 59t
Enalapril, 211–212
Enalapril maleate, 32–33
Enalaprilate, 211
Encainide, 106–109
Encephalopathy
hypertensive, 152–153
with thiazide therapy, 159
Endothelial cell-derived relaxation factor, 219–220
Endothelial cell-myocyte connection, 227f, 228
Endothelial cells, 219–220
fibrin deposition and, 258–259
inspissation of blood-borne material through, 259
lipoprotein receptors of, 267–268
prostacyclin from, 314
Enduron. *See* Methylclothiazide
Eosinophilia, 293
Ephedrine, 204
Epinephrine, 185
Epoprostenol sodium (Cyclo-Prostin), 255
ERP. *See* Effective refractory period
Erythrityl tetranitrate (Cardilate), 232, 235
Erythromycin, 44
Esidrix. *See* Hydrochlorothiazide
Esmolol, 118–119
Essential hypertension. *See* Hypertension, primary
Estrogens, 297–298
adverse effects of, 298
Ethacrynic acid (Edecrin), 165
plus cisplatin, 170–171
plus warfarin and coumarin anticoagulants, 170
for severe edema with pulmonary congestion, 29
Ethinyl estradiol, 297–298
European Cooperative Study Group for Streptokinase Treatment in Acute Myocardial Infarction, 338–339
Exercise
diminished tolerance of, 1
in hyperlipoproteinemia, 277
Exna. *See* Benzthiazide
Extrasystoles, 87, 91, 96

Fab fagments of digoxin antibody, 42
Fats. *See also* Cholesterol; Fatty acids; Lipids; Lipoproteins
absorption and transport of, 263–264
interference with absorption of, 289
monounsaturated/polyunsaturated, 273–276
saturated, 273–276
Fatty acids
essential, 222f
fish oil-derived, 276–277
free, 263, 264, 268
long-chain, 286
nonessential, 276
Fetal malformation, 113
Fibrillation, 111. *See also* Atrial fibrillation; Ventricular fibrillation
Fibrin, 307, 346
breakdown of, 306
deposits, 258–259
formation of, 334
specificity of, 341
Fibrinogen, 304, 307, 341
Fibrinolysis, 337–338
Fibrinolytic system, 306–307, 334–335
Fibrinolytics, 343–344
adverse effects of, 344
anticoagulation and, 340
contraindications for, 339
indications for, 343–344
intracoronary, 336–338
intravenous, 338–339
specific agents, 345–347
status of, 342–343
Fibrinopeptides, 304
Fish, 276
Fish oil, 276–277
in anti-restenosis treatment, 349
Flecainide acetate, 108–110
Fluid retention, 28–30, 196, 198. *See also* Water retention
Folate deficiency, 289, 291
Frank-Starling relationship, 4, 5f, 14
Free radicals, 227–228
scavengers, 348
Furosemide (Lasix, SK-Furosemide), 153
for acute congestive heart failure, 7–8
adverse effects of, 164
plus beta blockers, 185
plus captopril, 212
for dilutional hyponatremia, 29
dosages of, 28, 164–165
for intractable edema and severe ansarca, 29
pharmacokinetics of, 164
for severe edema with pulmonary congestion, 28–29
side effects of, 7

Gallbladder disease, 287
Gallstones, 285
Gastro-hypersecretion, 188
Gemfibrozil (Lopid), 279, 286–288
GISSI study, 338–339

Glomerular filtration, 4, 41
Glucose tolerance, 158, 299
Glycinexylide (GX), 99
Glycogenolysis, 112–113
Glycoproteins, 265, 306
Glycosaminoglycans, 349
Glycosides. *See also* Cardiotonic glycosides; Digitalis glycosides
   source and chemical characteristics of, 16–17
Guanabenz (Wytensin), 197–198
Guanadrel (Hylorel), 192–194
   plus alpha-agonists, 203
   plus chlorpromazine, 202
   plus desipramine, 202
   plus dextroamphetamine, 202–203
   plus insulin, 203
   plus mazindol, 203
   plus minoxidil, 203
   plus monoamine oxidase inhibitors, 203
Guanethidine (Ismelin), 191–192
   in combination therapy, 202–203
   in monotherapy, 149
Guanfacine, 198–199
Guanosine triphosphate, 219
Guanylate cyclase, 220
   intracellular, activation of, 219, 231

Hair growth, excessive, 207–208
Halothane, 186
HDL. *See* Lipoproteins, high-density
Heart
   in beta blockers and, 173–175
   calcium channel antagonists effects on, 213
   changes in with hypertension, 143–144
   coordinated pump function of, 62–63
   electrical activation of, 62–63
   electrical and mechanical properties of, 59–62
   oxygen extraction by, 218
   size and efficiency of, 4
   transplantation of, 229
Heart beats
   coupled, 96
   triggered, 69
Heart block
   digitalis toxicity and, 41
   with esmolol, 118
   with verapamil, 252
Heart disease, 5. *See also* Coronary heart disease; Ischemic heart disease; Valvular heart disease
   digitalis toxicity and, 41
Heart failure. 115–116, 118. *See also* Congestive heart failure
Heart rate, 1
   autonomic control of, 67–69
   decreased, 239
   reduction of, 14–16

Heart valves, prosthetic, 333
Helsinki Heart Study, 271
Hemodynamics
   in atherosclerosis, 259–260
   monitoring of, 240
Hemorrhage
   with heparin, 316–317
   with long-term anticoagulants, 335*t*
   management of, 343
   with thrombolytics, 343
   with vitamin K antagonists, 321
Heparin
   abortion rates and, 322
   adverse effects of, 316–317
   for angina, 331–332
   plus coumadin, 328
   dosages of, 317, 318–319
   monitoring of, 318
   for myocardial infarction, 330
   pharmacokinetics of, 316
   in platelet inhibition, 348
   precautions with, 317
   for prevention of reocclusions, 342
   for prevention of thrombosis, 329–330
   resistance to, 9
   uses and actions of, 316
   plus warfarin sodium, 327
Heparin calcium (Calciparine), 319
Heparin sodium (Liquaemin sodium), 319
Heparin-mediated response, treatment of, 319–320
Hepatitis, 89, 104, 252
Hepatomegaly, 294
Histamine, hypersensitivity to, 247
HMG-CoA reductase, 260, 294
   inhibition of, 266, 295
Hormone therapy, 296–299
Hydralazine (Apresoline), 8, 153, 205–207
   blood pressure effects of, 149
   in chronic congestive heart failure treatment, 31
   dosages of, 29, 207
   for primary hypertension, 151
Hydrochlorothiazide (Esidrix, Hydrodiuril, Oretic), 28, 160, 169
   in combination therapy, 151, 169
Hydrodiuril. *See* Hydrochlorothiazide
Hydroflumethiazide (Diurcardin, Saluron), 161
Hydromox. *See* Quinethazone
Hydromox-R, 189
Hydropres-25–50, 190
Hydroxychloroquine sulfate, 44
Hydroxymethylmexiletine, 104
4-Hydroxypropranolol, 116
Hygroton. *See* Chlorthalidone
Hylorel. *See* Guanadrel
Hypercalcemia, 41
Hypercholesterolemia
   atherosclerosis and, 260

LDL receptor encoding defects in, 265–266
  treatment of, 292
  type II, treatment of, 294–296
Hyperglycemia, 158, 164
Hyperkalemia, 42, 167
Hyperlipidemia, 158–159, 286–288
Hyperlipoproteinemia
  diet and, 272–277
  phenotypes of, 268, 270
  secondary, 268
  treatment of, 288–290, 294, 296, 298
    criterion for, 271
    drug, 277–296
    hormonal, 296–299
  types of, 278–279
Hypermagnesemia, 42
Hyperparathyroidism, 41
Hyperproteinemia, 283–286
Hypersensitivity reactions
  to diltiazem, 253
  to heparin, 317
  to procainamide, 92
  to protamine sulfate, 320
  to quinidine, 89
  to streptokinase, 344
  to sulfinpyrazone, 312
Hypertension
  arterial
    drug therapy for, 154–216
    emergencies of, 152–153
    pathophysiology of primary, 141–145
    resistant, 154
    treatment of, 148–152
    types of, 145–148
    urgencies of, 153
  in blacks vs. whites, 151
  complications of, 154
  diagnosis and classification of, 146–147
  hyperkinetic, 177
  malignant, 146, 150, 152
  neuroendocrine processes in, 141–143
  nutritional therapy for, 148
  ophthalmoscopic criteria for, 146t
  primary, 150–152
    drugs for, 148–149
    in elderly, 151
    pathophysiology of, 141–145
    remission of, 151
    treatment of, 148–152
  rebound, 195–198
  therapy for, 187
    in black patients, 208
    goals of, 147–148
  vasodilators for, 205
Hypertensive encephalopathy, 152–153
Hyperthyroidism, 41, 122, 298
Hypertrichosis, 207–208
Hypertriglyceridemia, 286–288

Hyperuricemia, 158
Hypocalcemia, 41, 55
Hypochloremic alkalosis, 29, 164
Hypocholesterolemia, 283
Hypoglycemia, 113–114
  insulin-induced, 112–113
  with pindolol, 115
  with propranolol, 116
  with timolol, 117
Hypokalemia, 55
  clinically significant, 157
  digitalis toxicity and, 39–41
  diuretic-induced, 29, 156–157, 164, 166–167
  prevention of, 44
Hypomagnesemia, 55
  digitalis toxicity and, 40–41
  with thiazide therapy, 157–158
Hyponatremia, 29, 159
Hypoparathyroidism, 41
Hypoprothrombinemia, 289, 325
Hypotension
  with bretylium, 124
  with calcium channel antagonists, 215
  with captopril-chlorpromazine, 212
  with diltiazem, 126
  with dipyridamole, 311
  with diuretics, 164
  with esmolol, 118
  with lorcainide, 111
  with nitrates, 234
  orthostatic, 232
    in elderly, 29
    with hydralazine, 31
    induction of, 9
    with niacin, 282
    with phentolamine, 32
    with verapamil, 252
  postural, 193–195, 199–200
  vasodilators and, 30
Hypothyroidism, 41, 122
Hypouricemia, 164
Hypoxanthine, 228

Ibopamine, 48
Ibuprofen, 44
IDL. *See* Lipoproteins, intermediate density
Impedance phlebographic technique, 328
Impotence, 188
Indandione, 321
  derivative of, 320
Indapamide (Lozol), 162–163
Inderal. *See* Propranolol
Inderide. *See* Propranolol hydrochloride-hydrochlorothiazide tablets
Indomethacin, 31
  plus beta blockers, 185
  with digitalis, 47
  plus prazosin, 204

Indomethacin—*Continued*
  prostaglandin production with, 224
  plus thiazides, 169
  plus triamterene, 171
Infants. *See also* Children
  deslanoside dosages for, 35–36
  digoxin dosages for, 34–35
Inflammatory reaction, 224
Inosine, 85
Inotropic agents, 12, 47–48
  nonglycoside, 21–26, 47–50
Insulin
  plus beta blockers, 185–186
  plus guanethidine/guanadrel, 203
Intraluminal pressure, precompressed, 219
Intramural arteries, 248
ISA, 173–174, 176
ISAM (Federal Republic of Germany) streptokinase trial, 338–339
Ischemic heart disease, 41, 299, 313
Ismelin. *See* Guanethidine
Isoproterenol, 23
  dosage for, 8
Isoptin. *See* Verapamil
Isordil. *See* Isosorbide dinitrate
Isosorbide dinitrate (Dilatrate-SR, Isordil, Sorbitrate), 232–233, 236
  dosages of, 234–235
5-Isosorbide mononitrate (5-ISMN), 232
Italian Group for the Study of Streptokinase in Myocardial Infarction (GISSI study), 338–339

Kabinkinase. *See* Streptokinase
Kaolin-pectin, 44
Kidney
  changes in with hypertension, 145
  in congestive heart failure, 3–4
  digitalis toxicity and, 41
  dysfunction of with gemfibrozil, 287
Kinins
  activation of, 224
  convergence of, 307–308
Konakion. *See* Phytonadione

Labetalol (Normodyne, Trandate), 153, 177–179
  plus cimetidine, 185
  plus halothane, 186
Lactation
  anticoagulants during, 322
  cholestyramine resin during, 289
  clofibrate during, 285
  colestipol during, 291
  dextrothyroxine during, 298
  gemfibrozil during, 288
  heparin during, 317
  probucol during, 293
Lanatoside, 17*f*
Lasix. *See* Furosemide

LCAT. *See* Lecithin-cholesterol acyltransferase
LDL. *See* Lipoproteins, low-density
Lecithin-cholesterol acyltransferase, 267
Leukopenia, 106, 194
Levodopa, 48
  plus reserpine, 204
Lidocaine, 91, 98–100
  analog of, 104. *See also* Tocainide
  congener of, 102. *See also* Mexiletine
  for digitalis toxicity, 42
Lipase, 264, 265
Lipid profile, 175–176
Lipid Research Clinics Coronary Primary Prevention Trial (LRF-CPPT), 258
Lipids. *See also* Fats; Lipoproteins
  abnormalities of, 265, 268
  antihypertensive drug effects on, 147
  peroxidation, limitation of, 348
  removal of from cells, 267
  solubility of beta blockers in, 176
Lipophobic beta blockers, 177
Lipoprotein lipase, 277
Lipoproteins. *See also* Cholesterol; Hyperlipidemia; Lipids
  atherosclerosis and, 265–268
  composition and size of, 262*t*
  electrophoretic mobility of, 262*t*
  fish oil-derived fatty acids and, 276–277
  high-density, 113, 262, 264–265, 275
    antihypertensive drug effects on, 147
    mediated reduction of, 292–294
    with prazosin, 199
    with thiazide therapy, 159
  inspissated, 259
  intermediate density, 264
  low-density, 113, 262, 264–265
    catabolism of, 275, 297
    intracellular cholesterol homeostasis and, 265–267
    mediated reduction of, 283–286, 292–294
    modulation of absorption of, 288–290
    with prazosin, 199
    receptors for, 267, 278, 290–292, 298
    thiazide diuretics and, 147, 158
  phenotypes of, 269–270*t*
  plasma, 261–262
    hormone modulation of, 264–265
    metabolic pathways of, 263–264
  removal of from cells, 267
  uptake of by endothelial and atheromatous lesions, 267–268
  very-low-density, 113, 262–264, 265

mediated reduction of, 279–282, 283
receptors for, 267–268
Liquaemin Sodium. *See* Heparin sodium
Lithium, plus diuretics, 169–170
Liver
  beta blocker metabolism of, 178
  disease of, 116, 287
Loniten. *See* Minoxidil
Loop diuretics, 153, 163–166
  mechanism and site of action of, 164
  in combination therapy, 170, 212
Lopid. *See* Gemfibrozil
Lopressor. *See* Metoprolol
Lopressor HCT. *See* Metoprolol tartrate-hydrochlorothiazide tablets
Lorcainide hydrochloride, 110–112
Lorelco. *See* Probucol
Lozol. *See* Indapamide

Macroglobulin, 306
Magnesium, 42, 143
  deficiency of, 157–158
Magnesium aspartate, 41
Magnesium hydroxide, 44
Magnesium sulfate, 41
Magnesium trisilicate, 44
Mazindol, 203
Meat, fats in, 275–276
MEGX, 99
Membrane stabilization, 176
Menadiol Sodium Diphosphate. *See* Phytonadione
Menadion. *See* Phytonadione
Mephyton. *See* Phytonadione
Metahydrin. *See* Trichlormethiazide
Metatensin, 190
Methemoglobinemia, 234
Methenamine, 198
Methylclothiazide (Aquatensen, Enduron), 161
Methyldopa, 148–149, 151
  plus norepinephrine, 204
α-Methyldopa (Aldomet), 194–195
Methyldopa-chlorothiazide tablets (Aldoclor), 201
Methyldopa-hydrochlorothiazide tablets (Aldoril), 202
α-Methylnorepinephrine, 195
Metoclopramide hydrochloride, 44–45
Metolazone (Diulo, Zaroxyolyn), 163
  recycling of, 159
Metoprolol (Lopressor), 49, 178–180
  benefits of, 242
  plus cimetidine, 185
  dosages of, 244–245
  plus pentobarbital/rifampin, 186
Metoprolol in Acute Myocardial Infarction (MIAMI) trial, 240–242

Metoprolol tartrate-hydrochlorothiazide tablets (Lopressor HCT), 183
Mevinolin, 278, 294–295
Mexiletine, 46, 102–104
MIAMI trial, 240–242. *See also* Metoprolol, Myocardial infarction
Milrinone, 50
Minipress. *See* Prazosin
Minoxidil (Loniten), 31, 205, 207–208
  plus guanethidine/guanadrel, 203
Miradon. *See* Anisidone
Mirador. *See* Amiloride
MODE, 107
Monoamine oxidase inhibitors, 203–204
Monoethylglycinexylidide. *See* MEGX
Monounsaturated fats colloquium, 273
Morphine sulfate, 8–9
Myalgia, 295
Myocardial contractile response, 62–63
Myocardial contractility, 1
  digitalis stimulation of, 73
  impaired, 121
  with ischemia, 229–230
  modulation of, 12–21
    digitalis glycoside dosages for, 33–42
    digitalis-drug interactions in, 42–47
    drugs for, 21–26
    mechanism of action of, 21–23
    nonglycosidic drugs for, 23–26, 47–50
  reduced, 239
Myocardial infarction
  acute
    intracoronary fibrinolytic therapy with, 336–338
    thrombogenesis and, 335–336
  anticoagulants for, 330
  antiplatelet agents for, 331
  aspirin for, 309
  with beta blocker withdrawal, 114–116, 188
  beta blockers for, 12, 240–242
  calcium channel blockers for, 248–249
  clofibrate with, 285
  digitalis toxicity and, 41
  early recurrence of, 330
  mortality with, 240–242
  non-Q-wave, 248–249
  pathophysiology of, 223–224
  prostaglandin production change with, 224–228
  reinfarction following, 330
  repolarization and, 55
  sympathetic discharge and, 228–229
  thrombi and, 313
  thrombolytics for, 345–349

Myocardial infarction—*Continued*
  treatment of, 99, 329–331
    drug, 230–255
Myocardial inotropy,
    digitalis-mediated, 13–14
Myocardial ischemia
  critical time for reversing of, 336–337
  disturbed physiology with, 229–230
  drug treatment of, 230–255
  pathophysiology of, 223–224
    reperfusion injury in, 225–228
    prostaglandin production change with, 224–225
  reperfusion therapy rationale in, 229–230
  silent, 247–248
  and sympathetic discharge, 228–229
Myocardial oxygen, 24, 252
  consumption rate of, 218
  demand, reduced, 251
Myocardial reperfusion injury, 347–348
Myocardial rupture, 224
Myocarditis, 41
Myocardium
  β-adrenoceptors in, 23
  digitalis action on, 39–41
  dysfunction of, 5
  vasodilator effects on, 30
Myositis, 284, 295

N-acetylprocainamide. *See* NAPA
Nadolol (Corgard), 180, 245
Nadolol-bendroflumethiazide tablets (Corzide), 183
NADPH oxidase, 226*f*, 227
NAPA, 92–95
Naqua. *See* Trichlormethiazide
Naquival, 190
Natriuresis, 197, 205
Natriuresis-pressure relationship, 145
Naturetin. *See* Bendroflumethiazide
Neomycin sulfate, 45
Nephropathy, quinidine-induced, 89
Netherlands Sixty-Plus study, 330
Netherlands-Interuniversity streptokinase trial, 338
Neuroendocrine processes, 141–142
  aberrant, 141, 143
Neurohumoral systems, 2–3
Neurotransmitters
  depletion of, 188, 191, 193
  enhanced release of, 200
  receptors, 22*f*
  slowed synthesis of, 189
Neutropenia, 210
Niacin (Nicotinic acid, Nicolar), 278–282
Nicolar. *See* Niacin
Nicotinic acid. *See* Niacin
Nifedipine (Adalat, Procardia), 153, 213
  adverse effects of, 215
  before angioplasty, 249–250
  dosages of, 215–216, 251
  effects of, 84
  pharmacokinetics of, 214–215
  for silent myocardial ischemia, 248
  in stable angina, 246
  uses and actions of, 251
Nipride. *See* Sodium nitroprusside
Nitrates
  adverse effects of, 232
  for coronary artery spasm, 247
  dependence on, 233
  directions for intravenous infusion of, 9–10
  drug interactions of, 234
  for left ventricular diastolic dysfunction, 51
  mediation of effects of, 31
  nifedipine with, 250
  nitroglycerin storage requirements of, 234
  pharmacokinetics of, 231–232
  pharmacologic properties of, 231
  precautions for, 232–234
  specific agents, 234–238
  tolerance of, 232–233
  uses and actions of, 230–231
Nitric acid, free, 231
Nitrites, 231
Nitro-Bid. *See* Nitroglycerin, oral; Nitroglycerin, topical
Nitro-Bid IV. *See* Nitroglycerin, intravenous
Nitroglycerin, 8
  buccal, 235
  intravenous (Nitro-Bid IV, Nitrostat IV, Tridil), 237–238
    dosages of, 238
    directions for, 9–10
    tolerance of, 233
  lingual aerosol (Nitrolingual), 235
  oral (Nitro-Bid, Nitroglyn, Nitro-Stat SR, Nitrospan, Nitrong), 235
    dosages, 236
    tolerance of, 233
  short-acting, 233
  storage requirements of, 234
  sublingual (Nitrostat), 234
  topical (Nitro-Bid, Nitrol, Nitrong, Nitrostat), 237
  transcutaneous compounds of, 238*t*
  transdermal, 233
Nitroglycerin gradient, 231
Nitroglycerin-containing discs/patches, 237
Nitroglyn. *See* Nitroglycerin, oral
Nitrol. *See* Nitroglycerin, topical
Nitrolingual. *See* Nitroglycerin, lingual aerosol
Nitrong. *See* Nitroglycerin, oral; Nitroglycerin, topical

Index

Nitrospan. *See* Nitroglycerin, oral
Nitrostat. *See* Nitroglycerin, sublingual; Nitroglycerin, topical
Nitrostat IV. *See* Nitroglycerin, intravenous
Nitro-Stat SR. *See* Nitroglycerin, oral
Nonglycosidic drugs, 21–26, 47–50
Nonsteroidal anti-inflammatory agents, 348
Norepinephrine. *See also* Norepinephrine bitartrate
  effects of, 26
  high levels of, 2
  hypersensitivity to, 247
  interaction with receptors of, 141–142
  myocardial, release of, 228–229
  plus methyldopa, 204
  prostaglandins in release of, 221–222
  release of, 123, 142, 348
Norepinephrine bitartrate, 26
Norethindrone (Acetate-Aygestin, Norlutate), 279
  dosages of, 296–297
  uses and actions of, 296
Norlorcainide, 111
Norlutate. *See* Norethindrone
Normodyne. *See* Labetalol
Norwegian timolol study, 241–242, 245
Nutrition, 148. *See also* Diet

Occluded arteriovenous cannulae, 344
ODE, 107
Olive oil, 273–275
Omega-3 and -6 fatty acids, 276, 349
Open heart surgery, 249
Oretic. *See* Hydrochlorothiazide
Organic nitrates, 9–10
Osmoregulation, 3
Ototoxicity, 164–165
Oxandrolone (Anavar), 279, 297
Oxprenolol (Trasicor, Slow-Trasicor), 178, 180–181
  ISA in, 175
Oxygen
  myocardial, 225–228, 231
    exchange, 218
    extraction, 218

P cells, 62–63
  in heart rate control, 67, 68f
Pacemakers
  ectopic, 82
  indications for, 59t
  permanent, 58
PAI. *See* Plasminogen activator inhibitor
Panwarfin. *See* Warfarin sodium
Parahydroxymexiletine, 104
Parasympathetic predominance, 188, 194
Penicillamine, 45
Pentaerythritol tetranitrate (Pentritol, Peritrate), 232, 236

Pentobarbital, 186
Pentritol. *See* Pentaerythritol tetranitrate
Peripheral artery thrombosis, 344
Peripheral resistance
  with guanadrel, 193
  increased, 3
  reduced, 14, 197, 200, 214
Peripheral vascular disease, 114
Peripheral vasoconstriction, 115–117
Peripheral vasodilation, 126–127
Peritrate. *See* Pentaerythritol tetranitrate
Persantin. *See* Dipyridamole
PGI$_2$. *See* Prostacyclin
Phenelzine, 203
Phenobarbital, 45
Phentolamine, 31–32
Phenylphrine, 203
Phenytoin, 42,
  with clofibrate, 286
Phenytoin sodium (Dilantin, Diphenylan), 100–102
PHLA, 297
Phlebotomy, 6
Phosphodiesterase inhibitors, 49
Phospholipase activation, 347
Photosensitivity reactions, 121–122
Phytonadione (Mephyton, Menadion, Menadiol Sodium Diphosphate), 325–326
Pindolol (Visken), 181, 245
  adverse effects of, 115
  ISA in, 175
  lipid metabolism and, 265
  pharmacokinetics of, 115
  pharmacology of, 115
  preparations and dosages of, 116
Pindolol hydrochloride-hydrochlorothiazide tablets (Viskenzide), 183
Pirbuterol hydrochloride, 48
Plasma renin activity, 174
Plasma volume. *See* Volume depletion, Volume expansion
Plasmin, 306, 307
Plasminogen, 306, 307
  activators of, 307, 340–342, 346
  activator inhibitor of, 336
Plateau principle, 18–19
Platelet-inhibitor therapy, 342
Platelets, 308
  aggregation of, 220, 247, 258, 304, 308–309
  inhibition of, 253, 314, 348
  thrombin and, 258
PMNs. *See* Polymorphonuclear leukocytes, circulating
Pneumonitis, interstitial, 106
Polymorphonuclear leukocytes
  circulating, 224
  enzyme on, 226f, 227
Polythiazide (Renese), 161

Potassium, 41
  conservation mechanism of, 167
  plasma concentration of, 156–157
  in resting potential, 64–65
Potassium channel, 15–16
  in action potential, 64
Potassium chloride, 29, 42
Potassium-depleting diuretics, 43–44
Potassium-sparing diuretics, 41, 166
  adverse effects of, 167
  drug interactions of, 171
  mechanism of action of, 166–167
  specific agents, 167–168
  with thiazide diuretics, 158, 168–169
PR interval, 74
Prazosin (Minipress), 187, 199–200, 205
  in chronic congestive heart failure treatment, 32
  dosages of, 200–201
  plus indomethacin, 204
  for primary hypertension, 151
  plus propranolol, 204
Preexcitation syndrome, 55–57
Pregnancy
  anticoagulants during, 322
  beta blockers during, 113
  cholestyramine resin during, 289
  clofibrate during, 285
  colestipol during, 291
  dextrothyroxine during, 298
  gemfibrozil during, 288
  heparin during, 317, 322
  probucol during, 293
Preload, 1
  diuretic effect on, 7
  modulation of, 6–7, 8
  in children and adolescents, 28
  in geriatric patients, 29
  side effects in, 29
Premature ventricular contractions (PVCs), 108
  treatment of, 109, 114
Prenalterol, 48
Pressure-natriuresis relationship, 145
Prinzmetal's angina, 218
  calcium channel blockers for, 246–247
  silent ischemia in, 248
Proaqua. See Benzthiazide
Probenecid, 158
Probucol (Lorelco), 278, 292–294
Procainamide, 46, 90–93
  patient monitoring with, 92–93
Procardia. See Nifedipine
Propantheline bromide, 45
Propranolol (Inderal, Inderal LA, Detensol), 75
  adverse effects of, 116
  plus aminophylline/theophylline, 182–184
  antihypertensive action of, 172

  benefits of, 242
  in combination therapy, 184–186, 202, 204
  for digitalis toxicity, 42
  dosages of, 117, 181–182, 243
  hemodynamic effects of, 173
  for hypertension, 148, 153
  liver metabolism of, 178
  pharmacokinetics of, 116, 181
  renin inhibition of, 174
Propranolol hydrochloride-hydrochlorothiazide tablets (Inderide), 183
Propylbutyl dopamine, 48
Prostacyclin, 253, 277
  activation of, 4
  in platelet aggregation inhibition, 314
Prostaglandin-related agents, 253–255
Prostaglandins
  in congestive heart failure, 4
  in coronary artery blood flow, 221–222
  increased production of, 31, 209
  inhibited synthesis of, 169, 212, 312
  in modulation of digoxin effects, 44
  precursor of, 347
  production changes in with myocardial ischemia/infarction, 224–225
Prosthetic heart valves, 333
Protamine sulfate, 319–320
Protein C, 305, 306f, 323
Proteinuria, 210
Prothrombin, 258, 304
Prothrombin time, 315
  increased, 291
  with oral anticoagulants, 324
Protriptyline, 123
Pro-urokinase, recombinant, 335
Psychoses, 92
PTCA. See Angioplasty, percutaneous transluminal coronary
Pulmonary congestion, 1, 6
Pulmonary disease, 41
Pulmonary edema, 8
Pulmonary embolism
  diagnosis of, 328–329
  fibrinolytics for, 343
  treatment of, 327
Pulmonary fibrosis, 106, 121
Purkinje fiber
  conduction in, 77
  reentry in, 72
Purple toe syndrome, 322
PVC killers, 109

QRS complex, 86
QT interval
  prolonged, 54–55, 114
  quinidine effects on, 86, 88
Questran. See Cholestyramine resin

Index

Quinethazone (Hydromox), 163
Quinidine, 75, 91
  adverse effects of, 88–89
  autonomic effects of, 86–87
  interaction of with digitalis, 46
  patient monitoring with, 89
  pharmacokinetics of, 87–88
  pharmacology of, 86–87
  preparations and dosages of, 89–90
  therapeutic use of, 87
  with verapamil, 252
Quinidine gluconate, 90
Quinidine polygalacturonate, 89–90
Quinidine sulfate, 90
Quinidine syncope, 88
Quinine, 46
Q-wave infarctions, 249

Radiofibrinogen technique, 327
Rauwolfia serpentina, 187
Recombinant tissue plasminogen activator. *See* t-PA activator
Reentrant arrhythmias, reversal of, 77
Reentry, 71–72
  requirements for, 71–72
  reversal of, 77
Reflex cardiac stimulation, 205, 207
Reflex tachycardia, 30–32
Refractoriness
  abnormalities of, 71–73
  class I agents effect on, 81
  extended, 78
  postrepolarization, 78
Refractory period, 65. *See also* Effective refractory period
Regroton, 190
Renal insufficiency, 116
Renese. *See* Polythiazide
Renese-R, 190
Renin
  circulating, 142
  plasma activity of, 174, 208
  release of, 205
Renin-angiotensin system, 3, 29
Renin-angiotensin-aldosterone axis, 142, 208
Reperfusion myocardial injury, 225–228
Reperfusion therapy, 229–230
Repolarization, 54–55
Reserpine (Sandril, Serpasil, SK-Reserpine), 153, 187–189
  adverse effects of, 188
  with diuretics, 189–190
  dosages of, 189
  in monotherapy, 149
  plus chlorothiazide, 189
  plus ephedrine, 204
  plus levodopa, 204
  plus monoamine oxidase inhibitors, 204
  plus thiopental, 204

Respiratory distress, 1, 8
Resting potential, 64–65, 67
Restriction-fragment-length (RFLP) analysis, 268
Retrograde conduction, 77
Rheumatoid arthritislike syndrome, drug-induced, 206
Rhythm disturbances. *See* Arrhythmias; Tachycardia
Rifampin, 186

Salbutamol, 48
Salt restriction, 148
Salt retention, 194. *See also* Sodium, retention of
Saluron. *See* Hydroflumethiazide
Salutensin, 190
Salutensin-demi, 190
Sandril. *See* Reserpine
Saphenous vein grafting, 332
Sarcolemma breakdown, 226
Sectral. *See* Acebutolol
Serotonin, 220
  hypersensitivity to, 247
Serpasil. *See* Reserpine
Serpasil-esidrix, 190
Sexual dysfunction, 197
SGOT levels
  elevated, 284
  with mevinolin, 295
SGPT, elevated levels of, 284
Sick sinus syndrome, 57
  with verapamil, 252
Sinus bradycardia, 42, 119
Sinus nodal disease, 111
Sixty Plus Reinfarction Study (Netherlands), 330
SK-Chlorothiazide. *See* Chlorothiazide
SK-Furosemide. *See* Furosemide
Skin rash
  with captopril, 210
  with cholestyramine resin, 289
  with clofibrate, 285
  with colestipol, 291
  with vitamin K antagonists, 321
SK-Reserpine. *See* Reserpine
Sleep disturbances, 111
SLE-like syndrome, 92, 95
Slow-trasicor. *See* Oxprenolol
Smooth muscle relaxation, 219, 220t. *See also* Arterial Smooth Muscle
Sodium
  abnormal levels of in congestive heart failure, 3–4
  depletion of, 29, 212
  excretion of, 4
  intracellular concentration of, 14
  reduced, 156
  in resting potential, 64–65
  retention of, 205, 207
Sodium bicarbonate, 118

Sodium channel
  in action potential, 65–66
  antagonists, 108
  conduction rate and, 67
  drug association and dissociation with, 79–82
  impaired function of, 102–103
  inactivation of, 107
  states of, 79, 80*f*
Sodium pump, 13
Sodium nitroprusside (Nipride), 8, 10–11, 25, 31–32, 153
  calculation of infusion rates of, 12
  overdosage of, 11–12
Sorbitrate. See Isosorbide dinitrate
Sotalol, 83
Spironolactone (Aldactone), 167–168
  dosages of, 168
    for children, 28
  plus digoxin, 171
  drug interactions of, 171
    with digitalis, 46
  and hydrochlorothiazide, 169
  mechanism of action of, 166–167
ST interval, 86
Starr-Edwards model 6000 prosthesis, 333
Steatorrhea, 289, 291
Stokes-Adams syncope, 57
Streptase. See Streptokinase
Streptokinase (Kabinkinase, Streptase), 335, 336
  allergic reaction to, 344
  dosages of, 340, 345–346
  indications for, 343
  IV administration of, 345
  pharmacokinetics of, 345
  trials of, 338–339
ST-T depression
  asymptomatic, 247
  reduction of, 251
Succinylcholine chloride, 46
Sulfasalazine, 46
Sulfinpyrazone (Anturane), 312–313
Sulfonamides, 312
Superoxide dismutase (SOD), 225, 227
Supraventricular arrhythmias, 107
Supraventricular tachyarrhythmias
  paroxysmal, 125
  quinidine for, 87
Supraventricular tachycardia, 54
  digitalis treatment for, 73
  mechanisms underlying, 58
  paroxysmal, 54, 69, 120
  therapy for, 55*t*, 101, 120
Sympathetic depressant drugs, 148, 171–172
  adverse effects of, 177
  antihypertensive uses of, 176–177
  blood pressure effects of, 149
  with diuretics, 182–183
  drug interactions of, 183–186
  hemodynamic effects of, 173

mechanism of antihypertensive action of, 172–173
  organ systems in antihypertensive effects of, 173–174
  pharmacokinetics of, 178
  pharmacologic properties of, 174–176
  specific drugs, 178–182
  with thiazides, 155
Sympathetic nervous system
  depression of, 188
  digitalis and, 14–15
  response of to congestive heart failure, 1–2
Sympathetic nervous system depressant drugs, 186–187
  with diuretics, 201–202
  interactions of, 202–204
  properties of, 187–201
Sympathetic stimulation, reflex, 205
Sympathetic tone, increased, 82
Sympathoadrenal activity, enhanced, 208
Sympathomimetic amines, 48–49
Syncope, 232, 311
Systemic lupus erythematosus (SLE)
  drug-induced, 206
  procainamide-induced, 92
  quinidine-induced, 89
  treatment of, 91, 94

Tachyarrhythmias
  digitalis toxicity therapy for, 41
  treatment of, 87, 120
  ventricular, 114–118
Tachycardia
  atrial, treatment of, 87, 125
  AV junctional, 38
  AV nodal reentry, 87
  circus-movement, 58*t*
  with lorcainide, 111
  paroxysmal
    electrophysiologic effects of ATP on, 85
    treatment for, 73, 87, 96
  reflex, 213
    attenuation of, 239
    with calcium channel antagonists, 215
  supraventricular, 54
    digitalis treatment for, 73
    mechanisms underlying, 58
    paroxysmal, 69
    therapy for, 55*t*, 73, 101
  ventricular, treatment for, 38, 107, 123
Tachyphylaxis, 47, 49
Tenoretic. See Atenolol
Tenormin. See Atenolol
Terbutaline sulfate, 48
Tetracycline, 44
Theophylline, 49
  plus beta blockers, 184

Thiazides
    with ACE inhibitors, 209
    adverse effects of, 156–159
    effectiveness of, 29
    in hypertension treatment, 147, 151
    interactions of, 169–170
    long-acting, 28
    mechanism and site of action of, 155–156
    in monotherapy or combined therapy, 154–155
    pharmacokinetics of, 159
    with potassium-sparing diuretics, 168–169
Thiopental, plus reserpine, 204
Thrombin, 304, 305
    in atherosclerosis, 258
Thrombin-binding protein, 305
Thrombocytopenia, 194
    drug-induced immune, 316–317
    with mexiletine, 104
    quinidine-induced, 89
    with thiazide therapy, 159
Thromboembolism
    with estrogens, 298
    rates of with prosthetic valves, 333, 334t
    risk of, 224
Thrombogenesis
    intracoronary, 336
    intravascular, 304–306
    limiting of, 347–348
    management of hemorrhagic complications of, 343
    pathways for, 305f
    platelet aggregation in, 309
    processes of, 224
    sites of, 314–315
    tissue kinins and complement activation in, 307–308
Thrombolysis
    intravascular, 306–307
    mechanism of, 334–335
    preventing reocclusion after, 342
    tissue kinins and complement activation in, 307–308
Thrombolytics, 334–335. See also Fibrinolytics
    for acute myocardial infarction, 335–336
    pharmacologic and clinical features of, 343t
Thrombomodulin, 305
Thromboplastin, 304
Thromboplastin time
    activated partial, 315–316, 318
    partial, 318
Thrombosis
    deep vein, 327–328, 343–344
    peripheral artery, 344
    venous, 327
Thrombospondin, 341
Thrombotic disease, 309–313

Thromboxane A_2, 224, 253, 309
Thrombus(i), 313–314
    atherosclerosis and, 313
    deep saphenous vein, 328
    dissolution of, 304
    drugs to prevent, 330–331
    intravascular thrombogenesis sites and, 314–315
    sites of formation of, 314–315
    treatment of, 315–349
    types of, 313
    vascular endothelium and, 314
    venous, 327–328
Thyroid analogues, 298–299
Thyroid hormone
    interaction of with digitalis, 46–47
    plus propranolol, 186
TIMI trial, 341. See also t-PA
Timolide. See Timolol maleate-hydrochlorothiazide tablets
Timolol (Blocardren), 117–118, 182
    benefits of, 242
    dosages of, 245–246
Timolol maleate-hydrochlorothiazide tablets (Timolide), 183
Timolol-Norwegian study, 241–242, 245
Tissue injury, 307–308
    response to, 349
Tissue oxygen tension (tpO$_2$), 219
Tocainide, 104, 105–106
Tolbutamide, with clofibrate, 286
Tourniquets, rotating, 6
t-PA (Alteplase, Activase), 347
    activation of, 307
    activator, 335–336, 340–342
    current status of, 347
    double- and single-stranded, 341
    effects of, 342
    half-life of, 347
    pharmacokinetics of, 347
    in platelet inhibition, 348
    TIMI trial, 341
    uses and action of, 346
Trandate. See Labetalol
Trasicor. See Oxprenolol
Triamterene (Dyrenium), 166
    dosages of, 168
    drug interactions of, 171
    and hydrochlorothiazide, 169
    plus indomethacin, 171
    interaction of with digitalis, 46
    mechanism of action of, 167
Trichlormethiazide (Metahydrin, Naqua), 162
Tridil. See Nitroglycerin, intravenous
Triglycerides, 261
    elevated levels of, 271
        procedure to follow with, 272f
    fish oil-derived fatty acids and, 276–277
    reduction of, 297
    removal of, 268

Triglycerides—*Continued*
  with thiazide therapy, 158–159
  transport of, 263
Trimethaphan camsylate, 153

Urokinase (Abbokinase), 340
  dosages of, 346
  indications for, 343

Vagal activity, reduced, 86–87
Vagal maneuvers, 54
Vagal stimulation, 15–16
Valsalva maneuver, 54
Valvular heart disease, 333
Variant angina. *See* Prinzmetal's angina
Vascular endothelium, 314
Vascular smooth muscle, 144–145
Vasoconstriction, hypersensitivity to, 247
Vasoconstrictor fibers, 220–221
Vasodilation, 25, 200
  with calcium channel antagonists, 213
  mechanism of, 205
  with nitrates, 231
Vasodilators, 31–33, 148, 204–205.
    See also Nitrates; *specific agents*
  action and dosages of, 29, 30t
  blood pressure effects of, 149
  direct and indirect, 205
  for left ventricular diastolic dysfunction, 51
  mode of action and reflex responses to, 205
  specific agents, 206–208
  therapeutic use of, 29–31, 205
  with thiazides, 155
  triple therapy with, 205
Vasodilatory therapy, 8–12
  for children and adolescents, 8
Vasopressin, 4
Vasoreactive modifiers, 221t
Vegetable oils, 273–275, 276
Vegetarian diet, 271
Vein grafting, 332
Venodilation, 200
  with nitrate concentrations, 231
Venous return, reduced, 8
Venous thromboembolism, 330
  prevention of, 329
Ventricular action potential, 64f
  digitalis effects on, 73–74
Ventricular arrhythmias
  digitalis toxicity therapy for, 42
  procainamide for, 91
Ventricular diastolic dysfunction, left, 50–51
Ventricular ectopy, 54
  treatment of, 56t, 110
Ventricular fibrillation, 38
  treatment of, 91, 107, 123

Ventricular flutter, 91
Ventricular hypertrophy, left, 144
  cardiovascular disease risk and, 148
  reversal of, 199
Ventricular premature complexes, 87
Ventricular systolic dysfunction, left, 26–27, 51
  diuretics for, 28–29
  modulation of myocardial contractility in, 33–50
  modulation of preload and afterload in, 28–29
  therapeutic end points in, 27–28
  treatment of, 27
  vasodilators for, 29–33
Ventricular tachycardia, 38
Verapamil (Calan, Isoptin), 46, 75, 213
  adverse effects of, 127, 215, 252
  plus beta blockers, 184
  dosages of, 127, 216, 252
  drug interactions of, 252
  effects of, 83
  interaction of with digitalis, 47
  for left ventricular diastolic dysfunction, 51
  for myocardial ischemia, 251–252
  pharmacokinetics of, 126–127, 215
  pharmacology of, 125
  precautions with, 252
  uses and actions of, 125, 252
Virilization, 297
Visken. *See* Pindolol
Viskenzide. *See* Pindolol hydrochloride-hydrochlorothiazide tablets
Vitamin K
  analogues of, 325
  bleeding and, 321
  deficiency of, 289, 291
  oxidation of, 320–321
Vitamin K antagonists
  adverse effects of, 321–322
  contraindications for, 324
  dipyridamole and, 310
  dosages of, 322–323
  drug interactions of, 322
  monitoring of, 323–324
  pharmacokinetics of, 321
  precautions with, 322
  for prevention of thrombosis, 330
  specific agents, 324–325
  therapy of overdose of, 325–326
  use and actions of, 320–321
VLDL. *See* Lipoproteins, very-low-density
Volume depletion, 164
Volume expansion, 30–31, 188, 206–207

Warfarin, plus ethacrynic acid, 170
Warfarin potassium, 320–322

Warfarin sodium (Coumadin, Panwarfin), 320–322
  dosages of, 324–325
  plus heparin, 327
Water retention, 194. *See also* Edema
  in congestive heart failure, 3
  mechanisms of, 205
  with minoxidil, 207
Weight reduction, 148
Western Washington Intravenous Streptokinase Trial (WWIST), 338–339
White blood cell aggregation, 227
Wisken. *See* Pindolol

Wolf-Parkinson-White syndrome, 71, 109
  drug-induced arrhythmias in, 215
  treatment of, 120, 125
Wytensin. *See* Guanabenz

Xansterol, 48
Xanthine dehydrogenase, 228
Xanthine oxidase, 228
  inhibitor, 348
Xanthomas, 278, 279

Zaroxyolyn. *See* Metolazone